FORUM
ON
IMMUNOMODULATORS

British Library Cataloguing in Publication Data
A catalogue record for this book is available from the British Library.
ISBN 2-7420-0076-3

Éditions John Libbey Eurotext
127, avenue de la République, 92120 Montrouge, France
Tél. : (1) 46.73.06.60

John Libbey and Company Ltd
13, Smiths Yard, Summerley Street,
London SW18 4HR, England
Tel. : (1) 947.27.77

John Libbey CIC
Via L. Spallanzani, 11
00161, Rome, Italy
Tel. : (06) 862.289

© 1995, John Libbey Eurotext, Paris

Il est interdit de reproduire intégralement ou partiellement le présent ouvrage — loi du 11 mars 1957 — sans autorisation de l'éditeur ou du Centre Français du Copyright, 6 *bis*, rue Gabriel-Laumain, 75010 Paris, France.

FORUM ON IMMUNOMODULATORS

M. GUENOUNOU

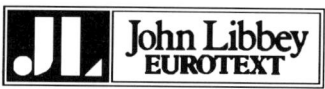

Contents

List of contributors VII

Foreword
W.H. Fridman IX

Introductive remarks
M. Guenounou XI

1. **Muramylpeptides as immunomodulators**
   A. Adam 1

2. **OK-432, a killed streptococcal preparation, in the treatment of animal and human cancer and its mechanisms of action**
   M. Saito 13

3. **Bestatin : immunopharmacology and clinical results**
   H. Blomgren 31

4. **Immunopharmacology of glucan phosphate**
   D.L. Williams, H.A. Pretus, I.W. Browder 43

5. **Immunomodulators from *Nocardia opaca***
   R. Barot-Ciorbaru, C. Bona 63

6. **Lentinan**
   R. Bomford 79

7. **RU 41740 (Biostim), an immunomodulating agent from bacterial origin**
   C. Bloy, M. Morales, M. Guenounou 85

8. **Immunostimulating lipopeptides**
   D. Migliore-Samour, P. Jollès 101

9. **The immunomodulating and therapeutic properties of AS 101**
   B. Sredni, M. Albeck, Y. Kalechman 123

10. **Levamisole**
    M. Roch-Arveiller 147

11. **Cyclosporine**
    F. de La Tour du Pin, H. Humbert, F. Devaux, H. Pham-Gia 161

12. **FK506 : a powerful new drug for T cell-directed immunointervention**
    A.W. Thomson, J. Woo, A. Zeevi, N. Murase, J.J. Fung, S. Todo, T.E. Starzl 175

13. **Antisense oligonucleotides as tools for immune regulation**
    S. Esnault, N. Benbernou, M. Guenounou 205

14. **Interferons**
    C. Billard 215

15. **Tumor necrosis factor and its inhibitors**
    W.S. Liao, B.B. Aggarwal 233

16. **Eicosanoids and immunomodulation**
    N. Gualde, M. Juzan 251

17. **Anti-inflammatory drugs and immunomodulation**
    L.F. Perrin, P.E. Laurent 275

18. **Immunological effects of neuropsychotropic substances**
    B. Deleplanque, P.J. Neveu 287

19. **An alternative concept of immunomodulation**
    M. Bastide, F. Boudard 303

List of contributors

Adam A., CNRS, URA 1116, Institut de Biochimie, Université de Paris-Sud, 91405 Orsay, France.
Aggarwal B.B., Department of Clinical Immunology and Biological Therapy, University of Texas, MD Anderson Cancer Center, Houston, Texas 77030, USA.
Albeck M., CAIR Institute, Department of Life Sciences, Bar-Ilan University, Ramat Gan, 59200 Israël.
Barot-Ciorbaru R., CNRS, URA 1116, Université Paris-Sud, Bâtiment 432, 91405 Orsay, France.
Bastide M., Laboratoire d'Immunologie, Faculté de Pharmacie, Université de Montpellier-I, 34060 Montpellier Cedex 1, France.
Benbernou N., Laboratoire d'Immunologie, Institut de Recherche Médicale André Demonchy, Université de Reims, 51100 Reims, France.
Billard C., INSERM U 365, Institut Curie, Section de Biologie, 26, rue d'Ulm, 75231 Paris Cedex 05, France.
Blomgren H., Department of General Oncology, Radiumhemmet, Karolinska Hospital, S-10401 Stockholm, Sweden.
Bloy C., Laboratoire Cassenne, 17, rue de Pontoise, 95520 Osny, France.
Bomford R., Unité d'Épidémiologie des Virus Oncogènes, Institut Pasteur, 28, rue du Docteur-Roux, 75724 Paris Cedex 15, France.
Bona C., Department of Microbiology, Mount Sinai School of Medicine, Mount Sinai Hospital, New York, 10029, USA.
Boudard F., Laboratoire d'Immunologie, Faculté de Pharmacie, Université de Montpellier-I, 34060 Montpellier Cedex 1, France.
Browder I.W., Department of Surgery, Quillen-Dishner College of Medicine, East Tennessee State University, Johnson City, Tennessee 37614-0002, USA.
Deleplanque B., INSERM U 259, Université de Bordeaux-II, Domaine de Carreire, rue Camille-Saint-Saëns, 33077 Bordeaux, France.
Devaux F., Laboratoires Sandoz, 14, boulevard Richelieu, 92500 Rueil-Malmaison, France.
Esnault S., Laboratoire d'Immunologie, Institut de Recherche Médicale André Demonchy, Université de Reims, 51100 Reims, France.
Fung J.J., Pittsburg Transplantation Institute and Department of Surgery and Pathology, University of Pittsburg School of Medicine, Pittsburg, Pennsylvania, USA.
Gualde N., Laboratoire d'Immunologie, CNRS, URA 1456, Université de Bordeaux-II, Fondation Bergonié, 33076 Bordeaux Cedex, France.
Guenounou M., Laboratoire d'Immunologie, Faculté de Pharmacie, 31, rue Cognacq-Jay, 51100 Reims, France.
Humbert H., Laboratoires Sandoz, 14, boulevard Richelieu, 92500 Rueil-Malmaison, France.
Jollès P., Laboratoire des Protéines, Université René-Descartes, CNRS Paris-V, 45, rue des Saints-Pères, 75270 Paris Cedex 06, France.
Juzan M., Laboratoire d'Immunologie, CNRS, URA 1456, Université de Bordeaux-II, Fondation Bergonié, 33076 Bordeaux Cedex, France.

Kalechman Y., CAIR Institute, Departement of Life Sciences, Bar-Ilan University, Ramat Gar, 59200 Israël.
La Tour du Pin F. de, Laboratoires Sandoz, 14, boulevard Richelieu, 92500 Rueil-Malmaison, France.
Laurent P.E., Institut Pasteur, Lyon, France.
Liao W.S.L., Department of Biochemistry and Molecular Biology, University of Texas, MD Anderson Cancer Center, Houston, Texas 77030, USA.
Migliore-Samour D., Laboratoire des Protéines, Université René-Descartes, CNRS Paris-V, 45, rue des Saints-Pères, 75270 Paris Cedex 06, France.
Morales M., Laboratoire Cassenne, 17, rue de Pontoise, 95520 Osny, France.
Murase N., Pittsburg Transplantation Institute and Department of Surgery Pathology, University of Pittsburg School of Medicine, Pittsburg, Pennsylvania, USA.
Neveu P.J., INSERM U 259, Université de Bordeaux-II, Domaine de Carreire, rue Camille-Saint-Saëns, 33077 Bordeaux, France.
Perrin L.F., Faculté des Sciences, Université Catholique, Lyon, France ; et Faculté de Médecine, Lyon, France.
Pham-Gia H., Laboratoires Sandoz, 14, boulevard Richelieu, 92500 Rueil-Malmaison, France.
Pretus H.A., Department of Physiology, Tulane University School of Medicine, 1430 Tulane Avenue, New Orleans, Louisiana 70112, USA.
Roch-Arveiller M., Départment de Pharmacologie, CNRS, URA 595, 27, rue du Faubourg-Saint-Jacques, 75674 Paris Cedex 14, France.
Saito M., Laboratory of Cancer and Hematological Disease, Chugai Pharmaceutical Co., Ltd., 41-8, Takada 3-chome, Toshima-Ku, Tokyo, Japan.
Sredni B., CAIR Institute, Department of Life Sciences, Bar-Ilan University, Ramat Gan, 59200 Israël.
Starzl T.E., Pittsburg Transplantation Institute and Department of Surgery and Pathology, University of Pittsburg School of Medicine, Pittsburg, Pennsylvania, USA.
Thomson A.W., Pittsburg Transplantation Institute and Department of Surgery and Pathology, University of Pittsburg School of Medicine, Pittsburg, Pennsylvania, USA.
Todo S., Pittsburg Transplantation Institute and Department of Surgery and Pathology, University of Pittsburg School of Medicine, Pittsburg, Pennsylvania, USA.
Williams D.L., Department of Surgery, Quillen-Dishner College of Medicine, East Tennessee State University, Johnson City, Tennessee 37614-0002, USA.
Woo J., Pittsburg Transplantation Institute and Department of Surgery and Pathology, University of Pittsburg School of Medicine, Pittsburg, Pennsylvania, USA.
Zeevi A., Pittsburg Transplantation Institute and Department of Surgery and Pathology, University of Pittsburg School of Medicine, Pittsburg, Pennsylvania, USA.

Foreword

The immune system, in interaction with the neuroendocrine networks, is responsible for the homeostasis of higher organisms. To exert its primary function of protecting against microbiological invaders, it has acquired a sophisticated recognition system, allowing discrimination between self and non-self, and a complex machinery controlling immune reactions. The immune system, as a result of a unique genetic mechanism based on the rearrangement of genes that code for antibody and T cell receptor, has a recognition repertoire of billions of antigens, and, therefore, « knows the unknown », *i.e.* most of the organic substances of the universe. During foetal life, it has been educated to tolerize self, the vast majority of scholar thymocytes dying during this merciless process. When immunocompetent cells encounter an antigen, to which they are not tolerant, they proliferate and differentiate into effector cells, under the control of activating or suppressive cytokines. Thereafter, they keep memory of this encounter, being even more effective when they meet again. Immunocompetent cells do not home in a single organ but are permanently produced in the bone marrow and circulate in lymph, blood and tissues, concentrating in thymus, spleen, lymph nodes or Peyer patches. For these reasons, the immune system can be seen as a « mobile brain ».

Not only is the immune system equipped with receptors allowing recognition of invaders but is has, through evolution, learned to cope with the biology of the latter, to utilize, for instance, bacterial membrane components as stimulants. In contrast, invaders have developed means to escape immune attack, by changing their antigenicity or producing suppressive molecules. The same is true for mutant cells of the organism, such as cancer cells, which are destroyed if the immune system locates them, and which hide and suppress it as long as possible.

The list of human diseases in which the immune system plays a direct, or indirect, role increases day after day. Infections, allergies, immune deficiencies and an increasing number of autoimmune diseases (systemic lupus erythematosis, multiple sclerosis, juvenile diabetes, rheumatoid arthritis, Alzheimer diseases...), but also cancer and aging. Controlling the immune system in organ transplantation is crucial and may open the way to use of xenogenic organs. Immunity is everywhere.

The immune system is a powerful, potentially dangerous, delicately tuned machine which appropriate modulation should have a tremendous medical impact. What is appropriate ? How not to overamplify the expected effects by hyperstimulating or depressing too low ? Should the natural, but pleiotropic, cytokines or rather bacterial or synthetic compounds be used ? These are central questions to which diverse responses are given to-day, but which condition the development of powerful immunopharmacology that will represent a major medical breakthrough and pharmaceutical market in the coming decades.

This *Forum on Immunomodulators* presents an almost comprehensive review on the different approaches — cytokines, bacterial derivatives, synthetic compounds, stimulatory and inhibitory factors — written by highly recognized authors in each field. It allows to understand the to-day's state of the art and to foresee the first steps of the future. Most of what is necessary to « keep in touch » is here.

Wolf H. Fridman

Introductive remarks

Immunomodulation means that one can stimulate or suppress immunity. This concept gives rise to the development of a great number of substances, of natural or synthetic origin, devoted to the treatment and the prevention of diseases with immunological imbalance. These substances are distinct from vaccines or antibiotics and are supposed to enhance host resistance towards malignant and infectious diseases, or to regulate abnormal immune response in allergic and auto-immune disorders. Immunosuppressive drugs can also be used to inhibit normal immune response, to prevent allogenic graft rejection. A wide variety of synthetic drugs, natural and microbial substances are, thus, needed for the management of the immune system. Microbial sources have provided several purified and chemically defined compounds with high immunotherapeutic potential, such as fungal glycan (lentinan, glycan...), bacterial lipopolysaccharide endotoxin, glycoproteins extracts and active mycobacterial cell wall analogues such as muramyldipeptides (MDP). It is known that the immune system produces its own regulatory factors. Cytokines constitute a wide family of proteins and glycoproteins specialized in delivering signals from one cell to another. This sophisticated network is playing a major role in the physiological interactions within the immune system and in fact between cells of the whole organism. Recombinant cytokines are now available in a highly purified form allowing their use in human therapy. Cytokines are multipotent molecules and possess a high therapeutic potential. Many of them are used in cancer therapy and bone marrow reconstitution.

This Forum represents a selection of important examples of immunomodulating agents readily usable in human therapy. Several potential applications of cytokines or antisense to cytokines as immunomodulators as well as synthetic products are also presented.

The book is addressed to physicians as well as to students and to scientists interested in the applications of immunomodulating agents to human therapy.

Many individuals have helped in producing this Forum. First and foremost, I have to thank Dr Claudine Brossard for initiating and maintaining the contact between the contributors. Without her constant « devotion », this would not come to achievement.

I would like to express my gratitude and special appreciation to my colleagues for their important contribution and productive discussions for the achievement of this project.

Professor M. Guenounou
Editor

1

Muramylpeptides as immunomodulators

Arlette ADAM

CNRS, URA 1116, Institut de Biochimie, Université de Paris-Sud, 91405 Orsay, France.

Muramylpeptides

The possibility of replacing mycobacteria in Freund's complete adjuvant by a simple synthetic compound has attracted many researchers to this field and led to the publication of more than a thousand papers. Because comprehensively covering this field is impossible, I have selected some of the findings that reflect the properties of muramylpeptides which are of potential interest in the context of this book. Reviews and recently published papers have been chosen in order to provide reference sources.

From Freund's adjuvant to muramyl dipeptide

The most potent adjuvant still in use today was developed in the thirties as a result of the early observations of Ramon, Dienes and Coulaud. Freund's incomplete adjuvant (FIA) is a water-in-oil emulsion containing mineral oil and an emulsifier such as Arlacel A. Antigens administered in FIA elicit high antibody levels. Freund's complete adjuvant (FCA) contains in addition killed tubercle bacilli. The mycobacterial component further increases antibody levels and induces a cellular immune response.

It soon appeared that FCA can induce other effects as well, which can be either beneficial or harmful to the host. These include stimulation of the reticuloendothelial system, increase of nonspecific resistance to infectious agents and tumors, and damaging effects such as the induction of autoimmune diseases, sensitization to endotoxins, inflammatory and necrotizing reactions and fever.

The use of FCA had to be confined to laboratory animals. That is why many investigators have tried to propose a new formulation presenting the beneficial properties of FCA while showing reduced side effects. In an endeavor to identify the minimal chemical structure responsible for the adjuvant activity of mycobacterial cells, we have shown that natural muramylpeptides as well as the synthetic muramyl dipeptide (MDP) N-acetylmuramyl-L-alanyl-D-isoglutamine could replace all bacilli included in FCA [1].

Muramyl dipeptide and analogs

Muramyl dipeptide (MDP) presents a wide spectrum of biological effects; moreover, mineral oil or a substitute is essential for the full expression of the immunomodulatory properties of MDP *in vivo*. Therefore, several hundred derivatives of MDP have been synthesized in order to define the structure-activity relationship and with the goal of obtaining an analog of MDP which would be effective in the absence of mineral oil and present a reduced spectrum of biological effects [2-4]. Indeed, simple structural modifications can modulate the properties of the starting molecule.

I will mention only the most commonly used MDP derivatives:
— MDP(D-Ala) (N-acetylmuramyl-D-alanyl-D-isoglutamine) appears to be biologically inactive and it can even be antagonistic to MDP in adjuvant assays. MDP(D-Ala) has often been used as a negative control in experiments [2-4].
— Murabutide (N-acetylmuramyl-L-alanyl-D-glutamine-n-butylester) has been developed by Choay laboratories as a nonpyrogenic derivative of MDP, presenting most of the other properties of the parent molecule [5].
— Nor-MDP (N-acetyldesmethylmuramyl-L-alanyl-D-isoglutamine) has been successfully used in an antifertility vaccine, the paraffin oil of FIA being replaced by squalene, a precursor of cholesterol [6].
— Thr-MDP (N-acetylmuramyl-L-threonyl-D-isoglutamine), included in the « Syntex Adjuvant Formulation » (SAF), is proposed as a promising substitute for MDP in FIA for increasing both humoral and cellular immunity to a variety of antigens including viral and tumoral antigens. Similarly to MDP, Thr-MDP has to be included in an oily vehicle for an optimal adjuvant effect. A formulation with an efficacy comparable to that of FIA, but acceptable for clinical use, has been proposed: it consists of a stable oil-in-water emulsion of squalane, the saturated form of squalene, with pluronic polymer L121. SAF appears to be a very potent adjuvant which does not present the other biological properties of MDP and is devoid of major undesirable side effects [7]. Another alternative to the use of FIA is the encapsulation within multilamellar vesicles. In addition, the attachment of acyl side chains to muramyl peptides makes the molecule more lipophilic, resulting in a prolonged intracellular residence time. A number of acyl derivatives such as muroctasin (MDP-Lys-L-18) have been developed, essentially by Japanese laboratories [8].
— MTP-PE (MDP-L-alanyl-phosphatidylethanolamine) can be encapsulated within liposomes with a high degree of efficiency. A stable and reproducible preparation of liposomal MTP-PE has been produced for clinical use in humans by Ciba-Geigy laboratories [9].

Physicochemical studies

A nuclear magnetic resonance study has shown that MDP in dimethyl sulfoxide has an S-shaped conformation with two adjacent β-turns; murabutide has only one, and the adjuvant inactive MDP(D-Ala) has a cyclic structure. These conformational variations can be correlated with the different activities of the three molecules and may be of importance for the design of new structures [10].

Experimental studies

MDP or derivatives elicit a number of biological effects in the host which can sometimes be selectively exploited or, on the contrary, attenuated and even eliminated by the choice of the appropriate analog and vehicle. The main effects of muramylpeptides will be presented.

Toxicology

MDP is less toxic than all mycobacteria and devoid of the main side effects linked to the use of FCA including biotransformation of drugs. However, MDP is pyrogenic and it elicits uveitis in rabbits as well as arthritis in rats. Acute toxicity studies have shown important species differences in the sensitivity to MDP, LD_{50} being approximately 2 g/kg in mice and 100 mg/kg in dogs and monkeys. The administration of 5 mg/kg of MDP in dogs for up to 10 days elicited an acute systemic inflammatory reaction correlated with an excessive stimulation of the reticuloendothelial system and a marked activation of the liver functions [2, 7, 11].

The nonpyrogenic analog murabutide has been shown to be devoid of toxicity in humans in a phase I study [12].

NorMDP was generally well tolerated. Its chronic administration in mice at daily doses of up to 1 g/kg over a period of 3 months failed to create any significant toxicity [6].

Thr-MDP is nonpyrogenic and, moreover, it is the only analog that has been described as having no effect on the induction of anterior uveitis. In addition, it has a selective effect on the specific immunity to co-administered antigens and does not induce any other apparent side reactions [7].

MTP-PE is pyrogenic, it has vasculatory effects and induces inflammatory reactions. Its incorporation in liposomes, however, greatly reduced its toxicity and liposomal-MTP-PE has been produced for clinical use in humans [9].

MDP increases the susceptibility to endotoxins. At an early stage, the synergistic effect of endotoxin and MDP in the immunotherapy of line 10 hepatoma in strain 2 guinea pigs has been described. However, when guinea pigs were injected at the tumor site with 150 μg of endotoxin from *S. typhymurium*, trehalose dimycolate (TDM) and MDP(Ser), some died of an early shock suggesting a potentiation of the toxicity of endotoxin. Indeed, it has been shown that injection of 500 mg MDP by the intravenous route with sublethal doses of LPS (150 μg) increased the toxic effect of endotoxins, leading to the death of 100 % of treated guinea pigs. A similar toxic synergism has also been observed in mice. In contrast, murabutide appears to be devoid of any effect on the lethality of endotoxins [13].

Pharmacokinetics

MDP injected in saline in mice is cleared very rapidly. When 100 Mg of ^{14}C-MDP labeled on the C-1 of the lactyl group was injected i.v. or s.c., 50 % of the radiolabeled material was recovered unchanged in urine 30 minutes later. More than 90 % was recovered within 2 hours. Rapid elimination may account for the lack of activity of MDP on cell-mediated immunity and macrophage activation when it is injected in saline [2, 3, 14].

Encapsulation of MDP in multilamellar liposomes increases its remaining *in situ* and may explain its increased efficiency in activating macrophages both *in vitro* and *in vivo*. The attachment of acyl side chains to MDP makes the molecule more lipophilic resulting in a prolonged intracellular residence time and efficiency. Thus, the encapsulation of MTP-PE in liposomes has been shown to enhance the activation of macrophages and monocytes by 100-fold, as compared with free MDP [15].

Production of cytokines

MDP has been shown to affect multiple cells, either directly and/or through the secretion of various cytokines leading to an amplification of the initial stimulatory process.

Early results have demonstrated the enhancing effect of MDP on the production of IL-l (interleukin 1) by human monocytes and murine macrophage cell lines [16]. Because IL-l plays a central role in a wide range of biological phenomenons, some of the properties of MDP can be partially explained by its capacity to increase IL-l production.

Hemopoietic growth factors are produced by a number of cells including monocytes/macrophages. These latter produce TNF (tumor necrosis factor) and IL-l which can in turn stimulate growth factor production by endothelial cells. As a result, the stimulating effect of MDP on CSF (colony stimulating factor) production has been widely demonstrated but its mechanism of action was unknown. Recently, Broudy *et al* [17]. have shown that MDP induces the production of M-CSF (macrophages-CSF) and GM-CSF (granulocyte-CSF) by a mechanism independent of TNF .

Parant *et al*. [18] have reported the priming effect of MDP on TNF production by *in vivo*-stimulated mice upon triggering with LPS. It is noteworthy that in these experiments, MDP itself was inefficient in inducing TNF production whereas, in well-defined conditions, a 100-fold increase in TNF titers has been produced by costimulation.

Human monocytes appear to be more susceptible to MDP stimulation and Sanceau *et al*. [19] have reported that IL-l, TNF and IL-6 gene expression was increased by MDP , TNF having a cooperating effect for IL-6 secretion by MDP-stimulated monocytes.

Effect on hemopoiesis

MDP can stimulate hemopoiesis *in vivo* and *in vitro*. According to experimental conditions, it has been shown to affect myeloid progenitor cells, to stimulate the recruitment of commited stem cells, to increase the proliferation of multipotential stem cells and more generally to induce the production of a colony stimulating activity CSA [2]. It has been reported that MDP was effective also in C3H/HeJ mice, its injection resulted in the appearance of CSA in the serum within 4 hours in a dose dependent manner (10-500 μg/mouse). A Northern blot analysis was used to identify the growth factors induced by MDP treatment. It revealed the presence of transcripts for M-CSF and GM-CSF whereas mRNA for G-CSF, IL-3, IL-4 and IL-5 were not detected. Since IL-l mRNA but not TNF-mRNA was identified after MDP treatment, it has been concluded that MDP induces the production of M-CSF and GM-CSF by a mechanism independent of TNF ; however, IL-l could be implicated in the regulation of this CSF production [17].

Use as adjuvants for vaccines

Muramylpeptides have been used in experimental models to stimulate immunity to a variety of viral, bacterial, fungal and parasitic agents, as well as to tumor cell antigens [2-4]. At present, one of the most promising adjuvants seems to be the Syntex adjuvant (SAF) containing Thr-MDP. SAF has been shown to increase both humoral and cellular immunity, in a variety of animal species, to a wide variety of antigens such as IL-l, human IgM and antigens from infectious agents including simian acquired immunodeficiency syndrome oncovirus (SAIDS), influenza virus, hepatitis B virus, Epstein-Barr virus (EBV) and herpes simplex virus (HSV) [17].

Muramylpeptides have also been shown to increase the efficacy of subunit vaccines. A synthetic construct termed Tl-SP10 which contains B and T cell epitopes from HTLV (human T leukemia virus) envelope gpl20 which is recognized by neutralizing antibody, by Th cells and by MHC class I and class II CTL (cytotoxic T lymphocyte), was used to immunize rhesus monkeys. SAF was effective in eliciting an HIV-specific neutralizing antibody response and a proliferative response of peripheral blood mononuclear cells (PBMC) to the Tl-SP10 and to gpl20 [20]. Liposomal-MTP-PE has been administered with an acylpeptide containing a synthetic peptide corresponding to residues 1 to 23 of glycoprotein D of HSV-l ; the presence of MTP-PE increased antibody levels, stimulated cellular immunity and induced a 70 % protection of mice against lethal challenge [21]. It has been reported that MTP-PE in an oily formulation was as potent as FCA. Recombinant glycoprotein D of HSV-l termed rgDl was used as the antigen. Optimal results were obtained when guinea pigs were injected in footpads 4 weeks before viral challenge with FCA or MTP-PE emulsified with squalene and 0.008 % Tween 80. It is noteworthy that in these experiments MDP covalently conjugated to rgDl has shown little efficacy [22]. This is in contrast with other findings reporting the use of MDP-antigen conjugates as effective immunogens with built-in-adjuvanticity [23].

The pleitropism of muramylpeptides has been widely demonstrated and it is difficult to delineate which activities are directly responsible for the adjuvant effect. It is clear that macrophages, which play an important role in antigen processing and presentation and release a number of factors that are involved in the elaboration of an immune response, could be of importance for the mediation of the adjuvant effect. Thr-MDP, however, is a strong adjuvant and is reported as not being a macrophage activator [7].

It has been shown that purified B cells, cultivated in the presence of recombinant IL-2, can be stimulated by MDP to produce an optimal specific antibody response. In addition, MDP further increased the proliferation of polyclonally activated B cells. These findings suggest that B cells could be the essential target for the adjuvant effect of muramylpeptides [24]. This is in agreement with results showing that human tonsillar B cells could be immunized *in vitro* against various antigens in the presence of IL-2 provided that MDP was added to the culture [25]. Flow cytometric analyses have shown that, while MDP did not stimulate B cells to move out of the resting G0 state, it was able to act on once-stimulated B cells leading to an increased frequency of cells in the late G1 (G1B), S and G2/M phases of the cell cycle [26]. Furthermore, MDP has been shown to increase markedly LPS-induced expression of alkaline phosphatase activity suggesting that protein phosphorylation-dephosphorylation mechanisms could play an important role in MDP-mediated B cell activation [26].

Immunosuppression, inflammatory and autoimmune diseases

Muramylpeptides, as most immunomodulators, can exert positive as well as negative effects on both specific and nonspecific immunity. The final outcome depends on experimental conditions. Pretreatment by MDP and the use of large doses preferentially lead to an immunosuppression that can be partially explained by a regulation of interleukin-2 production. Two interesting examples are provided by the effect of MDP in skin allografts that resulted in prolonged graft survival and by streptozotocin-induced diabetes in which MDP prevented the autoimmune disease [2-4].

FCA induces inflammatory and necrotizing reactions at injection site, increased vascular permeability, arthritis and autoimmune diseases. Side effects of MDP, even when injected in mineral oil, are attenuated ; however, muramylpeptides stimulate or suppress autoimmune processes. This activity has been exploited in a number of experimental models to investigate the mechanism of autoimmunity. These include adjuvant arthritis and experimental encephalomyelitis [2-4]. A sensitive assay was developed by Syntex laboratories based on the induction of anterior uveitis in rabbits, its use has permitted to select Thr-MDP as an analog of MDP almost devoid of stimulating effect on autoimmune and inflammatory responses [7].

Stimulation of host resistance to infections

MDP and, even more, lipophilic derivatives stimulate natural host defence mechanisms. They are also effective in immunocompromised and immunodeficient hosts. Muramyldipeptides have been reported to increase protection against a number of pathogens including *Klebsiella pneumoniae, Escherichia coli, Staphylococcus pneumoniae, Salmonella thyphimurium, Mycobacterium tuberculosis, Pseudomonas aeruginosa, Candida albicans, Naeqleria fowleri, Trypanosoma cruzi* and *Toxoplasma gondii* [2-4].

The mechanism by which stimulation of nonspecific resistance occurs is thought to involve both activation of macrophages to a cytotoxic state and the release of cytokines including a chemotactic factor for polymorphonuclear cells [27]. This is in agreement with findings showing that the incorporation within liposomes and the use of lipophilic derivatives dramatically enhance the effectiveness of MDP. Ozaki *et al.* [28] have shown that MDP-Lys(L18) stimulated alveolar macrophages to phagocytize *P. aeruginosa* and stimulate the release of a neutrophil chemotactic factor *in vitro*. MDPLys(L18) enhanced the neutrophil response to inoculated *P. aeruginosa* in rats. As a result, this compound stimulated the neutrophil dependent defense system against *P. aeruginosa*.

TNF, a very potent anti-infectious agent, has been suggested to be the mediator of the anti-infectious activity of MDP because it could prime macrophages for an increased production of TNF upon stimulation. An example has been provided by Parant et al. [18]. Mice were infected with 2×10^7 colony-forming units of living BCG and challenged 2 weeks later with 25 µg LPS. The TNF levels in serum were measured 2 hours later. Mice treated 6 hours before LPS challenge with 300 µg/mouse MDP or analog exhibited a 100 fold increase in TNF titers.

MDP or analogs, alone or in combination with other agents, have been shown to confer resistance against a range of viruses including influenza, murine hepatitis, herpes simplex, Sendai, Semliki Forest and vaccinia viruses. Masihi et al. [29] have reported that MDP administration before or after lethal challenge with mouse hepatitis MHV-3 virus conferred hepatoprotection and significant survival of mice.

Recently, Masihi et al. [30] have reported the inhibitory activity of MDP on the replication of human HIV *in vitro*. The inhibition induced by a specific retroviral reverse transcriptase inhibitor (ddA) was, however, more important than that of MDP. Inhibition was measured on CD4+ and U937 monocytoid cells infected with HIV.

A synergistic effect of MDP with other immunomodulators has been reported by Wyde et al. [31]. MDP or murabutide when used alone were unable to protect mice from influenza virus infection. However sequential administration of MDP and poly(I :C) (polyinosinic-polycytidilic acid) which by themselves were ineffective, significantly reduced pulmonary influenza virus titers and protected mice from lethal disease. The mechanism of poly(I :C) plus MDP-induced protection does not appear to be due to an increased production of interferon and even to interferon itself because anti-interferon antibodies had no effect on the protective effect.

Liposomal MTP-PE exhibits prophylactic and therapeutic effects in a broad range of viral infections. Topical, intranasal, or oral administration could be effective even against viruses inoculated *via* a distant route. The mechanism of the antiviral activity of MTP-PE, administered within liposomes, is not yet clearly understood. MTP-PE is devoid of any direct antiviral activity for infected cells and is apparently unable to induce the production of interferon, although it could potentiate the effect of interferon inducers. *In situ* activation of macrophages, and natural killer cells, appears to be essential for antiviral activity. MTP-PE in micelle form in saline also showed antiviral activity in a variety of experimental models [32].

Stimulation of resistance to tumors

MDP and hydrosoluble analogs influence several macrophage functions and have often been used as a costimulator signal for macrophage activation *in vitro*. Comparable effects, however, have not been observed *in vivo*, probably because MDP has an extremely short half-life. Even when injected at very high doses, MDP fails to induce significant macrophage-mediated antitumor activity.

A promising approach to achieve macrophage activation *in situ* is the selective targeting to appropriate sites of action. Liposomes are biodegradable particles composed of natural phospholipids which generally have no intrinsic toxicity. Encapsulation in liposomes requires 1,000 times less MDP for an optimal stimulation, thus it greatly reduces side-effects. The incorporation of lipophilic derivatives of MDP leads to more stable and more active preparations ; for example liposomal MTP-PE is 3 times more effective than liposomal MDP. The antitumoral properties of liposomal MTP-PE has been widely demonstrated in experimental models. Macrophages from treated animals have tumoricidal activity. In addition, the systemic administration of liposomal MTP-PE has been shown to bring about regression of lymph nodes, lung and liver metastases [33].

The covalent linkage of MDP or MTP-PE to a carrier which can bind specifically to macrophages has been used to increase further the selective delivery to macrophages. Examples include monoclonal antibodies which bind to Fc receptors and facilitate endocytosis, acetylated low density lipoprotein (LDL) and mannosylated glycoproteins which bind to mannose receptors [2-4].

Neuropharmacological properties

The relationship between the neuroendocrine and immune systems is influenced by the microbial environment, examples are provided by muramylpeptides and endotoxins. MDP is pyrogenic, but endotoxin is about a thousand times more pyrogenic. Pyrogenicity is partially due to the release of endogenous pyrogen by macrophages but it is also due to a direct effect of MDP on brain structures. This was demonstrated by injecting MDP intracerebroventricularly ; under these conditions the effective dose was 10^5 times lower and was not mediated by endogenous pyrogen. Pyrogenicity, however, is not a prerequisite for the positive effect on immune response because immunostimulating derivatives such as murabutide and Thr-MDP are devoid of pyrogenicity [2-4, 7].

The discovery that endogenous sleep-promoting substances are muramylpeptides led to the finding that MDP itself is somnogenic [34]. When infused intracerebroventricularly, it induces an excess of slow-wave sleep but does not affect paradoxical sleep. Somnogenic analogs are generally pyrogenic, but the two effects are independent because antipyretic drugs suppress the febrile response while maintaining the somnogenic activity. In addition, some pyrogenic derivatives are totally devoid of effect on sleep. Somnogenicity appears to require amidation of the α-carboxyl group of glutamic acid. Thus, murabutide is not somnogenic. Somnogenic activity could be, at least partially, mediated by a local production of IL-1 by MDP-stimulated astrocytes and microglia cells. Indeed, IL-1 exhibited a more rapid effect on slow-wave sleep than MDP itself.

It has been proposed that the neurologic effects of MDP could be linked to a direct effect on central and peripheral serotonin-binding sites the turnover of which is increased by MDP. In agreement with these findings, it has been shown that serotonin agonists can mimic some effects of MDP and that serotonin does indeed compete for binding at MDP binding sites. More recently, another correlation has been established between sleep and MDP. It was shown that 100 % of narcoleptic patients express the MHC phenotype DR2,DQW1 and, in contrast to other phenotypes, B cells expressing DR2,DQW1 molecules failed to bind MDP [35].

Clinical studies

Murabutide has been administered to healthy volunteers and found to be safe but ineffective in increasing the immune response to tetanus toxoid [12].

MTP-PE in liposomes is currently undergoing clinical trials in cancer patients. In a phase I trial MTP-PE (0.5 to 12 mg/m^2) in phosphatidyl-serine : phosphatidylcholine liposomes (1 :250) was infused over 1 hour twice weekly up to 9 weeks. Various clinical parameters were monitored during treatment. The maximum-tolerated dose was 6 mg/m^2. Essentially, an increase of whole blood cell counts was induced, levels of acute phase reactants were increased, monocytes became tumoricidal and serum IL-1 was induced while serum cholesterol was significantly decreased. Technetium-99 labeled liposomes scanning revealed uptake of radiolabel in the liver, spleen, lung, nasopharynx, thyroid gland and tumor. However, despite a prolonged tumoricidal activity of monocytes *in vitro*, no antitumor activity could be recorded. This was explained by the fact that systemic macrophage-activation is not sufficient to get rid of large tumor burdens. Therefore, combination with other therapies should be used for optimally treating minimal residual disease [15].

Results of a similar phase I trial have been reported recently by Urba *et al.* [36]. A weekly 0.1 to 2.7 mg/m^2 dose was safe and well tolerated. The dose of 0.1 mg/m^2 appears to be above the maximal immunologically active dose. The C-reactive protein levels were increased and, interestingly, a consistent increase in serum neopterin levels has been found. It was suggested that neopterin levels could constitute a valuable indicator of the biological effect of MTP-PE in patients. Monocyte activation, however, failed to occur, suggesting the use of γ-interferon as a second signal for the optimal activation of monocytes to a tumoricidal state.

MTP-PE in liposomes administered to patients with advanced malignancies has been shown to increase IL-6 levels in sera. An early rise was observed with medium (0.25 and 0.5 mg/m^2) and high doses (1 up to 6 mg/m^2) which correlated with an increase in temperature. A maximal effect was recorded 2 and 4 hours after administration. These findings suggest that IL-6 which acts as an hepatocyte-stimulating factor could play a role in the modification of biological responses observed in MTP-PE-treated patients [37].

Concluding remarks

Muramylpeptides are multifunctional molecules that act on a variety of cells exerting either positive or negative effects depending on environmental factors and on the state of the target cell. Their activity is further amplified by their capacity to induce the production of cytokines, such as IL-1, TNF and IL-6, which play themselves a central role in inflammation and defense mechanisms. Muramylpeptides provide precious tools for basic immunologic research and some analogs, when used with an appropriate delivery system, are of potential interest for therapeutic use. At the present time, Thr-MDP is very promising for vaccines because it stimulates immunity, only to the co-administered antigen, whereas MTP-PE constitutes a potent and safe stimulator of nonspecific immunity.

References

1. Ellouz F, Adam A, Ciorbaru R, Lederer E. Minimal structural requirements for adjuvant-activity of bacterial peptidoglycan derivatives. *Biochem Biophys Res Commun* 1974 ; 59 : 1317.

2. Adam A. Synthetic adjuvants. In : Bona CA, ed. *Modern concepts in immunology*. Vol. 1, New York : Wiley-lnterscience Publication, 1985 : 1-239.
3. Adam A, Lederer E. Muramyl peptides : immunomodulators, sleep factors and vitamins. *Med Res Rev* 1984 ; 4 : 111.
4. Adam A, Lederer E. Muramylpeptides as immunomodulators. *ISI Atlas of Science Immunology* 1988 ; 1 : 205.
5. Chedid L, Parant MA, Audibert FM, Riveau GJ, Parant FJ, Lederer E, Choay JP, Lefrancier PL. Biological activity of a new synthetic muramyl dipeptide adjuvant devoid of pyrogenicity. *Infect Immun* 1982 ; 35 : 417.
6. Jones WR, Bradley J, Judd SJ, Denholm EH, Ing RMY, Mueller YW, Powell J, Griffin PD, Stevens YC. Phase I clinical trial of a world health organization birth control vaccine. *Lancet* 1988 ; 11 : 1295.
7. Eppstein DA, Byars NE, Allison AC. New adjuvants for vaccines containing purified protein antigens. *Adv Drug Delivery Rev* 1990 ; 4 : 233.
8. Azuma I, Yamamura Y. Immunoadjuvants for vaccine. *Adv Immunopharmacol* 1989 ; 4 : 149.
9. Van Hoogevest P, Frankhauser A. An industrial liposomal dosage form for muramyl-tripeptide-phosphatidyl-sthanolamine (MTP-PE). In : Lopez-Berestein G, Fidler IJ, eds. *Liposomes in the therapy of infectious diseases and cancer*, vol. 89. New York : Liss, 1989 : 117-25.
10. Sizun P, Perly B, Level M, Lefrancier P, Fermandjian S. Solution conformations of the immunomodulator muramyl peptides. *Tetrahedron* 1988 ; 44 : 991.
11. Masek K. Relationship between the pharmacological and toxicological effects of immunomodulators. In : Bizzini B, Bonmassar E, eds. *Adv Immunomodulation,* Roma : Pythagora Press ; 1988 : 245-50.
12. Telzak E, Wolff SM, Dinarello CA, Conlon T, El Kholy A, Bahr GM, Choay JP, Morin A, Chedid L. Clinical evaluation of the immunoadjuvant murabutide, a derivative of MDP, administered with a tetanus toxoid vaccine. *J Infect Dis* 1986 ; 153 : 628.
13. Parant M, Chedid L. Various aspects of synergism between endotoxin and MDPs. *Adv Exp Med Biol* 1990 ; 256 : 537
14. Williams JF. Pharmacokinetics of immunomodulators. *Immunopharmacol Rev* 1990 ; 1 : 65.
15. Murray JL, Kleinerman ES, Cunningham JE, Tatom JR, Andrejcio K, Lepe-Zuniga J, Lamki LM, Rosenblum MG, Frost H, Gutterman JU, Fidler IJ, Krakoff IH. Phase I trial of liposomal muramyl tripeptide phosphatidylethanolamine in cancer patients. *J Clin Oncol* 1989 ; 7 : 1915.
16. Oppenheim JJ, Togawa A, Chedid L, Mizel S. Components of mycobacteria and muramyl dipeptide with adjuvant activity induce lymphocyte activating factor. *Cell Immunol* 1980 ; 50 : 71.
17. Broudy YC, Kaushansky K, Shoemaker SG, Aggarwal BB, Adamson JW. Muramyl dipeptide induces production of hemopoietic growth factors *in vivo* by a mechanism independent of tumor necrosis factor. *J Immunol* 1990 ; 144 : 3789.
18. Parant M, Parant F, Vinit MA, Jupin C, Noso Y, Chedid L. Priming effect of muramyl peptides for induction by lipopolysaccharide of tumor necrosis factor production in mice. *J Leukocyte Biol* 1990 ; 47 : 164.
19. Sanceau J, Falcoff R, Beranger F, Carter DB, Wietzerbin J. Secretion of interleukin-6 (IL-6) by human monocytes stimulated by muramyl dipeptide and tumor necrosis factor alpha. *Immunology* 1990 ; 69 : 52.
20. Hart MK, Palker TJ, Matthews, TJ, Langlois AJ, Lerche NW, Martln ME, Scearce RM, McDanal C, Bolognesi DP, Haynes, BF. Synthetic peptides containing T and B cell epitopes from human immunodeficiency virus envelope gp 120 induce anti-HlV proliferative responses and high titers of neutralizing antibodies in rhesus monkeys. *J Immunol* 1990 ; 145 : 2677.

21. Brynestad K, Babbitt B, Huang L, Rouse BT. Influence of peptide acylation, liposome incorporation, and synthetic immunomodulators on theImmunogenicity of a 1-23 peptide of glycoprotein D of Herpes simplex virus : implications for subunit vaccines. *J Virol* 1990 ; 64 : 680.
22. Sanchez-Pescador L, Burke RL, Ott G, Van Nest G. The effects of adjuvants on the efficacy of a recombinant herpes simplex virus glycoprotein vaccine. *J Immunol* 1988 ; 141 : 1720.
23. Shapira M, Jolivet M, Arnon R. A synthetic vaccine against influenza with built-in adjuvanticity. *Int J Immmunopharmacol* 1985 ; 7 : 719.
24. Souvannavong V, Brown S, Adam A. Muramyl dipeptide (MDP) synergizes with interleukin 2 and interleukin 4 to stimulate, respectively, the differentiation and proliferation of B cells. *Cell Immunol* 1990 ; 126 : 106
25. Carroll K, Prosser E, O'Kennedy R. Parameters involved in the *in vitro* immunization of tonsillar lymphocytes : effects of IL-2 and muramyl dipeptide. *Hybridoma* 1990 ; 9 : 81.
26. Souvannavong V, Adam A. Increased expression of alkaline phosphatase activity in stimulated B lymphocytes by muramyl dipeptide. *Immunol Lett* 1990 ; 29 : 247.
27. Nagao S, Nakanishi M, Kutsukake H, Yagawa K, Kusumoto S, Shiba T, Tanaka A, Kotani S. Macrophages are stimulated by muramyl dipeptide to induce polymorphonuclear leukocyte accumulation in the peritoneal cavities of guinea pigs. *Infect Immun* 1990 ; 58 : 536.
28. Ozaki T, Maeda M, Hayashi H, Nakamura Y, Moriguchi H, Kamei T, Yasuoka S, Ogura T. Role of alveolar macrophages in the neutrophil-dependent defense system against *Pseudomonas aeruginosa* infection in the lower respiratory tract. Amplifying effect of muramyl dipeptide analog. *Am Rev Respir Dis* 1989 ; 140 : 1595.
29. Masihi KN, Kroger H, Lange W, Chedid L. Muramyl peptides confer hepatoprotection against murine viral hepatitis. *Int J Immunopharmacol* 1989 ; 11 : 879.
30. Masihi KN, Lange W, Rohde-Schulz B, Chedid L. Muramyl dipeptide inhibits replication of human immunodeficiency virus *in vitro*. *AIDS Res Hum Retrovir* 1990 ; 6 : 393.
31. Wyde PR, Six HR, Ambrose MW, Throop BJ. Muramyl peptides and polyinosinic-polycytodylic acid given to mice prior to influenza virus challenge reduces pulmonary disease and mortality. *J Biol Resp Modif* 1990 ; 9 : 98.
32. Dietrich FM, Hochkeppel HK, Lukas B. Enhancement of host resistance against virus infections by MTP-PE, a synthetic lipophilic muramyl peptide. 1. Increased survival in mice and guinea pigs after single drug administration prior to infection and the effect of MTP-PE on interferon levels in sera and lungs. *Int J Immunopharmacol* 1986 ; 8 : 931.
33. Fidler IJ. Systemic activation of macrophages by liposomes containing muramyltripeptide phosphatidylethanolamine for therapy of cancer metastasis. *J Liposome Res* 1990 ; I : 461.
34. Krueger JM, Pappenheimer JR, Karnovsky ML. Sleep-promoting effects of muramyl peptides. *Proc Natl Acad Sci USA* 1982 ; 79 : 6102.
35. Silverman DH, Sayegh MH, Alvarez CE, Johnson TS, Milford EL, Karnovsky ML. HLA class II-restricted binding of muramyl peptides to B lymphocytes of normal and narcoleptic subjects. *Hum Immunol* 1990 ; 27 : 145.
36. Urba WJ, Hartmann LC, Longo DL, Steis RG, Smith II JW, Kedar I, Creekmore S, Sznol M, Conlon K, Kopp WC, Huber C, Herold M, Alvord WG, Snow S, Clark JW. Phase I and immunomodulatory study of a muramyl peptide, muramyl tripeptide phosphatidylethanolamine. *Cancer Res* 1990 ; 50 : 2979.
37. Frost H, Murray JL, Chaudri HA, Van Damme J. Interleukin-6 induction by a muramyltripeptide derivative in cancer patients. *J Biol Resp Modif* 1990 ; 9 : 160.

2

OK-432, a killed streptococcal preparation, in the treatment of animal and human cancer and its mechanisms of action

M. SAITO

Laboratory of Cancer and Hematological Disease, Chugai Pharmaceutical Co., Ltd., 41-8, Takada 3-chome, Toshima-ku, Tokyo, Japan.

OK-432, a streptococcal preparation, as a potent biological response modifier (BRM) [1], first studied by Drs Okamoto and Koshimura at Kanazawa University (Japan), became commercially available in Japan in 1975 [2], and during the 17 years since then, a significant amount of data obtained by both experimental and clinical studies has been reported.

Early studies indicated that OK-432 may exhibit its antitumor effect by direct action on tumor cells [3], while other studies suggested that the mode of action was host-mediated and hence characterized OK-432 as a potent interferon inducer [4]. Further studies disclosed ability of OK-432 to induce other cytokines, including IL-1, IL-2 and IL-6 [5, 6]. In accordance with these findings, OK-432 has also been shown to augment natural killer (NK) cell activity [7], to induce antitumor macrophages [8], to activate antitumor neutrophils [9], and to induce cytotoxic T lymphocytes (CTL) [10]. The tumor growth inhibitory effect of OK-432 has been attributed to these OK-432 induced enhancements.

Properties

In order to produce OK-432, attenuated Streptococcus pyogenes Su strain is treated with H_2O_2, and the cocci are suspended in Bernheimer's basal medium containing penicillin G [2]. The suspension is then kept at 37 °C for 30 min and at 45 °C for another 20 min to eliminate the capability of producing streptolysin S (SLS), and freeze-dried to form the finished streptococcal preparation. This preparation

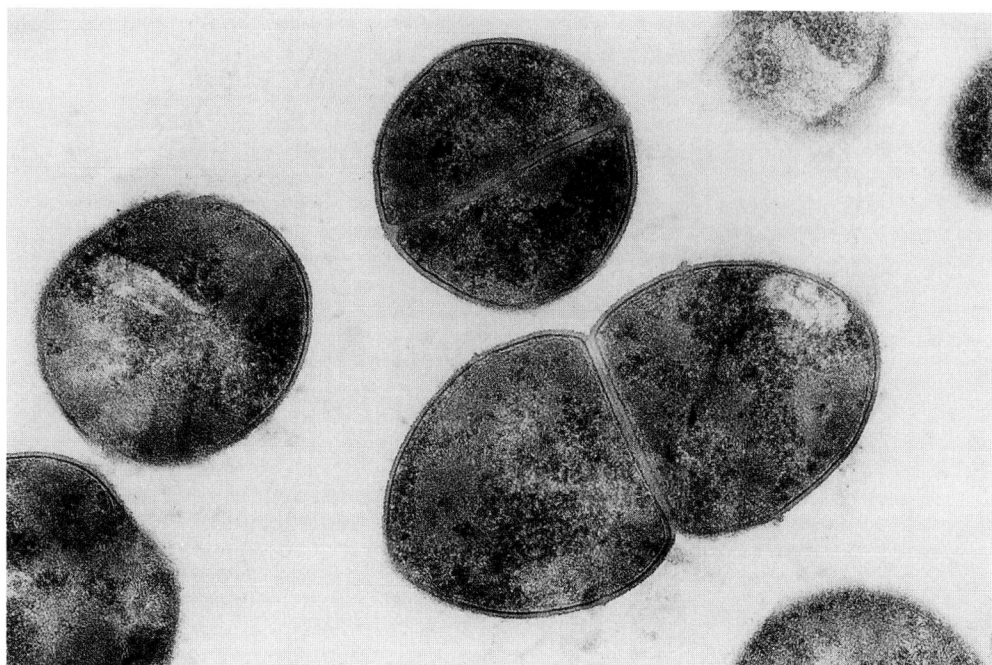

Figure 1. Electromicrograph of OK-432 (Picibanil®), a Streptococcal preparation (TEM, ×50,000).

contains no live cells, but the killed cells contained are similar to live cells with regard to form and size, although the cells are devoid of capsule and have a rather damaged cell wall, as demonstrated by electron microscopy (Figure 1). The similarity between live and killed cells seems to be significant in the manifestation of the antitumor effect of OK-432. Klinische Einheit (KE) is used as the unit of measure for OK-432 doses for clinical use ; 1 KE corresponds to 0.1 mg of dried streptococci.

Toxicity

LD_{50} of OK-432 is similar in mice and rats. LD_{50} values for intravenous (i.v.), intraperitoneal (i.p.) and subcutaneous (s.c.) administration are 250 KE/kg, 1,500 KE/kg, and 2,000 KE/kg, respectively. However, antitumor activity is present at 1/30 of the dose of LD_{50} i.p., *i.e.* 50 KE/kg. The optimal effective dose is 1 KE/animal for mice. In both rats and humans, the effective dose is 1-5 KE. OK-432 is clinically effective at a low dose in comparison with the corresponding doses in animal experiments, but the dose-effect relationship in human subjects is not as clear as in experimental animals.

Normally, in clinical practice, OK-432 is administered in doses of 2-5 KE once or twice a week when given by systemic administration (intradermally, subcutaneously, or intramuscularly), and in doses of 5-10 KE once or twice a week when given by either intracavitary or intratumoral injection.

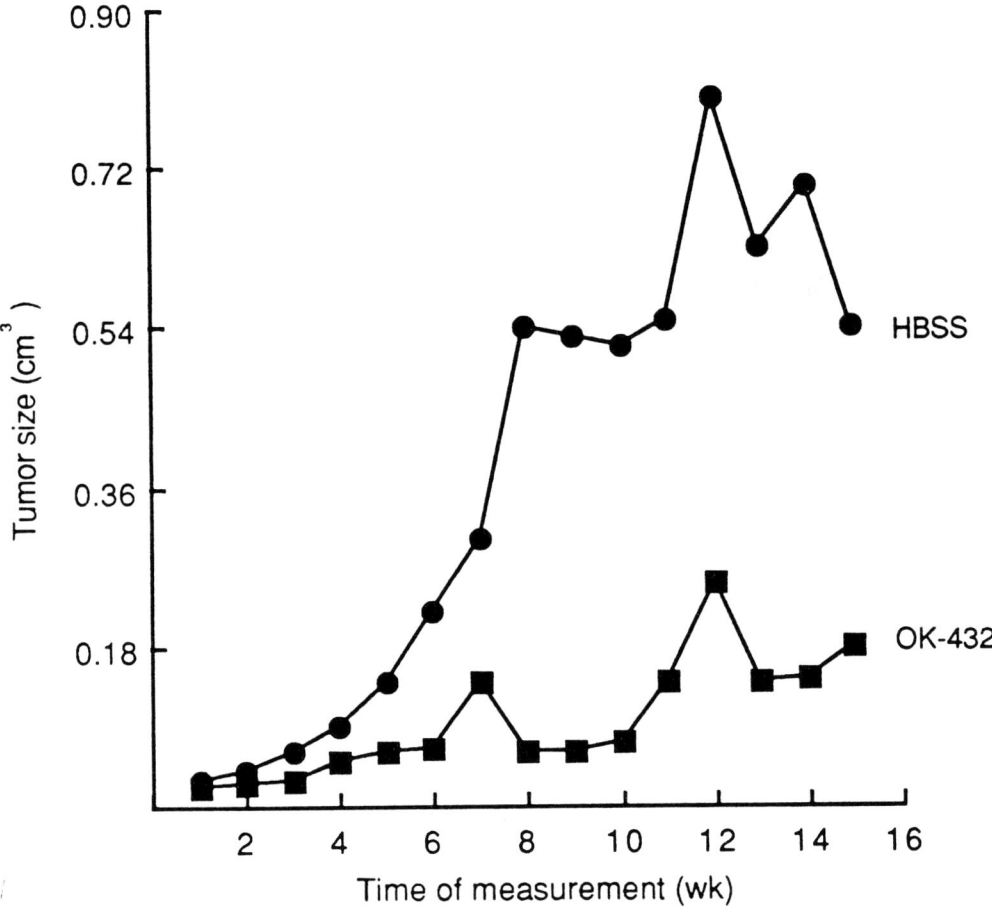

Figure 2. Effect of systemic administration of OK-432 on growth of primary autochthonous UV radiation-induced skin cancers. The size of primary skin neoplasms in BALB/c mice was monitored weekly by measuring the tumor diameter in two dimensions. Tumor volume was calculated by the formula for a prolated sphere $(0.5 \times a \times b^2)$. The difference in growth kinetics between saline treated (●) and OK-432 treated (■) mice was significant ($p = 0.014$).

When the toxicities of OK-432 is considered, pyrogenicity is the greatest issue. In rabbits, an intramuscular (i.m.) dose of 1.5 KE/kg or more or an i.p. dose of 0.3 KE/kg or more induces fever. It is not clear whether the rise in temperature is derived from the direct stimulation of the heat regulatory center by OK-432 or stimulation of the center by OK-432-induced IL-1. Clinically, tolerance to OK-432-induced fever occurs after repeated injection, and the patient shows no further febrile response.

In rabbits, intramuscular administration of OK-432 induces acute local inflammation at the injection site. A dose of more than 5 KE causes a small abscess with accumulation of polymorphonuclear leukocytes in its center. OK-432 induces no anaphylaxis in guinea pigs. Additionally no teratogenic effects, drug-associated embryonic deaths or abnormal effects on pregnant animals have been seen in either rabbits or rats.

Antitumor effects on experimental tumors in animals

It has been shown that OK-432 exerts an antitumor effect on UV-induced skin cancer and various transplantable syngeneic tumors. The antitumor effect is more distinct in animals sensitized with OK-432 than in non-sensitized animals, and similar findings have also been obtained in clinical cases. This section will give an outline of the published data on antitumor effects and metastasis-inhibitory effects observed after administration of OK-432 alone and in combined therapy with other chemotherapeutic agents and irradiation.

Effects on autochthonous tumors

OK-432 showed a tumor growth-inhibitory effect in *in vivo* antitumor experiments using various tumor models. UV-induced skin tumor of the BALB/c mouse was among such models [11]. Clear inhibition of tumor growth was observed after i.v. or intratumoral (i.t.) administration of OK-432 in mice bearing UV-induced tumors measuring 2-3 mm in diameter (Figure 2) [11]. Similarly, antitumor and life-prolonging effects were also noted after i.p. or i.t. administration of OK-432 in animals bearing methylcholanthrene-induced skin tumors.

Effects on syngeneic tumors

The antitumor activity of OK-432 has been confirmed in a number of syngeneic tumor models used in *in vivo* experiments. After s.c. transplantation of either Lewis lung carcinoma or B/6 melanoma in C57BL/6 mice, OK-432 administered by interaperitoneal or intratumoral route was found to inhibit tumor growth [12]. In addition, i.v. administration of this agent showed metastasis-inhibitory and life-prolonging effects in Lewis lung carcinoma-bearing mice [12]. A marked antitumor effect was also observed in BALB/c mice given i.p. administration of OK-432 after s.c. transplantation of M109 lung carcinoma, with complete response being obtained in 40 % of the tumor-bearing mice [13]. Additionally, a marked antitumor effect of OK-432 on ascitic tumor has also been reported [14]. When BAMC-l tumor was transplanted intraperitoneally into BALB/c mice, followed by i.p. administration of OK-432 at a dose of 0.1mg/mouse, all animals were still alive at 40 days after transplantation (Figure 3) [14]. The antitumor effect of OK-432 has also been demonstrated in mouse syngeneic MM2, MCA-F and KKN-l tumors.

The efficacy of OK-432 in rat syngeneic tumors has also been reported. When OK-432 was given i.p. to ACI rats which had received s.c. transplantation of syngeneic BC-47 urinary bladder carcinoma, the tumor completely regressed 28 days after transplantation [10]. When F344/N rats were given i.p. administration of OK-432 on the day following i.p. transplantation of syngeneic MADB106 mammary carcinoma, 60 % of the animals showed complete cure [15].

The antitumor effect of OK-432 was examined in Hartley/F guinea pigs after s.c. transplantation of syngeneic U-l tumor. In sensitized guinea pigs in which pretreatment with OK-432 had induced a positive skin reaction to the OK-432 derived Su-protein, i.t. administration of OK-432 starting 7 days after tumor transplantation

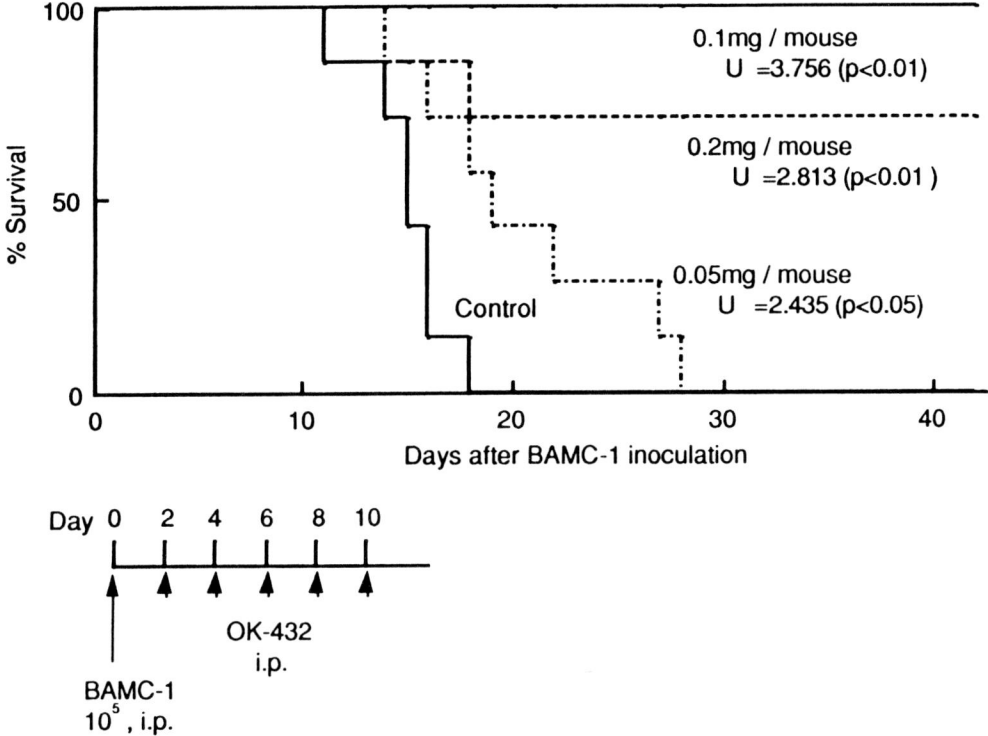

Figure 3. Dose effect of i.p. OK-432 on the survival of BALB/c mice bearing BAMC-1 tumor cells in ascilic form. BAMC-1 (1×10^5) were injected i.p. on day 0 to BALB/c mice. Five consecutive (once every 2 days) i.p. injections of OK-432 in 0.1 ml saline were performed as illustrated by the time schedule (below).

resulted in complete regression of the tumor [16]. However, the antitumor effects of OK-432 were not found in OK-432 non-sensitized guinea pigs [16]. This finding suggests that sensitization of the host with OK-432 is required for the manifestation of the antitumor effect of this agent. Similar findings have been obtained in clinical cases.

Inhibition of metastasis

Currently the most effective therapy for the treatment of cancer is surgical removal of the tumor. However, at present, significant problems remain in the inhibition of subsequent metastasis or recurrence. Metastasis of tumor is known to occur mainly *via* the hematogenous or lymphogenous route. Several reports have documented the efficacy of OK-432 in experimental models of these metastases. Lymph node metastasis of syngeneic MH-134 tumor and hepatic metastasis of Lewis lung carcinoma in C3H/He mice were markedly inhibited by OK-432 [17]. Intravenous administration of OK-432 after i.v. transplantation of mouse M109 tumor or B16 melanoma also markedly inhibited hepatic metastasis of the tumor [18]. Similarly, hepatic metastasis of MRMT-l cells in rats was markedly inhibited by pretreatment with OK-432 [19]. These metastasis-inhibitory effects of OK-432 have been attributed to the activation of NK cells. Intravenous administration of OK-432 before and after i.v. transplantation of U-l tumor in guinea pigs also resulted in evident inhibition of hepatic metastasis. The inhibition of metastasis was seen only in animals positive to the skin test with OK-432-derived Su-protein ; no inhibition was found in those with negative reaction [16].

Thus, since OK-432 inhibits metastasis of tumor, this drug seems to be highly useful for increase in survival period of patients after surgery.

Combined use with chemotherapeutic agents and irradiation

When antitumor agents with different mechanisms of action are administered combinedly, their effects are strengthened. In this regard, the use of OK-432 in combination with chemotherapeutic agents has been investigated. Favorable combined effects with OK-432 and various chemotherapeutic agents such as Mitomycin-C (MMC), 5-Fluruouracil (5FU) and adriamycin were observed in animal models. It has been demonstrated that timing is important in combined use of OK-432 with other chemotherapeutic agents. For example, a marked combined effect was obtained when OK-432 was given 2-3 days after administration of adriamycin, whereas no synergistic effect was seen when OK-432 was given before adriamycin [20]. Furthermore, a remarkable antitumor effect has also been demonstrated after the use of OK-432 combined with radiotherapy.

Mechanism of action

Induction of cytokines by OK-432

• *Induction of interferon (IFN)*

Ten years have already elapsed since OK-432, a streptococcal preparation, was established as an IFN inducer [4]. Initially it was reported that OK-432 induced IFN in serum in mice and in clinical cases [4, 21]. Additionally, IFN was detected in *in vitro* culture supernatant of lymphocyte stimulated with OK-432 [22]. Consequently, after a high titer of IFN-γ was detected in OK-432-presensitized animals, this agent was categorized as an IFN-γ inducer [23].

• *Induction of IL-1 and IL-2*

In 1982, Oppenheim *et al.* [24] and Farrar *et al.* [25] published the macrophage-T cell lymphokine cascade reaction theory, according to which the induction of cytotoxic T lymphocytes (CTL) involves cytokines interaction. Cytokines specified in the theory were IL-1 (macrophage-derived), IL-2 (helper T cell-derived) and immune interferon (IFN-γ). In light of their reports, splenocytes obtained from BALB/c mice were cultured *in vitro* with OK-432, and the IL-1 and IL-2 activities in the culture supernatant were determined. As in the case of IFN-γ production, the IL-1 and IL-2 activities were higher in the splenocytes of the mice which had been presensitized with *in vivo* administration of OK-432. There was no decrease in the level of these activities during successive OK-432 administration for 22 weeks from the level of activities observed after the first OK-432 administration. This indicated that the mice given OK-432 weekly were prepared to produce high levels of IL-2. This result also showed that the mice given boosters of the same antigen did not develop tolerance, indicating a characteristic feature of OK-432 differing from other extrinsic antigens.

- *Multi-cytokine inducer*

Thus, it was demonstrated that OK-432 induces IFN, IL-1 and IL-2 (1980-1982) [4, 5, 21], and in successive researches the induction of other cytokines also became apparent. Specifically, it was gradually found that OK-432 induces the production of effector molecules, such as TNF [26], NK cytotoxic factor [27], macrophage cytotoxic factor [27], neutrophil activating factor (NAF) [28], colony stimulating factor, (CSF) [29], NK cell chemotactic factor (NKCF) [30] and IL-6 [6]. Recent experiments have also shown that i.p. administration of OK-432 in mice results in the production of macrophage chemotactic factor (MCF) [31].

Table I. Biological activities of OK-432.

Induction of cytokines
  Interferon-alpha, beta and gamma
  Interleukin-1
  Interleukin-2
  Interleukin-6
  Colony-stimulating factor (CSF)
  Tumor necrosis factor (TNF)
  Natural killer cell-activating factor (NKAF)
  Natural killer cytotoxic factor
  Monocyte cytotoxic factor
  Neutrophil-activating factor (NAF)
  NK cell chemotactic factor (NKCF)
  Macrophage chemotactic factor (MCF)

Augmentation of cytotoxicity and/or cytostasis
  Cytotoxic T lymphocytes (CTL)
  Natural killer cells (NK)
  Fresh autotumor killer cells (ATK)
  Monocytes
  Macrophages
  Neutrophils
  Lymphokine-activated killer cells (LAK)

Enhancement of immune response
  Circulating lymphocytosis
  Phytomitogen blastogenesis of lymphocytes
  Reduction of suppressor T cells
  Reduction of suppressor macrophages
  Activation of complement

Others
  Metastasis prohibiting effect
  Combination effect with chemotherapy
  Direct tumoricidal effect
  Protection of bone marrow chemical damage
  Enhancement CFU-S colony formation

OK-432 is a multi-cytokine inducer which induces various cytokines, as shown in Table I. For the manifestation of antitumor activity of OK-432, it is necessary that these cytokines be induced at the proper time, for the proper duration and at the proper site, in accordance with sequence and tempo, hence elevating the host's immune responses, as shown in Table I, and thereby activating effector cells induced by these cytokines to act against cancer cells.

Analysis of the mechanism of action in mouse tumor cell system highly sensitive to OK-432

- *Standard experimental system*

When BAMC-l (10^5 cells), methylcholanthren-induced fibrosarcoma in BALB/c mice, was transplanted intraperitoneally into BALB/c mice, all the control mice died, whereas none of the mice given 5 i.p. administrations of OK-432 (0.1 mg/mouse) every other day after transplantation. In this experimental system, the optimal dose was 0.1 mg, and OK-432 was found to be less effective at either a higher or a lower dose, reflecting the characteristic feature common to all known BRMs. In these surviving mice, no recurrence was noted even at 3 to 6 months after transplantation, and re-transplanted BAMC-l was rejected completely, indicating that cytotoxic killer T cells were induced and immunological memory persisted [14, 32].

- *Appearance and involvement of polymorphonuclear neutrophils* (PMN) — *the starting runner in a relay for complete disappearance of tumor*

When OK-432 is administered intraperitoneally to BAMC-1 tumor-bearing mice, PMN are induced immediately, followed by an increase in macrophages, and then in T cells. Three hours after OK-432 administration, PMN account for more than 85 % of peritoneal exudate cells (PEC), corresponding to a level about 20-fold higher than the resident. These neutrophils serve as the starting runner essential for complete disappearance of tumor.

— **Characteristic of the antitumor action of PMN** : Tumor-inhibitory potentials of PMN were investigated using the Winn-neutralization assay. Admixture of PEC obtained 3 and 15 hours after i.p. administration of OK-432 and BAMC-1 tumor cells were transplanted subcutaneously into BALB/c mice. The results of the assay showed that PEC obtained at 3 hours (PMN accounted for more than 85 %) completely inhibited the growth of tumor in euthymic mice, whereas there was only transitory inhibition of tumor growth in athymic nude mice [33]. This result indicates that the contribution made by T cells is essential for complete inhibition of tumor growth by OK-432. PMN obtained at 15 hours after i.p. administration of OK-432 were found to have induced almost no inhibition of tumor growth, indicating that the starting runner, large PMN appearing at 3 hours, soon disappeared from the peritoneal cavity.

— **Cytokines produced by PMN** [31] : From the above-mentioned findings, it became apparent that PMN induced during the initial stage after OK-432 administration play the role of the starting runner. Based on the assumption that communication between PMN (the first runner : 3h after OK-432 administration) and subsequently appearing macrophages (the second runner) and T cells (the third runner) exist, the ability of these cells to produce cytokines was investigated.

PEC obtained 3h after OK-432 administration were cultured in 1 % BALB/c mouse serum-supplemented RPMI-1640 medium for 16 h, and the supernatant was injected intraperitoneally into mice. Morphological examination of PEC obtained at 24 hours after injection of culture-supernatant revealed large macrophages (*i.e.* in comparison to resident macrophages) in increased numbers. Since the presence of macrophage chemotactic factor (MCF) was suspected, the MCF activity of the supernatant was determined. Accordingly, the supernatant was found to have markedly high MCF activity [31]. IL-1 and IL-6 activity was also noted. IL-6 is known to be produced by human splenocytes after *in vitro* stimulation with OK-432 [6].

— **IL-6 stimulates liver cells to produce alpha-1 acid glycoprotein** : IL-6 stimulates liver cells to produce alpha-1 acid glycoprotein (alpha-1 AG) and C-reactive protein (CRP), *i.e.* inflammatory proteins. Therefore, as signified by the production of IL-6 after OK-432 administration, tumor-bearing animals given i.p. administration of OK-432 develop inflammation.

• *Involvement of macrophages (the second runner following PMN)*

Macrophages, which are induced following PMN in the peritoneal cavities of mice given OK-432 administration, serve as the second runner. The Winn assay was carried out after *in vitro* OK-432 stimulation of thioglycollate-induced peritoneal macrophages or OK-432 induced peritoneal macrophages obtained 4 days after i.p. administration of OK-432. Tumor growth was completely inhibited in euthymic mice, whereas only transitory inhibition was noted in athymic *nude* mice [34]. When anti-macrophage antiserum was administered to mice 2-4 days after tumor transplantation, the antitumor effect of OK-432 completely disappeared, showing that macrophages play an important role at this stage.

The above results indicate that the appearance of the second runner macrophages is necessary for the manifestation of the antitumor effect of OK-432. It is also clear from the experiment in nude mice that complete cure cannot be achieved in athymic *nude* mice without the appearance of a third runner, probably T cells.

• *Involvement of T cells (the third and fourth runners following macrophages)*

— *In vivo* **effects** : Through the examination of the antitumor effect of OK-432 in the standard experimental system using euthymic mice and athymic nude mice, antitumor activity of OK-432 was confirmed in euthymic mice. However, no complete cure was obtained in any of the athymic nude mice treated with OK-432, although there was a survival-prolonging effect [14]. This result shows that the antitumor effect of OK-432 requires the involvement of T cells.

— **Induction of helper T cells (the third runner)** : The mechanism of tumor elimination by OK-432 was then investigated in two experimental systems using athymic *nude* and euthymic mice. PEC obtained from OK-432 treated, tumor-bearing euthymic mice 3, 7 or 9 days after transplantation were transferred into the peritoneal cavities of tumor-bearing athymic *nude* mice treated with OK-432. Tumor cells gradually decreased on day 14 and completely disappeared later on in nude mice given PEC at 7 or 9 days. When PEC were treated with anti-L3T4 antibody and complements before transfer, such activity was completely abolished [35]. This result indicates that helper T cells play an important role at about 7-9 days after tumor transplantation, suggesting the involvement of IL-2 and IFN-γ at this stage. Recently, Ozaki et al [36] established the process for producing antigen-specific helper T cell clones for OK-432 and demonstrated that these cloned helper T cells attack tumor cells in the presence of OK-432, hence suggesting the importance of helper T cells [36].

— **Induction of non-specific killer T cells (the fourth runner)** : To examine effects of OK-432 on killer cells, PECs were collected from the tumor site, and their *in vitro* killer activity was investigated using syngeneic BAMC-1, NK-sensitive or NK-insensitive tumor as target. As a result, PEC obtained 12 days after BAMC-1 transplantation (2 days after the last injection of OK-432 therapy which consisted of 5 injections in total) showed non-specific killer activity on syngeneic BAMC-1, NK sensitive and NK insensitive tumor target cells in ^{51}Chromium release test [14]. The *in vivo* effects of these pantropic killer cells were then examined in adoptive immunotherapy. When 1×10^7 pantropic killer cells were transferred intravenously 1 h after administration of cyclophosphamide (CPA) 4 mg/kg on the fifth day following subcutaneous transplantation of 1×10^6 BAMC-1 or Meth-A tumor cells, the tumor subsequently disappeared [32]. These results indicate that non-specific killer cells, so-called pantropic killer cells (PKCs), effective under both *in vitro* and *in vivo* conditions were induced at the tumor site in mice after the administration of OK-432. When the PKCs were treated either with anti-Thy1 antibody and complement or anti-AsGM 1 antibody and complement, both the *in vivo* and *in vitro* killer activity of the PKCs was completely abolished, suggesting the coexistence of NK-LAK and T-LAK [32].

In conclusion, the appearance of the first runner (or PMNs) seems to be a prerequisite for the appearance of the second runner (or macrophages). The second runner (macrophages) also seems to be a prerequisite for appearance of the third and the fourth runner and such a sequential emergence of runners (or effector cells) at a definite tempo is required to achieve complete cure in OK-432-treated mice.

OK-432 clinical results

Clinical experiences with OK-432, during the past ten years, such as tumor reduction induced by intratumoral administration of OK-432 and life prolongation associated with systemic administration of OK-432 are reported in this section.

Efficacy in tumor reduction

Tumor reduction achieved by local administration of OK-432 in tumor tissue has been verified in patients with gastric [37], hepatic [38], colorectal [39], thyroid gland [40], head and neck [41], and lung cancers [42].

In a study involving 9 patients with inoperable gastric cancer [37], OK-432 was administered endoscopically to each patient, intratumorally and/or peritumorally. Tumor shrinkage was observed in 3 of the patients in this study. Moreover, in a study with 27 patients suffering from inoperable hepatoma [38], who were treated with OK-432 under ultrasonic, tumor reduction was identified in 22 of them.

Table II. Tumor-reducing effects of OK-432 in head and neck cancer patients.

Case No.	Sex	Age	Primary organ	Histology	TNM	Immunotherapy 432 Times of local injection	Total KE	Immunotherapy response
1. TO	M	49	Tongue oral floor	SCC	$T_2N_1M_0$	1	5	PR
2. KO	M	81	Oral floor	Epidermoid Ca.	$T_4N_2M_0$	6	70	PR
3. AI	F	33	Tongue	SCC	$T_2N_0M_0$	2	6	CR
4. JT	M	55	Buccal mucosa	SCC	$T_1N_1M_0$	11	71	PR
5. TS	M	78	Fauces	Mucoepidermoid Ca.	$T_4N_0M_1$	20	113.7	CR
6. KH	M	63	Oral floor	SCC	$T_1N_2M_0$	8	74	CR
7. FM	M	77	Tongue	SCC	$T_3N_0M_0$	12	117	PR
8. KE	M	63	Maxilla	SCC	$T_4N_1M_0$	9	66	PR
9. KK	M	62	Mandibula oral floor	SCC	$T_4N_1M_0$	1	5	NC
10. YN	M	62	Maxilla	Undifferentiated Ca.	$T_4N_0M_0$	31	374.5	PR (tempor.) followed by PD
11. RS	F	45	Maxilla	Adenoid cystic Ca.	$T_4N_0M_0$	13	88	PR
12. YY	M	58	Tongue	SCC	$T_2N_0M_0$	4	4	CR
13. KS	F	72	Oropharyngeal area	Adenoid cystic Ca.	$cT_4N_0M_0$	(2 ~ 3 KE/2 W) 6	21	PR
14. MN	F	66	Buccal mucosa	SCC	$cT_4N_3M_0$	(5 KE/2 W) 2	10	PR
15. SO	M	58	Maxilla	SCC	$cT_4N_2M_0$	(2/5 KE/W) 4	20	PR
16. TO	F	68	Buccal mucosa	SCC	$cT_1N_0M_0$	(2 ~ 5 KE/W) 5	20	PR
17. KS	F	58	Gingiva	SCC	$cT_4N_0M_0$	(5 KE/W) 2	10	MR
18. KW	M	52	Gingiva Mandibula, oral floor	SCC	$cT_4N_2M_0$	(2 ~ 5 KE/W) 12	60	MR (tempor.) followed by NC
19. MK	M	35	Oropharyngeal area	Malignant Fibrous Histiocytoma	$cT_4N_1M_0$	(10 KE/W) 1	10	MR
20. HK	F	60	Maxilla	SCC	$cT_4N_3M_0$	(5 KE/W) 2	10	PR

Evidence of tumor-reducing effect of OK-432 was also obtained in head and neck cancer patients who received OK-432 combination therapy with intravenous injections for 3 days, followed by intratumoral administrations [41]. As shown in Table II, CR or PR was seen in 80 % of the patients. The typical induction pattern of cytokines, *i.e.* TNF-α, IFN-α, and IFN-γ, was observed in the serum of patients who had responded well to OK-432 therapy.

It has also been reported that intracavitary administration of OK-432 is effective in patients with cancerous pleural effusion and/or ascites. In a study of 53 patients with carcinomatous pleurisy, where OK-432 was administered intrathoracically through tube drainage, the disappearance of pleural effusion for at least 4 weeks in 39 cases and a remarkable decrease in pleural effusion in 10 cases were observed [43]. Furthermore, in this study, a prolongation of survival period was achieved in the patients who experienced the disappearance or reduction of pleural effusion.

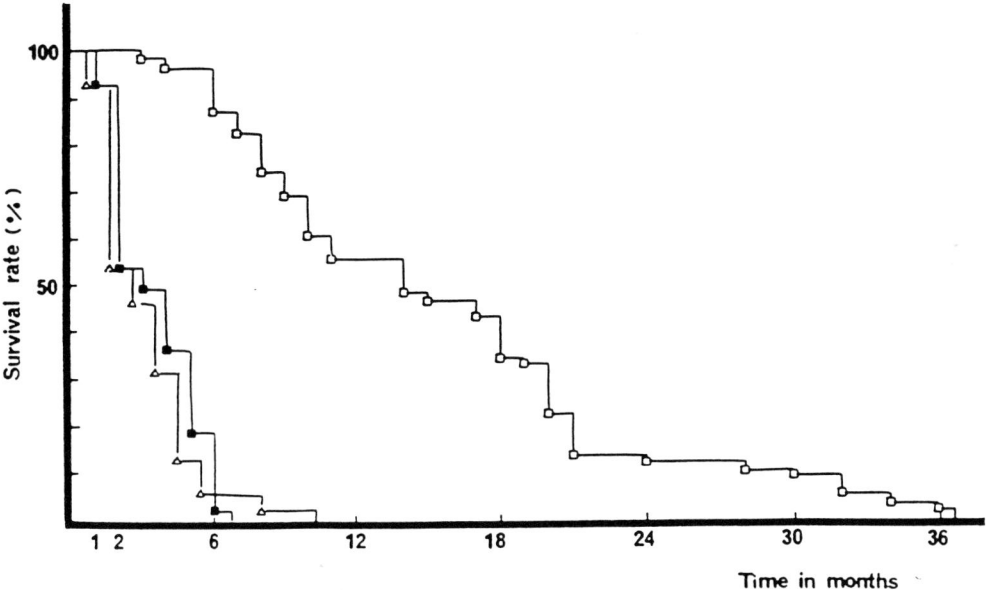

Figure 4. Comparison of survival rate between groups treated with and without OK-432. *Solid squares*, palliative therapy group (48 patients) ; *open squares*, group responsive to OK-432 therapy (58 patients) ; *triangles*, group non responsive to OK-432 therapy (41 patients).

Similar results were obtained in patients with carcinomatous ascites, who received intraperitoneal administrations of OK-432 once a week [44]. The disappearance or reduction of the ascites was noted in 62.7 % of patients. These effects were particularly remarkable in the patients with tumor cells in the ascites. The average survival period of the patient group which received OK-432 administrations was 10.2 months, while that of the control group was significantly lower (3.1 months) (Figure 4). In addition, in those who responded to OK-432 in this study, improvement in immune response, such as increase in serum protein, elevation of peripheral blood T-cells, and increase in delayed skin reaction, was observed. Upon dynamic histological study of the ascitic cells, it was observed that immediately after administration of OK-432 a number of neutrophils migrate to surround the tumor cells, consequently inflicting damage to the cells. Neutrophil activation is then followed concurrently by an increase in the number of macrophages and T-cells and a marked decrease in the number of tumor cells, which is accompanied by inhibition of DNA synthesis in the tumor cells [45].

As demonstrated in the above-mentioned studies, OK-432 shows remarkable effect when injected locally into either the tumor tissue or the vicinity of the tumor of cancerous peritonitis or carcinomatous pleurisy.

The effect of preoperative, intratumoral administration of OK-432 in gastric [46] and colorectal cancer patients [39] was recently observed. Histological examination of cancer tissue, surgically resected from patients who had received OK-432 through intratumoral administration (5-1OKE) prior to surgery, revealed the presence of OK-432 in the regional lymph nodes of the tumor tissue, as well as remarkable infiltration of lymphocytes into the tumor.

Moreover, the killer activity of the lymphocytes at the lymph nodes were shown to be enhanced. Considering the remarkable metastatic inhibition and life prolongation achieved in these studies, it is expected that further evidence of the clinical usefulness of preoperative OK-432 administration will be obtained.

Effect on survival

Efficacy of OK-432 in combination therapy with chemotherapeutic agents are reviewed by cancer cell type with particular focus on the life-prolonging effects.

- *Gastric cancer*

Survival prolongation attributable to OK-432 has been demonstrated in patients who have undergone surgery, including non curative resections and non-resections [47-49], and patients with inoperable cancer [50], although these life prolonging effects have been found to vary slightly with the degree of resection. In general practice, OK-432 (5 KE 1-2 times/week) is concomitantly administered either intramuscularly or intradermally with intravenous injections of chemotherapeutic agents, primarily MMC and 5-FU, from the period immediately following surgery. Subsequently, as maintenance therapy, the patient receives oral administrations of 5-FU derivatives, such as Tegafur, in combination with OK-432 injections which are consistently administered, if possible, on a permanent basis. While this method has generally proved successful in prolonging survival time, it has been suggested that the life prolonging effects of OK-432 are not obtainable in long-term combination therapy with aggressive chemotherapeutic agents, such as combination of MMC, 5-FU and cyclophosphamide (MFC) therapy [49].

- *Lung cancer*

It is widely accepted that the therapeutic approach to lung cancer must vary in accordance with the histological features and stage of the disease. However, it has been demonstrated that combination treatment with OK-432 and chemotherapy results in increased survival time in both non-small cell and small cell lung cancer patients.

In one such study, OK-432 was administered in combination with chemotherapeutic agents as postoperative therapy in a randomized comparison, involving a total of 311 non-small cell lung cancer patients. OK-432 was administered intramuscularly at a dose of 2 KE once a week for 3 years. The accompanying chemotherapy treatment, mainly composed of cyclophosphamide (CPA) and adriamycin (ADM), was intermittently applied every 3-6 months. A significantly longer survival period was noted in the patient group treated with OK-432 in comparison with the control group. The life-prolonging effect of OK-432 was also found to be significant when comparing the patients in the two groups by cancer stage and by type of operation (with or without resection [51].

Similarly, in the small cell lung cancer patients, it was demonstrated that OK-432, when administered in combination with chemotherapeutic agents, prolonged both mean duration of responses (CR and PR) and median survival time [52].

- *Other cancer types*

In colorectal cancer patients, treated with OK-432 as part of a postoperative chemotherapy regimen, inhibition of cancer recurrence and prolongation of survival time has been noted [53]. Similarly, increased survival time attributed to OK-432 has been documented in hepatoma patients who have received combined drug therapy with OK-432 and 5-FU after undergoing transcatheter arterial embolization [54].

Focusing on the combined usage of OK-432 and radiation therapy in cervical cancer treatment, researchers performed a controlled study investigating the rate of cancer recurrence and the length of remission [55]. In the treatment group, radiation therapy for 5-8 weeks at the initiation of the study was supplemented by OK-432 therapy, which was applied once every 1-2 weeks for at least two years by intradermal administration ; no chemotherapy was used during this time. At the end of 5 years of observation, the OK-432 treatment group showed significantly higher non-recurrence and survival rates than the control group, which had been treated only with the 5-8 week radiation therapy. As a result, it was concluded that the long-term administration of OK-432 led to remarkable inhibition of recurrence of cervical cancer [56].

In other combination drug-radiation therapy research concerning intratumoral administration of OK-432, evidence of the agent's efficacy in unresectable and inoperable esophageal carcinomas has been reported. In one such study, involving 26 patients, 20 were classified as CR and 6 as PR, *i.e.* 100 % of study subjects responded to the OK-432 and radiation therapy regimen. At one year after the start of treatment, the survival rate was recorded at 57.0 % ; the two-year survival rate was 31.6 % [57].

Calling for autologous transplantation of tumor infiltrating lymphocytes (TIL), which have been isolated from surgically extracted tumor and then activated *in vitro* by IL-2, etc., adaptive immunotherapy (AIT) has recently come into practice worldwide. When this therapy was combined with OK-432 treatment in liver metastasis arising from breast cancer, excellent clinical results were obtained with 9 out of the 19 cases recorded as PR in one representative study [58]. Evidence of life prolonging effects of OK-432 in head and neck cancer [59] and malignant lymphoma [60, 61] has also been obtained.

- *Summary of clinical results*

As discussed, it has been shown that OK-432 when used either alone or in combination with chemotherapy or radiation therapy exhibits marked effect in prolonging the survival time of patients suffering from various cancers. Recently, review on the therapeutic efficacy of OK-432 has been published by Abel and Vogler [62]. It should be emphasized here that long-term treatment with OK-432, exceeding one year, has been shown to be particularly beneficial. Furthermore, it has been demonstrated that effect of OK-432 emerges through activation of the immunological defense mechanism of the host, attributable to the interaction between time-sequential appearance of effector cells, such as neutrophil → macrophage → helper T-cell → LAK cell → CTL and induced cytokines. In comparing the OK-432 after-treatment results in carcinomatous ascites, for example, in both preclinical and clinical studies, the effector cells and effector molecules involved in the agent's mechanisms of action were clearly specified (Table III).

Table III. Effector mechanisms of OK-432. Ascitic maligancy.

			Exp. Animals		Patients	
			Effector cells	Cytokines	Effector cells	Cytokines
OK-432 i.p. → → → →	PMN MØ	Phase I	PMN MØ	MCF IL-6 IL-1	PMN MØ	(NK-CF)
L3T4	LAK	Phase II	L3T4 T-LAK NK-LAK	IFNγ IL-2	CD4 LAK	IFN
	CTL	Phase III	CTL ? Specific Immunity			

MCF : MØ chemotactic factor.
NK-CF : NK chemotactic factor.

In order to carry out a deliberate regimen of cancer treatment, involving aggressive surgery, chemotherapy, radiation therapy, or a combination of these methods, it is necessary to prevent the deterioration of patient's immune system. If this objective is accomplished, total kill of the tumor cells becomes possible. No matter what approach to cancer treatment is chosen, the enhancement of the host's immunological condition and the maintenance of the host-defense system is considered to be fundamental, and it is in this context that clinical usefulness of OK-432 is most apparent.

References

1. Talmage IE, Herberman, RB. Evaluation of immunomodulatory and therapeutic properties of biological response modifiers. *Cancer Treat Rep* 1986 ; 70 : 171-82.
2. Okamoto H, *et al.* Experimental anticancer studies. Part XXXI. On the streptococcal preparation having potent anticancer activity. *Jpn J Exp Med* 1966 ; 36 : 175-86.
3. Ono T, *et al.* Inhibitory effect of a streptococcal preparation (OK-432) on nucleic synthesis in tumor cells *in vitro*. *Gann* 1973 ; 64 : 59-69.
4. Saito M, *et al.* Induction of IFN-gamma in mouse spleen cells by OK-432, a preparation of *Streptococcus pyogenes*. *Cell Immunol* 1982 ; 68 : 187-92.
5. Ichimura O, *et al.* Augmentation of IL-1 and IL-2 production by OK-432. *Int J Immunopharmacol* 1985 ; 7: 263-70.
6. Fukui H, Koishihara Y, Nagamuta M, *et al.* Production of IL-6 by human spleen cells stimulated with streptococcal preparation OK-432. *Immunol Lett* 1989 ; 21 : 127-30.
7. Uchida A, Micksche M. *In vitro* augmentation of natural killing activity by OK-432. *Int J Immunopharmacol* 1981 ; 3 : 365-75.
8. Saito M, *et al.* Activated macrophages are responsible for the tumor-inhibitory effect in mice receiving intravenous injection of OK-432. *Int J Cancer* 1984 ; 33 : 271-6.
9. Watabe S, *et al.* Activation of cytotoxic polymorphonuclear leukocytes by *in vivo* administration of a streptococcal preparation, OK-432. *J Natl Cancer Inst* 1984 ; 72 : 1365-70.
10. Hojo H, Hashimoto Y. Cytotoxic cells induced in tumor-bearing rats by a streptococcal preparation (OK-432). *Gann* 1981 ; 72 : 692-9.
11. Talmadge JE, *et al.* The therapeutic properties for transplantable and autochthonous tumors. In : Ishida N, ed. *Mechanisms of antitumor effects of OK-432*. Tokyo : Excerpta Medica, 1986.
12. Micksche M, *et al.* Experimental and clinical studies with OK-432. A streptococcal preparation with immunomodulation properties. In : Serrou B, *et al.*, ed. *Human cancer immunology*. Amsterdam : Elsevier/North Holland, 1982.
13. Inaba S, *et al.* The therapeutic effect of picibanil given on Madison lung tumor bearing mice. *Jpn J Cancer Chemother* 1981 ; 8 : 974-8.
14. Saito M, Ichimura O, Kataoka M, *et al.* Pronounced antitumor effect of LAK-like cells induced in the peritoneal cavity of mice after intraperitoneal injection of OK-432, a killed streptococcal preparation. *Cancer Immunol Immunother* 1986 ; 22 : 161-8.
15. Fukui H, Reynolds CW. Antitumor activity of streptococcus pyogenes preparation (OK-432) I. Sequential effector mechanisms following a single OK-432 injection in F344 rats leading to the rejection of syngeneic MADB106 tumor cells. *JNCI* 1987 ; 79(3) : 1011-7.
16. Honjou M. Augmentation of cellular immunity to guinea pig tumor by antitumor agent OK-432 (picibanil). In : Hoshino T, ed. OK-432, Proceedings of the 13th International Congress of Chemotherapy. Tokyo : Excerpta Medica, 1984 ; 197-201.
17. Fujii G, *et al.* Effect of regional administration of nonspecific immunopotentiators on the lymph node metastasis. In : Torisu M, Yoshida T, eds. *Basic mechanisms and clinical treatment of tumor metastasis*. London : Academic Press, 1985 ; 223-53.
18. Chirigos MA, *et al.* The immunomodulatory and therapeutic activity of Picibanil (OK-432). In : Ishida N, ed. *Mechanisms of antitumor effect of OK-432*. Tokyo : Excerpta Medica, 1986 : 1-9.
19. Tanemura H, *et al.* Influence of operative stress on cancer bearers and effect of immunopotentiators. Experimental and clinical studies. *J Jpn Surg Society* ; 83(12) : 1359-68.
20. Saito M, *et al.* Combined effect of intraperitoneally administered adriamycin and OK-432 against Meth-A ascites tumor. *Jpn J Cancer Chemother* 1976 ; 6 : 1101-7.
21. Wakasugi H, *et al. In vitro* potentiation of human natural killer cell activity by a streptococcal preparation, OK-432 : interferon and interleukin-2 participation in stimulation with OK-432. *J Natl Cancer Inst* 1982 ; 69 : 807-12.
22. Noda T, *et al.* IFN-gamma induction in human peripheral blood mononuclear cells by

OK-432, a killed preparation of *Streptococcus pyogenes*. *Microbiol Immunol* 1983 ; 78 : 379-86.
23. Saito M, et al. In vitro production of immune interferon (IFN-gamma) by murine spleen cells when different sensitizing antigens are used *in vitro*. *Cell Immunol* 1983 ; 78 : 379-86.
24. Oppenheim JJ, et al. Circuit cytokine-cell interaction that regulate immunological and inflammatory reactions. Self-defense mechanisms. Role of macrophages. Mizuno D, ed. University of Tokyo Press, Elsevier Biochemical, 1982 : 127-36.
25. Farrar JJ, et al. The biochemistry, biology and role of interleukin 2 in the induction of cytotoxic T cell and antibody forming B cell response. *Immunol Rev* 1982 ; 63 : 129-66.
26. Kato M, et al. Antitumor therapy by induction of endogenous TNF. *Lancet* 1985 ; 8449 : 270.
27. Uchida A, Klein E. Activation of human blood lymphocytes and monocytes by the Streptococcal preparation OK-432 : enhanced generation of soluble cytotoxic factors. *Immunol Lett* 1985 ; 10 : 177-81.
28. Watabe S, et al. Activation of cytotoxic polymorphonuclear leukocytes by *in vivo* administration of a streptococcal preparation, OK-432. *J Natl Cancer Inst* 1984 ; 72 : 1365-70.
29. Hiraoka A, et al. Effect of a streptococcal preparation, OK-432, on murine hematopoietic stem cells. *Cancer Res* 1981 ; 41 : 2954-8.
30. Hayashi Y, Torisu M. New approach to management of malignant ascites with a streptococcal preparation OK-432 III — OK-432 attracts natural killer cells through a chemotactic factor diffused from activated neutrophils. *Surgery* 1990 ; 107 : 74-8.
31. Oikawa K, et al. Neutrophils induced by OK-432 produce a macrophage chemotactic factor. (In Japanese) *Biotherapy* 1991 ; 5 : 666-70.
32. Saito M, et al. Adoptive immunotherapy by pantropic killer cells recovered from OK-432-injected tumor sites in mice. *Cancer Res* 1988 ; 48 : 4163-7.
33. Kamijo E, et al. Role of polynuclear leukocytes in relation to the antitumor effect of OK-432. *J Clin Exp Med* (Igaku no ayumi) 1991 ; 158 : 875-6.
34. Nanjo M, et al. Antitumor effect of OK-432 (3). Mechanisms of tumor growth inhibition by OK-432 induced activated macrophages. *Jpn J Cancer Chemother* 1985 ; 12(4) : 887-93.
35. Moriya Y, et al. Induction of antitumor L3T4-positive T cells by OK-432 at tumor sites in mice. *Cancer Immunol Immunother* 1993 ; 36 : 245-50.
36. Ozaki S, Suginosita S. Biological response modifier as antigen : OK-432 specific T-cell clone as an antitumor effector cells. *Cell Immunol* 1989 ; 120 : 447-81.
37. Ochiai M, Amano H, Sugiue K, et al. Effect of endoscopic intratumoral administration of OK-432 in unresectable stomach cancer. (In Japanese) *Prog Med* 1988 ; 8(1) : 183-8.
38. Takada T, Yasuda H, Uchiyama K, et al. Intratumoral injections of the immunopotentiator OK-432 in the treatment of unresectable liver cancers. *Southeast Asian J Surgery* 1987 ; 10(2) : 93-8.
39. Monden T, Morimoto H, Shimano T, et al. Use of fibrinogen to enhance the antitumor effect of OK-432. *Cancer* 1992 ; 69 : 636-42.
40. Sugenoya A, Usuda N, Adachi W, et al. Immunohistochemical studies on local antitumor effects of streptococcal immunopotentiator, OK-432, in human solid malignant tumors. *Arch Pathol Lab Med* 1988 ; 112 : 545-9.
41. Umezu Y, Nagayama M, Nagasaka T, et al. Experimental and clinical study of OK-432 combination therapy. (In Japanese) *Biotherapy* 1990 ; 4(2) : 199-208.
42. Suzuki Y. Studies concerning the effects of presensitization on the antitumor activity of OK-432 (Picibanil, a streptococcal preparation) in terminal lung cancer patients. In : OK-432, Proceedings of an international symposium held at the 13th International Congress of Chemotherapy. Hoshino T, ed. Tokyo : Excerpta Medica, 1984 : 290-9.
43. Nagao K, Sugita T, Takizawa H, et al. Treatment of pleural carcinomatosis with intracavitary OK-432. In : Ota K, ed. *Clinical application of OK-432 for control of cancer.* Tokyo : Excerpta Medica, 1986 : 161-6.

44. Torisu M, Katano M, Kimura Y, et al. New approach to management of malignant ascites with a streptococcal preparation, OK-432. I. Important of host immunity and prolongation of survival. *Surgery* 1983 ; 93(3) : 357-64.
45. Katano M, Torisu M. New approach to management of malignant ascites with a streptococcal preparation, OK-432 II. Intraperitoneal inflammatory cell-mediated tumor cell destruction. *Surgery* 1983 ; 93(3) : 365-73.
46. Orita K, Gochi A. Usefulness of preoperative intratumoral OK-432 injection for lymph node metastasis. (In Japanese) *Biotherapy* 1990 ; 4(2) : 176-81.
47. Yagawa H, Ogawa K, Otani Y, et al. Immunochemotherapy for gastric cancer after surgical treatment. In : OK-432, Proceedings of an international symposium held at the 13th International Congress of Chemotherapy. Hoshino T, ed. Tokyo : Excerpta Medica, 1984 : 290-9.
48. Sakabe T, Fujii M, Takamatsu K, et al. Effect of OK-432 on progressive stomach cancer. Reexamination by randomized controlled study. (In Japanese) *J Med Pharm Sci* 1987 ; 18(6) : 1907-12.
49. Yasue M, Murakami M, Nakazato H, et al. A controlled study of maintenance chemoimmunotherapy vs immunotherapy alone immediately following palliative gastrectomy and induction chemoimmunotherapy for advanced gastric cancer. *Cancer Chemother Pharmacol* 1981 ; 7 : 5-10.
50. Uchida A, Hoshino T. Clinical studies on cell-mediated immunity in patients with malignant disease. 1. Effect of immunotherapy with OK-432 on lymphocyte subpopulation and phytomitogen responsiveness *in vitro*. *Cancer* 1980 ; 45 : 476-83.
51. Watanabe Y, Iwa T. Clinical value of immunotherapy with the streptococcal preparation OK-432 in non-small cell lung cancer. *J Biol Response Modif* 1987 ; 6 : 169-80.
52. Miyamoto H, Takaoka K, Ito M, et al. Immunotherapy using OK-432, a streptococcal preparation, for small-cell carcinoma of the lung. In : Ota K, ed. *Clinical application of OK-432 for control of cancer*. Tokyo : Excerpta Medica, 1986 : 120-6.
53. Kikkawa N, Kawahara T. Study on adjuvant immunochemotherapy with long-term OK-432 administration for colorectal cancer. *Jpn J Cancer Chemother* 1988 ; 15(6) : 1881-5.
54. Kubo Y, Hirai K, Horie Y, et al. A randomized clinical trial of immunochemotherapy and chemotherapy by carmofur with and without OK-432 in patients with hepatocellular carcinoma treated with transcatheter arterial embolization. (In Japanese) *Oncologia* 1989 ; 22(3) : 109-17.
55. Cervical cancer immunotherapy study group : immunotherapy using the streptococcal preparation OK-432 for the treatment of uterine cervical cancer. *Gynecologic Oncology* 1989 ; 35 : 367-72.
56. Cervical cancer immunotherapy study group : immunotherapy using the streptococcal preparation OK-432 for the treatment of uterine cervical cancer. *Cancer* 1987 ; 60 : 2394-402.
57. Mukai M, Morita S, Tsunemoto H. Combined therapy of local administration of OK-432 and radiation for esophageal cancer. *Int J Radiation Oncology Biol Phys* 1992 ; 22 : 1047-59.
58. Okino T, Kan N, Nakanishi M, et al. The therapeutic effect of OK-432-combined adoptive immunotherapy against liver metastasis from breast cancer. *J Cancer Res Clin Oncol* 1990 ; 116 : 197-202.
59. Ogasawara H, Kumoi T, Sawaki S, et al. A randomized controlled study of OK-432 for head and neck cancer. *Head and Neck Cancer* 1989 ; 15(2) : 183-6.
60. Uchino H, Shirakawa S, Nishikori M. Effectiveness of OK-432, a streptococcal preparation, as remission maintenance therapy for malignant lymphoma. (In Japanese) *Jpn Arch Int Med* 1988 ; 35(1) : 1-9.
61. Shirakawa S, Kita K, Tanaka T, et al. Immunopotentiating action of OK-432 and its clinical usefulness immunotherapy of malignant lymphoma. In : Ota K, ed. *Clinical application of OK-432 for control of cancer*. Tokyo : Excerpta Medica, 1986 : 217-28.
62. Abel U, Vogler S. Das Streptokokkenpraparat OK-432 in der Therapie maligner Tunoren. *Tumordiagn u Ther* 1992 ; 13 : 43-8.

3

Bestatin: immunopharmacology and clinical results

H. BLOMGREN

Department of General Oncology, Radiumhemmet, Karolinska Hospital, S-10401 Stockholm, Sweden.

Historic

In 1976 Umezawa *et al.* isolated a metabolite from culture media of *Streptomyces olivoreticuli*, strain MD976-C7, which acted as a potent competitive inhibitor of amino peptidase B. The metabolite, which was termed Bestatin, also appeared to inhibit leucine amino peptidase but not other enzymes such as aminopeptidase A, trypsin, chymotrypsin, elastase, papain or pepsin [1, 2]. Since aminopeptidase B and leucine amino peptidase are exopeptidases which are present on several types of mammalian cells, it was considered of interest to examine the biological effect of Bestatin. As described later, this inhibitor was found to modulate several functions of lymphoid and myeloid cells.

Chemical structure

The structure of Bestatin was found to be ((2S,3R)-3-amino-2-hydroxy-4-phenyl-butanoyl)-L-leucine (abbreviated ((2S,3R)-AHPA-L-Leu)). It is now being synthesized in large scale under the trade name Ubenimex [3].

Toxicology

Bestatin appeared to be extremely nontoxic for mice, rats, and dogs when administered subcutaneously, intraperitoneally or orally. There were no deaths in any species following oral administration of single doses ranging from 1.0-4.0 g/kg body weight.

In man, Bestatin has been given by the oral route at daily doses ranging from 10-800 mg for 7 consecutive days without causing any undue side effects [4].

In a series of leukemic patients who were treated with 30 mg of Bestatin daily, a few of them experienced a rash, itchiness or numbness, which might have been caused by Bestatin therapy [5]. In another series comprising 181 patients with head and neck cancer, possible side effects were reported in 6. Three of them experienced a rash, 1 had diarrhoea, 1 partial hair loss and 1 had a facial edema [6]. At our department, we have treated more than 200 cancer patients with oral Bestatin (usually 10 mg 3 times daily) without observing any side effects in spite of the fact that some of them had taken the drug daily for more than 7 years.

Pharmacokinetics

Bestatin is absorbed relatively rapidly following oral administration. Peak serum levels in man are reached within 2 hours followed by a biexponential decay with halflives of the α- and β-phases of around 1 and 5 hours respectively. Most of the drug is excreted into the urine in an unchanged form and a minor fraction as p-OH-Bestatin and as (2S,3R)APHA ([7] and Koyama et al., unpublished results).

P-OH-Bestatin, but not (2S, 3R)AHPA, exhibits aminopeptidase inhibitory activity and may enhance several functions of lymphocytes and macrophages (Abe et al., unpublished results).

Autoradiographic studies of mice injected with ^{3}H-Bestatin indicated that the compound binds to macrophages, the medulla of thymus and lymph nodes and the red pulp of the spleen. It was also localized on hepatocytes, bile duct epithelium, proximal straight tubules of the kidney and intestinal epithelium [8].

Influence of Bestatin on lymphoid cells *in vitro*

Binding to specific membrane receptors, *e.g.* exopeptidases, seems to be a prerequisite for the immunomodulatory effects of Bestatin. Isotope labeled drug binds rapidly to various lymphoid cells *in vitro*. Mouse peritoneal macrophages bind approximately $1\,400 \times 10^4$ molecules/cell, T-cells 250×10^4 and B-cells 90×10^4. A high binding was also reported to unfractionated bone marrow cells and the mouse lymphoma line L 5178Y. Highest binding of Bestatin was observed during the S/G2phase. The complex between Bestatin and its membrane receptor does not seem to be sequestered into the cells [9, 10].

Bestatin increases ^{3}H-thymidine incorporation, DNA polymerase activity and terminal deoxynucleotidyl transferase in mouse T-cells but not B-cells [11] and there was an opposite effect in rat hepatocytes stimulated with insulin or epidermal growth factor [12].

The observation that stimulation of T-cells by Bestatin does not occur in the absence of adherent cells may suggest that the effect is mediated by monocytes-macrophages [13].

Bestatin also stimulates *in vitro* colony formation of human bone marrow cells. This stimulation, however, seems to be dependent on T-cells rather than macrophages [14]. Recent studies have shown that Bestatin stimulated the release of colony stimulating factors [15, 16].

Splenic lymphocytes from mice and guinea pigs cultured with PHA, ConA or allogeneic lymphocytes or LPS exhibit enhanced mitogenic responses in the presence of Bestatin [17-19]. Such potentiations, however, were not detected in human blood lymphocyte cultures [20]. On the other hand, Bestatin augments the release of Il-2 of mitogen stimulated lymphocytes from both man and rodents [8, 21-23] and it potentiates Il-2 responses of T-cells [22, 23].

There is also evidence that Bestatin exposure of blood lymphoid cells from both healthy subjects and cancer patients may augment NK-activity. The effect, however, is relatively small [20, 24].

Macrophages from mouse peritoneal exudate may become cytotoxic for tumor cells after exposure to Bestatin *in vitro*. This activation is not T-cell dependent [19, 25, 26]. Bestatin treatment of mouse macrophages also stimulates their release of Il-1 [8], certain lysosomal enzymes and prostaglandins [26] and it augments the phagocytic activity of human monocytes and granulocytes [27, 28].

Bestatin may also change the expression and turn-over of membrane structures of lymphocytes such as receptors for SRBC and IgG [29, 30].

Influence of Bestatin treatment on immunological responses *in vivo*

Studies in animals

Treatment of mice with Bestatin enhances delayed type hypersensitivity reactions to a number of antigenes [26, 31-34] antibody production [31, 34] and it activates monocytes-macrophages [8, 19, 25, 26, 31]. There are also reports showing that NK-activity of lymphocytes may be increased in Bestatin treated mice [8, 26, 35]. Contradictory results have been published concerning the effects on ADCC [31, 35]. Bestatin may also reduce the generation and action of suppressor cells [8]. Moreover, a number of studies have shown that Bestatin treatment may retard growth or metastasis formation of transplanted allogeneic or syngeneic tumors [8, 19, 26, 33, 36-38]. The antitumor activity of cytotoxic agents like mitomycin C, 5fluorouracil and bleomycin may be potentiated by Bestatin [8, 33, 35, 36].

The most pronounced anti-tumor activity of Bestatin was observed in animals inoculated with small numbers of tumor cells [33, 35] and it was not observed at all in *nude* mice [8, 35, 37]. The latter finding strongly indicates that Bestatin augments antitumor responses of T-cells. This conclusion is in agreement with the results of other experiments showing that Bestatin induced tumor growth inhibitory activity of mouse spleen cells (Winn assay) disappeared upon removal of T-cells [8].

Repeated injections of mice with Bestatin was reported to significantly reduce the incidence of spontaneous tumors [31] and to retard the induction of skin cancer by 20-methylcholanthrene [33]. In addition, it suppressed the development of gastric cancer in rats fed N-methyl-N'-nitro-N-nitrosoguanidine [8].

Bestatin treatment of mice infected with *S.typhimurium* reduced the number of bacterial colonies and necrotic foci in the spleens and livers. This protective activity correlated to the extent of delayed hypersensitivity elicited by these bacteria [26].

A similar protection was observed in mice infected with a strain of *E.coli* causing pyelonephritis [26] and in mice injected with *Listeria monocytogenes* [39].

Studies in man

Bestatin treatment of cancer patients does not significantly change the absolute lymphocyte or monocyte counts in the blood. However, it may change the cellular composition or expression of certain membrane structures used for identifying subsets of lymphocytes. For instance, there was a significantly increased proportion of SRBC-rosette forming lymphocytes 2 weeks after daily, oral Bestatin (30mg) treatment of patients with advanced solid tumors. This increase was still present after 4-7 weeks of Bestatin treatment. The proportion of lymphocytes expressing membrane receptors for the Fc-part of IgG or C'3, however, was not changed [40]. More recent studies, using monoclonal antibodies to identify lymphocyte subsets, showed that Bestatin treatment (30 mg daily) of cancer patients increased the proportion of T-helper cells whereas T-suppressor cells were reduced [41].These authors also observed that the proportion of HNK-1+ cells (NK cells) increased. The latter finding may provide an explanation for the augmentation of NK-activity in cancer patients treated with Bestatin [24, 40].

PHA- and PPD-responses of blood lymphocytes, as measured by ^{3}H-thymidine incorporation, was not significantly changed during Bestatin treatment of patients with solid tumors [24, 40]. However, skin reactions to these substances increased in patients with leukemia and lymphoma [42]. Patients with rheumatoid arthritis who were treated with 10-60 mg of Bestatin every second day displayed an increased proportion of activated T-cells in the blood and the superoxide release from monocytes increased [43].

Oral administration of 10 or 40 mg of Bestatin to patients with cancer or recurrent furunculosis significantly increased the capacity of blood granulocytes to ingest yeast particles *in vitro*. This increase was most pronounced 3 h after Bestatin administration [28, 44]. A similar increase was noted for peripheral monocytes [45].

A prospective randomized trial was performed in our department to determine the clinical value of adjuvant Bestatin treatment in full-dose irradiated patients with bladder cancer *(see below)*. Bestatin treatment started at the time of the most extensive radiation-induced immunosuppression, *e.g.* at completion of irradiation [46]. It was observed that radiation therapy sharply reduced the size of the lymphocyte population without significantly changing its cellular composition. Recovery of the lymphocyte counts was not accelerated in the patients randomized to Bestatin treatment (10 mg 3 times daily without breaks for at least 1 year). However, the frequency of lymphocytes forming rosettes with SRBC was significantly increased after 1 month of Bestatin treatment, but decreased upon continuation of treatment. Other lymphocyte subsets, as detected by various rosetting techniques, were not changed during the observation period of 24 months. NK-activity of the blood lymphocyte population was significantly augmented in those Bestatin treated patients who survived for more than 18 months [47]. Further studies showed that the radiation induced suppressions of PHA- and PPD-responses of lymphocytes and PWM-triggered IgM-secretion *in vitro* were rapidly reverted by Bestatin treatment [48]. Such an augmentation was not observed in other cancer patients who had not been immunosuppressed by radiation [40]. The results of these studies indicate that Bestatin therapy may accelerate the recovery of immunological functions which have been suppressed by irradiation.

Optimal Bestatin dose and intervals of administration

In an attempt to determine the optimal daily dose of Bestatin, Majima [49] studied the changes of certain immunological parameters. Cancer patients received daily doses of Bestatin ranging from 10-900 mg. It was observed that the frequency of blood lymphocytes binding SRBC and ConA responses increased in patients receiving 30 and 60 mg, but not in those who received higher doses.

The optimal time interval of Bestatin administration is a matter of debate. The observation that the Bestatin-induced enhancement of SRBC-receptor expression of blood lymphocytes vains after prolonged daily Bestatin treatment [47] may suggest that the drug should be given intermittently rather than continuously. The data of Schorlemmer *et al.* [25] also suggested that the drug should be given intermittently. These investigators showed that injection of mice with Bestatin rendered peritoneal macrophages cytotoxic for tumor cells with an optimal activation on day 4. Daily injections, however, reduced the activation. In experimental infections with *S. typhimurium*, Schorlemmer *et al.* observed that injections of Bestatin every second day was more protective than daily applications [26]. As stated earlier in this review, daily Bestatin treatment of irradiated bladder cancer patients enhanced the recovery of mitogenic responses and PWMtriggered IgM-secretion of blood lymphocytes. These enhancements did not seem to be exhausted upon prolonged daily Bestatin medication.

It must be concluded that the optimal dose and time intervals of Bestatin medication are not yet definitely established.

Clinical studies

A number of trials have been conducted to examine the possible clinical value of Bestatin treatment in malignant and non-malignant diseases.

Non-malignant diseases

The clinical value of Bestatin treatment (60 mg every second day for 3 months) has been studied in a group of 36 patients with chronic urinary tract infections. Prior to start of Bestatin treatment, all these patients had experienced more than 6 episodes of infection during the last 6 months. The results showed that only 4 out of 17 patients with cystitis, without anatomic changes of the urinary tract, relapsed during Bestatin therapy. Patients suffering from cystitis due to anatomical changes of the urinary tract, patients with chronic epididymitis and chronic prostatitis did not seem to benefit from Bestatin treatment [26].

A study has also been performed in 10 patients with chronic polyarthritis. They were all refractory to conventional treatments such as anti-inflammatory drugs and gold. The Bestatin dose was escalated to 60 mg which was given every second day. Five of the patients experienced a drastic decrease of disease activity during Bestatin therapy, two had stable disease and it was aggravated in 3 patients. Shortly after withdrawal of Bestatin therapy, the disease activity returned to pretreatment levels [26].

Malignant diseases

Several trials have been conducted to examine the possible clinical value of adjuvant Bestatin treatment in patients with various types of solid tumors. No convincing beneficial effects of Bestatin have been obtained in squamous cell carcinoma of the skin (Ishihara and Ikeda, personal communication), squamous cell carcinoma of the head and neck (Inuyama et al. personal communication) and oesophagus cancer [50]. Statistically significant beneficial effects of adjuvant Bestatin treatment, however, have been observed in other types of malignant disease.

- *Gastric cancer*

The Cooperative Study Group of Surgical Adjuvant Chemotherapy for Gastric Cancer in Japan has performed a prospective randomized study in which patients with macroscopically radically operated gastric cancer were randomized into two treatment arms : one group received postoperative chemotherapy only, whereas the other group received chemotherapy plus 60 mg of daily Bestatin for 1 year. The results could not demonstrate any significant difference in survival between the two groups (96 evaluable patients). However, it was observed that patients with serosal invasion and those with stage III and IV disease benefited from Bestatin treatment. For instance, patients with serosal invasion without Bestatin had a 7-year survival rate of 13 % compared to 48 % in the Bestatin group [51].

- *Lung cancer*

A prospective randomized trial in patients with inoperable lung cancer has shown that 30 mg of daily Bestatin in addition to chemotherapy or radiotherapy significantly prolonged survival of patients with squamous cell cancer ($n=76$) whereas Bestatin had no significant effect on survival in patients with adenocarcinoma, small cell or large cell cancer [52].

A similar beneficial effect of adjuvant Bestatin treatment has been reported in patients with resected squamous cell carcinoma of the lung ($n=70$). No significant impact on survival was noted in patients with other histological tumor types [53].

- *Bladder cancer*

Patients with biopsy proven bladder cancer received full-dose local radiation therapy. Before start of this treatment, the patients, stratified according to T-category of the tumors, were randomized to receive Bestatin or no further adjuvant treatment. Bestatin therapy, 10 mg capsules 3 times daily for at least 1 year, was started on the day after completion of irradiation. The first interim analysis was made when a total of 176 patients had entered the trial [46]. A number of 151 of these patients were included in the analysis. It was observed that the disease-free survival of the Bestatin treated patients ($n=75$) was longer than that of the controls ($n=76$) ($p<0.05$). The results indicated that favorable characteristics for Bestatin treatment were superficial tumor growth and a low malignancy grade. Moreover, men seem to benefit more from Bestatin treatment than women. Overall survival was not increased ; a finding which was confirmed later [54].

- *Malignant melanoma*

Patients with malignant melanoma stage Ib and ll were randomized into two treatment arms following surgery : 30 mg of daily oral Bestatin for 6 months or no further treatment. The authors reported a statistically significant prolongation of disease-free interval and overall survival in the Bestatin treated patients. The results, however, should be interpreted with caution since the number of evaluable patients was small ($n=69$) and the clinical follow-up period short (around 30 months) [55].

- *Leukemia*

Perhaps the most convincing positive results of adjuvant Bestatin therapy have been obtained in patients with acute nonlymphocytic leukemia (ANLL) in adults [5]. In this multicenter study, patients received remission induction therapy with a combination of chemotherapeutic drugs followed by 3 courses of consolidation therapy. Thereafter, the patients, stratified according to age and type of ANLL (myelogenous or monocytic), were randomly allocated to Bestatin (30mg daily) or no Bestatin treatment.

Maintenance chemotherapy was given every 5 weeks during Bestatin treatment. There were 48 evaluable patients in the Bestatin group and 53 in the control group. The mean remission duration of the Bestatin treated patients was 21 months and 12 months in the control group. The difference between the two groups was not statistically significant. The mean survival time, which was 33 and 19 months in the Bestatin and control groups respectively, however, was statistically significant with a p-value of 0.02 using the Generalized Wilcoxon test and 0.007 using the Cox Mantel test. The 4-year survival was 46 % in the Bestatin treated patients and 26 % in the control group. This suggests that Bestatin therapy may actually contribute to the cure of patients with ANLL. Further analysis of this patient material suggested that patients aged $5 \sim 65$ years were those who benefitted most from Bestatin treatment.

- *Myelodysplastic syndrome*

Most remarkable effects of Bestatin treatment (30 mg daily) have been observed in patients with myelodysplastic syndromes with more than 60 % responders, some of which have achieved complete remissions [56].

Conclusion

Bestatin belongs to a new generation of immunomodulating substances with great potential. Several clinical trials have already indicated that this non-toxic drug increases the resistance to infections and may improve survival in patients with malignant disease. Further studies, however, are necessary to determine optimal Bestatin doses and intervals of administration.

LIST OF ABBREVIATIONS
ADCC : antibody dependent cellular cytotoxicity
B-cell : bone marrow derived lymphocyte, dependent on Bursa of Fabricius in birds
C'3 : complement factor 3
ConA : concanavalin A
CFS : colony stimulating factor
IgG : immunoglobulin G
IgM : immunoglobulin M
Il-1 : interleukin 1
Il-2 : interleukin 2
LPS : lipopolysaccharide
NK-cell : natural killer cell
PHA : phytohemagglutinin
PPD : purified protein derivative of tuberculin
SRBC : sheep red blood cell
T-cell : thymus dependent lymphocyte

References

1. Suda H, Aoyagi T, Takeuchi T, Umezawa H. Inhibition of aminopeptidase B and leucine aminopeptidase by Bestatin and its stereoisomer. *Arch Biochem Biophys* 1976 ; 177 : 196-200.
2. Umezawa H, Aoyagi T, Suda H, Hamada M, Takeuchi T. Bestatin, an inhibitor of aminopeptidase B, produced by actinomycetes. *J Antibiotics* 1976 ; 29 : 97-9.
3. Nishizawa R, Saino T, Suzuki M, Fuji T, Shirai T, Aoyagi T, Umezawa H. A facile synthesis of Bestatin. *J Antibiotics* 1983 ; 36 : 695-7.
4. Saito K, Miysato H, Tajima K, Ikeda S. Phase I study of Bestatin. A clinical study on determination of an optimal dose of Bestatin. *Jpn J Cancer Chemother* 1983 ; 10 : 211-7.
5. Ota K, Kurita S, Yamada K, Masaoka T, Uzuka Y, Ogawa N. Immunotherapy with Bestatin for acute nonlymphocytic leukemia in adults. *Cancer Immunol Immunother* 1986 ; 23 : 5-10.
6. Inuyama Y, Miyake H, Horiuchi M, Taketa L. Adjuvant therapy with Bestatin for squamous cell carcinoma of the head and neck. In : Umezawa H, ed. *Recent results of Bestatin 1985. A biological response modifier*. Japan Antibiotics Research Association. T & T. Co., Ltd. 1985 : 91-100.
7. Miyazaki H. Pharmacokinetics and metabolism of Bestatin in humans and rats by gas chromatography-mass spectrometry. In : Umezawa H, ed. *Small molecular immunomodifiers of microbial origin. Fundamental and clinical studies of Bestatin*. Tokyo : Japan Scientific Societies Press, 1981 : 217-29.
8. Ishizuka M, Takeuchi T, Umezawa H. Effect of Bestatin on immune system and experimental animal tumors. In : Umezawa H, ed. *Recent results of Bestatin 1985. A biological response modifier*. Japan Antibiotics Research Association. T&T. Co., Ltd. 1985 : 1-12.

9. Leyhausen G, Cramzow M, Zahn RK, Steffen R, Umezawa H, Muller WEG. Immunochemical identification of cell surface bound leucine aminopeptidase, the target enzyme for the immunostimulant Bestatin. *J Antibiotics* 1983 ; 36 : 729-34.
10. Müller WEG, Schuster DK, Zahn RK, Maidhof A, Leuhauser G, Flake D, Koren R, Umezawa H. Properties and specificity of binding sites for the immunomodulator Bestatin on the surface of mammalian cells. *Int J Immunopharmacol* 1982 ; 4 : 393-400.
11. Müller WEG, Zahn RK, Arendes J, Munsch N, Umezawa H. Activation of DNA metabolism in T-cells by Bestatin. *Biochemical Pharmacol* 1979 ; 28 : 3131-7.
12. Takahashi K, Kato H, Seki T, Noguchi T, Naito H, Aoyagi T, Umezawa H. Bestatin, a microbial aminopeptidase inhibitor, inhibits DNA-synthesis induced by insulin or epidermal growth factor in primary cultured rat hepatocytes. *J Antibiotics* 1985 ; 38 : 1767-73.
13. Weissman N, Leyhausen G, Maidhof A, Tanaka W, Umezawa H, Müller EG. Mitogenic potentials of Bestatin, Amastin, Arphamenines A and B, FK-156 and FK-565 on spleen lymphocytes. *J Antibiotics* 1985 ; 38 : 772-8.
14. Maekawa T, Sonoda Y, Okamoto Y, Tsuda S, Nishida K, Taniwaki M, Abe T, Takino T. Effect of Bestatin on human granulocyte-macrophage progenitor cells (CFU-C) *in vitro* and its possible mechanism of action. *J Kyoto Pref Univ Med* 1984 ; 93 :1039-44.
15. Tsunogake S, Furusawa S, Takano N, Enokihara H, Shishida H, Abe F. Effect of Ubenimex on the proliferation of normal human hematopoietic cells and myeloid leukemia cells. In : Rubinstein E, Adam D, eds. *Recent advances in chemotherapy*. Proceedings of the 16th International Congress of Chemotherapy, 1989 : 764.1-764.2.
16. Okamura S, Omori F, Haga K, Baba H, Kawasaki C, Tanaka T, Sugimachi K, Niho Y. Ubenimex stimulates production of colony stimulating factor from human peripheral mononuclear cells *in vitro*. In : Rubinstein E, Adam D, eds. *Recent advances in chemotherapy*. Proceedings of the 16th International Congress of Chemotherapy, 1989 : 759.1-759.3.
17. Saito M, Aoyagai T, Umezawa H, Nagai Y. Bestatin, a new specific inhibitor of aminopeptidases, enhances activation of small lymphocytes by concanavalin A. *Biochem Biophys Res Commun* 1977 ; 76 : 526-33.
18. Saito M, Takegositi K, Aoyagi T, Umezawa H, Nagai Y. Stimulating effect of Bestatin, a new specific inhibitor of aminopeptidases, on the blastogenesis of guinea pig lymphocytes. *Cellular Immunol* 1978 ; 40 : 247-62.
19. Talmadge JE. Immunomodulatory and therapeutic characteristics of Bestatin. In : Umezawa H, ed. *Recent result of Bestatin. A biological response modifier*. Japan Antibiotics Research Association. T.&T. Co., Ltd. 1985 : 55-66.
20. Blomgren H, Strender LE, Edsmyr F. The influence of Bestatin on the lymphoid system in the human. In : Umezawa H, ed. *Small molecular immunodifiers of microbial origin. Fundamental and clinical studies of Bestatin*. Tokyo : Japan Scientific Societies Press, 1981 : 71-96.
21. Blomgren H. Bestatin, a new immunomodulator, augments the release of mitogenic factors from PHA-stimulated human lymphocytes. *Biomedicine* 1981 ; 34 : 188-92.
22. Kishter S, Hoffman FA, Pizo PO. Production of and response to interleukin-2 by cultivated T-cells : effects of lithium chloride and other putative modulators. *J Biol Response Modifiers* 1985 ; 4 : 185-94.
23. Noma T, Klein B, Cupissol D, Yata J, Serrou B. Increased sensibility of II-2-dependent cultured T-cells and enhancement of *in vitro* II-2 production by human lymphocytes treated with Bestatin. *Int J Immunopharmacol* 1984 ; 6 : 87-92.
24. Aoike A, Tanaka Y, Hosokawa T, Yamaguchi N, Kawai K. Effect of Bestatin on natural killer activity. In : Umezawa H, ed. *Small molecular immunodifiers of microbial origin. Fundamental and clinical studies of Bestatin*. Tokyo : Japan Scientific Societies Press, 1981 : 101-8.
25. Schorlemmer HU, Bosslet K, Sedlacek HH. Ability of the immunomodulating dipeptide Bestatin to activate cytotoxic mononuclear phagocytes. *Cancer Res* 1983 ; 43 : 4148-53.
26. Schorlemmer HU, Dickneite G, Bosslet K, Widman E, Hilfenhaus J, Luben G, Sedlacek HH. Immunomodulating effect, antitumor activity and effect of Bestatin on infec-

tious diseases. In : Umezawa H, ed. *Recent results of Bestatin 1985. A biological response modifier.* T.&T. Co., Ltd. 1985 : 13-28.
27. Jarstrand C, Blomgren H. Bestatin, a new immunomodulator, enhances migration and phagocytosis of human granulocytes *in vitro*. *J Clin Lab Immunol* 1981 ; 5 : 67-9.
28. Jarstrand C, Blomgren H. Increased granulocyte phagocytosis after oral administration of Bestatin, a new immunomodulator. *J Clin Lab Immunol* 1982 ; 7 : 115-8.
29. Blomgren H. Influence of Bestatin, a new immunomodulator, on the expression of Fc receptors on human lymphocytes *in vitro*. *Hum Lymphoc Differ* 1981 ; 1 : 159-66.
30. Blomgren H, Wasserman J. Bestatin treatment of human lymphocytes increases the frequency of sheep red blood cell binding cells. *Cancer Lett* 1981 ; 11 : 303-8.
31. Bruley-Rosset M, Florentin I, Kiger N, Schulz J, Mathe G. Restoration of impaired immune functions of aged animals by chronic Bestatin treatment. *Immunology* 1979 ; 38 : 75-83.
32. Ishizuka M, Aoyagi T, Takeuchi T, Umezawa H. Activity of Bestatin : enhancement of immune responses and antitumor effect. In : Umezawa H, ed. *Small molecular immunomodifiers of microbial origin. Fundamental and clinical studies of Bestatin*. Tokyo : Japan Scientific Societies Press, 1981 : 17-38.
33. Ishizuka MI, Masuda T, Kanbayashi N, Fukasawa S, Takeuchi T, Aoyagi T, Umezawa H. Effect of Bestatin on mouse immune system and experimental tumors. *J Antibiotics* 1980 ; 33 : 642-52.
34. Umezawa H, Ishizuka M, Aoyagi T, Takeuchi T. Enhancement of delayed type hypersensitivity by Bestatin, an inhibitor of aminopeptidase B and leucine aminopeptidase. *J Antibiotics* 1976 ; 29 : 857-9.
35. Abe F, Shibuya K, Ashizawa J, Takahashi K, Horinishi H, Matsuda A, Ishizuka M, Takeuchi T, Umezawa H. Enhancement of antitumor effect of cytotoxic agents by Bestatin. *J Antibiotics* 1985 ; 38 : 411-4.
36. Aoyagi T, Ishizuka M, Takeuchi T, Umezawa H. Enzyme inhibitors in relation to cancer therapy. *J Antibiotics* 1977 ; 30 : 121-32.
37. Sonoyama T, Terata N, Matsumoto H, Nozaki A, Kimura K, Kurioka H, Hashimoto I, Tsunoda F, Kodama M. Study on the antitumor effect of an inhibitor against cell surface enzyme (Bestatin). *J Jpn Soc Cancer Ther* 1982 ; 17 : 1264-69.
38. Tsuruo T, Naganuma K, Lida H, Yamori T, Tsukagoshi S, Sakurai Y. Inhibition of lymph node metastasis of P388 leukemia by Bestatin in mice. *J Antibiotics* 1981 ; 34 : 120-9.
39. Harada Y, Kajiki A, Higuchi K, Ishibashi T, Takamoto M. The mode of immunopotentiating action of Bestatin : enhanced resistance to Listeria monocytogenes infection. *J Antibiotics* 1983 ; 36 : 1411-4.
40. Blomgren H, Strender LE, Edsmyr F. Changes of the blood lymphocyte population in cancer patients treated with Bestatin, a new immunomodulator. A phase I study. *Biomed Pharmacother* 1980 ; 32 : 178-85.
41. Kamano N, Suzuki S, Oizumi K, Konno K, Himori T, Matachi Y, Wakui A. Imbalance of T-cell subsets in cancer patients and its modification with Bestatin, a small molecular immunomodifier. *Tohoku J Exp Med* 1985 ; 147 : 125-33.
42. Arimori S, Nagao T, Shimizu Y, Watanabe K, Komatsuda M. The effect of Bestatin on patients with acute and chronic leukemia and malignant lymphoma. *Tokai J Exp Clin Med* 1980 ; 5 : 63-71.
43. Meske S, Vogt P, Maly FE, Seitz M, Muller W. Erste Ergebnisse der klinischen Anwendung des Immunostimulants Bestatin bei patienten mit chronischer Polyarthritis. *Z Reumatol* 1985 ; 44 : 231-6.
44. Mattsson L, Blomgren H, Holmgren B, Jarstrand C. Bestatin treatment for the correction of granulocyte dysfunction in patients with recurrent furunculosis. *Infection* 1983 ; 11 : 205-7.
45. Jarstrand C, Blomgren H. Influence of Bestatin, a new immunomodulator, on various functions of human monocytes. *J Clin Lab Immunol* 1982 ; 9 : 193-8.

46. Blomgren H, Näslund I, Esposti PL, Johansen L, Aaskoven O. Adjuvant Bestatin immunotherapy in patients with transitional cell carcinoma of the bladder. Clinical results of a prospective randomized trial. *Cancer Immunol Immunother* 1987 ; 25 : 41-6.
47. Blomgren H, Edsmyr F, Esposti PL, Näslund I. Immunological and hematological monitoring in bladder cancer patients receiving adjuvant Bestatin treatment following radiation therapy. A prospective randomized trial. *Biomed Pharmacother* 1984 ; 38 : 143-9.
48. Blomgren H, Edsmyr F, von Stedingk LV, Wasserman J. Bestatin treatment enhances the recovery of radiation induced impairments of immunological reactivity of the blood lymphocyte population in bladder cancer patients. *Biomed Pharmacother* 1986 ; 40 : 50-4.
49. Majima H. Phase I clinical study of Bestatin. In : Umezawa H, ed. *Recent results of Bestatin 1985. A biological response modifier*. Japan Antibiotics Research Association. T. & T. Co., Ltd. 1985 : 67-72.
50. Isono K. Effect of Bestatin on primary tumor and prognosis in patients with oesophageal carcinoma. In : Umezawa H, ed. *Recent results of Bestatin. A biological response modifier*. Japan Antibiotics Research Association. T. & T. Co., Ltd. 1985 : 101-10.
51. Hattori T, Niimoto M, Saeki T. Prospective randomized study on Bestatin in resectable gastric cancer. In : *Recent advances in chemotherapy*. Proceedings of the 16th International Congress of Chemotherapy, 1989 : 769.1-769.3.
52. Takada M, Fukuoka M. Controlled study of Ubenimex on operable lung cancer. In : *Recent advances in chemotherapy*. Proceedings of the 16th International Congress of Chemotherapy, 1989 : 771.1-771.3.
53. Yasumisu T, Ohshima S, Nakano N, Kotake Y. In : Rubinstein E, Adam D, eds. *Recent advances in chemotherapy*. Proceedings of the 16th International Congress of Chemotherapy, 1989 : 772.1-772.3.
54. Blomgren H, Esposti PL, Näslund I, Johansen L, Lemming O. Adjuvant Bestatin (Ubenimex) treatment following full-dose local irradiation for bladder cancer. In : *Recent advances in chemotherapy*. Proceedings of the 16th International Congress of Chemotherapy, 1989 : 767.1-767.3.
55. Ikeda, S, Ishihara K. Randomized controlled study of Bestatin in the treatment of stage Ib and II malignant melanoma. *Int J Immunotherapy* 1986 ; 2 : 73-9.
56. Saito Y, Uzuka Y. Bestatin treatment of patients with myelodysplastic syndromes. In : Rubinstein E, Adam D, eds. *Recent advances in chemotherapy*. Proceedings of the 16th International Congress of Chemotherapy, 1989 : 766.1-766-2.

4

Immunopharmacology of glucan phosphate

D.L. WILLIAMS[1], H.A. PRETUS[2], I.W. BROWDER[1]

[1] Department of Surgery, Quillen-Dishner College of Medicine, East Tennessee State University, Johnson City, Tennessee 37614-0002, USA.
[2] Department of Physiology, Tulane University School of Medicine, 1430 Tulane Avenue, New Orleans, Louisiana 70112, USA.

Product

Historical background

The ability of naturally occurring complex polysaccharide polymers to modulate immunity has been well documented [1-5]. In 1957, Benacerraf and Sebestyn demonstrated that zymosan, a glucomannan isolated from *Saccharomyces cerevisiae*, would produce marked hyperplasia and hyperfunctionality of the reticuloendothelial or fixed tissue macrophage system [6]. Di Luzio [7] and Cutler [8] confirmed and extended the work of Benacerraf and Sebestyn. In 1961, Riggi and Di Luzio demonstrated that glucan, a β-1,3-linked glucopyranose polymer, was the macrophage stimulating agent in zymosan. Since that time, numerous studies have shown that β-D-glucan biological response modifiers (BRMs) will enhance the functional status of macrophages [9, 10], T and B lymphocytes [5] and neutrophils [11]. Glucan will also modify immunosuppression [12, 13], exert an anti-neoplastic effect [14] and increase resistance to microbial challenge [15]. These observations have stimulated investigation into the potential biomedical applications of polymeric β-D-glucan BRMs [5, 14]. However, there were certain technical problems associated with the application of these agents. By way of example, β-D-glucan is a micro-particulate (~1-2μ) upon initial isolation from *S. cerevisiae*. While topical or intralesional administration of micro-particulate glucan induces no toxicity [16], systemic administration of the micro-particulate form is associated with hepatosplenomegaly [17], granuloma formation [14], micro-embolization and enhanced endotoxin sensitivity [18, 19]. If β-D-glucan BRMs were to become clinically applicable, they had to be converted to a water soluble form that could be safely and effectively administered *via* the systemic route. Numerous reports exist which describe isolation methodology and immunologic effects of water soluble polymeric β-D-glucan BRMs isolated from a variety of plant and microbial sources [3, 20]. Specific examples include Lentinan [4], Krestin [21], schizophyllan [22], aminated β-D-glucan [23], Grifolan [24] and SSG [20]. While all of these compounds possess immune stimulatory activity to a greater or lesser extent, many still exhibit significant toxicity, including vasodilatation [4], microvascular hemorrhage [4] and circulatory collapse [25]. Clearly, there was a need for development of a process for the solubilization of micro-particulate β-D-glucans.

Based on the therapeutic potential of these agents, our laboratory undertook studies to develop methodology for the conversion of water insoluble β-D-glucan to a safe, effective water soluble form. We have successfully developed a process for the solubilization of micro-particulate β-D-glucan which satisfies these criteria. This simple and efficient process involves a phosphorylation reaction. Our model system has employed insoluble β-1,3-D-glucan isolated from the inner cell wall of *S. cerevisiae* as the starting material. Soluble phosphorylated glucan (hereafter referred to as glucan phosphate) is a non-toxic [26], immune stimulant [27-29] that is suitable for parenteral administration to humans [30] and animals [26]. This work reviews the development, characterization, preclinical and clinical evaluation of glucan phosphate.

Chemical and physicochemical properties

Elemental analysis indicates that glucan phosphate is composed of 34.66 % carbon, 6.29 % hydrogen, 42.83 % oxygen and 2.23 % phosphorus. Based on the elemental composition, glucan phosphate was determined to have an empirical formula of $(C_6H_{10}O_5)_7,PO_3H_2$, indicating a phosphate group substitution every seventh glucose sub-unit. Molecular weight averages, polydispersity and intrinsic viscosity were established by aqueous high performance size exclusion chromatography (SEC) with on-line multi-angle laser light scattering (MALLS) photometry and differential viscometry (DV) [31]. Two polymer peaks were resolved. Peak 1, the high MW peak represents ~2 % of the total polymers, while peak 2 comprises ~98 % of polymers (Table I).

Table I. Molecular weight averages, polydispersity and intrinsic viscosity of glucan phosphate [1].

Parameter	Peak 1	Peak 2
M_n (number-average MW)	1.28×10^6	2.52×10^4
M_w (weigh-average MW)	3.57×10^6	1.10×10^5
M_z (z-average MW)	12.23×10^6	3.04×10^6
I (polydispersity)	3.2	6.2
[η] (intrinsic viscosity)	—	0.29 g/dl
% of total polymers	~ 2 %	~ 98 %

[1] Molecular weight expressed in g/mol.

The average molecular weights (MWs), polydispersity and intrinsic viscosity of glucan phosphate are presented in Table I. The weight average MW (Mw), expressed in g/mol, represents the average MW of the polymers in each peak. The number average MW (Mn) is indicative of the proportion of low MW polymers. Z-average MW (Mz) reflects the proportion of high molecular weight polymers. The polydispersity number (I) reflects polymer homogeneity (*i.e.* the lower the I, the more homogeneous the polymers with regard to MW).

The conformational structure of glucan phosphate was determined by the method of Ogawa and Hatano [32]. This technique assesses the absorption maxima of polymers in solution complexed with congo red in the presence of varying concentrations of hydroxide ion. The presence of a triple-helical polymer is indicated by a shift in the absorption maxima of the solution as NaOH concentration increases, indicating disruption of intramolecular hydrogen bonds with subsequent relaxation of the helix (*i.e.* helix melting). A random coil polymer does not show the shift in absorption maxima. Glucan phosphate exhibits a triple helical conformation as denoted by a shift in the absorption maxima between 0.2 and 0.3 M NaOH (Figure 1). Laminarin served as the triple-helical control. A 40,000 D dextran served as the random coil control. Congo red in NaOH served as the negative control.

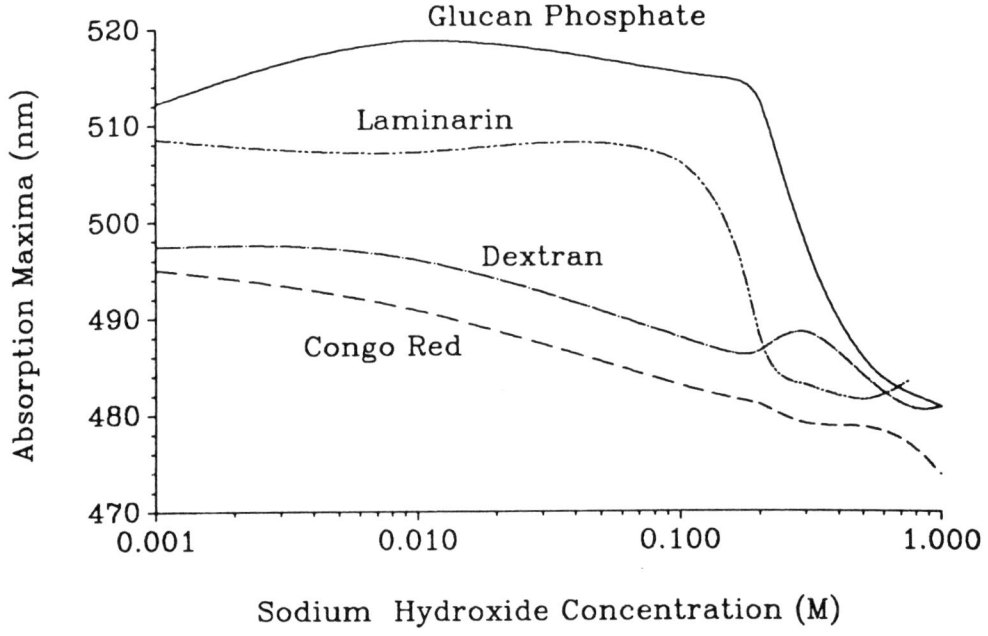

Figure 1. Helix-coil transition of glucan phosphate in the presence of congo red and varying concentrations of NaOH. Glucan phosphate exhibits a shift to a lower lambda $_{max}$ between 0.2 and 0.4 M NaOH, indicating disruption of the ordered (triple helical) conformation. Laminarin served as the β-1,3-linked triple helical control. Dextran (40,000 D) served as the random coil control. Congo red in NaOH served as the negative control.

To confirm the type of interchain linkages associated with glucan phosphate, samples were analyzed by ^{13}C-NMR in deuterated dimethyl sulfoxide (DMSO-d_6). This allows elucidation of the polymer backbone [24] and can also be employed to evaluate the type of side-chain branching, if any, along the backbone [24]. The ^{13}C-NMR spectrum of insoluble β-D-glucan isolated from *S. cerevisiae* and water soluble glucan phosphate prepared from the insoluble material are presented in Figure 2. Laminarin, a triple helical β-1,3-linked glucopyranose, in DMSO-d_6 served as control. Comparison of the β-D-glucan peaks shows excellent correspondence with

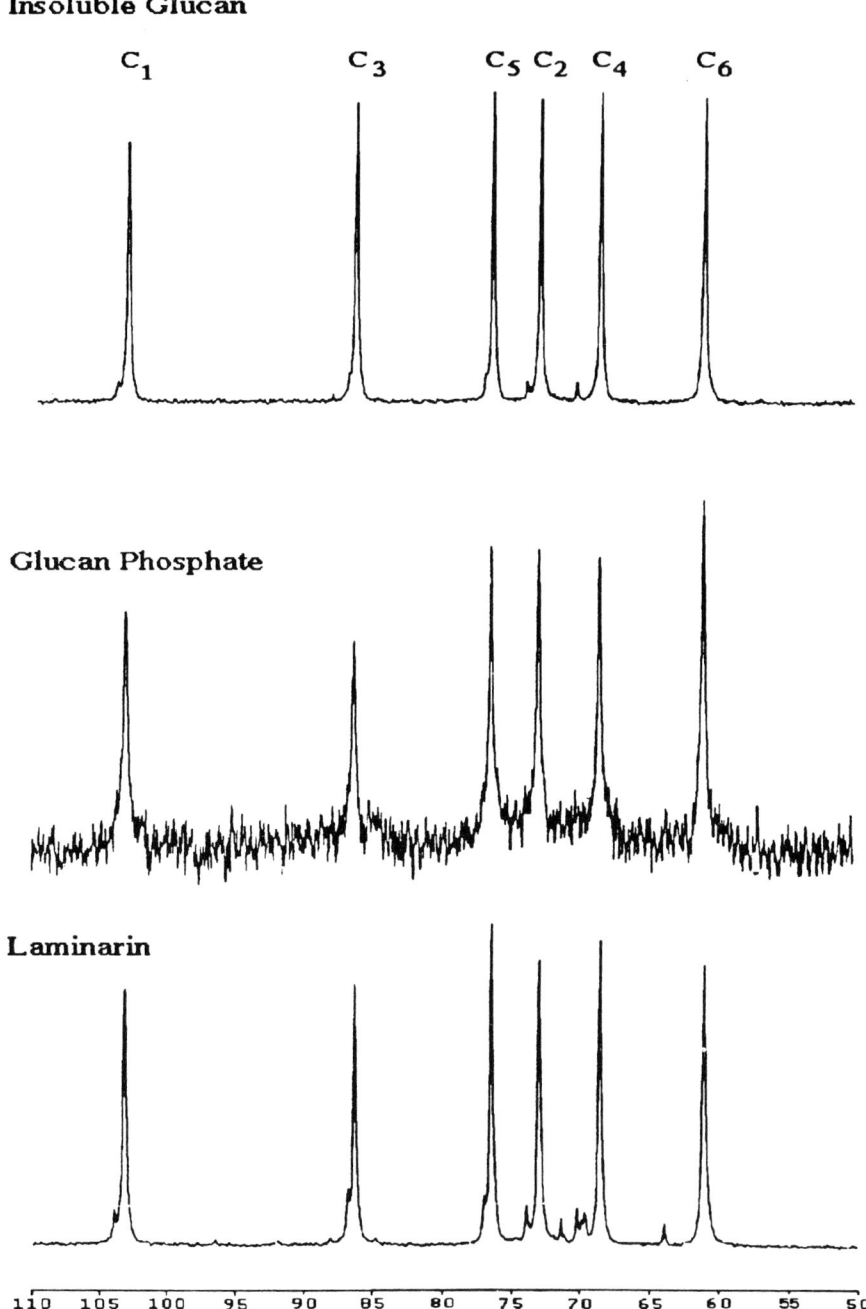

Figure 2. ^{13}C-NMR spectra of insoluble β-glucan (15,433 scans) and glucan phosphate (15,694 scans). Laminarin served as the β-1,3-linked triple helical control (15,685 scans). All samples were dissolved in dimethyl sulfoxide-d_6 at 50 mg/ml. Spectra were obtained at 50 Mhz.

laminarin and confirms the β-1,3 assignment and the lack of β-1,6 branches. These data also indicate that the solubilization procedure does not substantially alter the basic molecule. ^{31}P-NMR analysis of glucan phosphate was undertaken to confirm the presence of the phosphate group. A single phosphorus peak was observed (data not shown). We speculate that the phosphate group is substituted at the C_6 position and that it extends away from the triple-helical glucopyranose backbone.

Experimental and preclinical studies

Toxicology

Williams et al. [26] have examined the pre-clinical safety of glucan phosphate. The pre-clinical safety evaluation of glucan phosphate was studied in mice, rats, guinea pigs and rabbits. ICR/HSD mice and Harlan Sprague-Dawley rats received single intravenous injections of glucan phosphate in doses ranging from 40 to 1,000 mg/kg. Glucan phosphate administration did not induce mortality, appearance or behavioral changes in mice or rats. In subsequent studies, mice and guinea pigs were injected intraperitoneally with glucan phosphate (250 mg/kg) for 7 consecutive days. ICR/HSD mice gained weight at the same rate as did the saline-treated controls. In contrast, guinea pigs receiving intraperitoneal injections of glucan phosphate showed a mild, but statistically significant, 10-13 % decrease in weight gain over the 7 day period. No other toxicologic, behavioral or appearance changes were noted. To examine chronic toxicity, glucan phosphate was administered twice weekly for a period of 30 or 60 days to ICR/HSD mice in the dose of 40, 200 or 1,000 mg/kg. No deaths were observed in any group. Chronic glucan phosphate administration did not alter body weight, liver, lung or kidney weight. However, a significant splenomegaly was observed in both the 30 and 60 day study. Histopathologic examination showed no tissue alterations at 40 or 200 mg/kg. However, at 1,000 mg/kg a mononuclear infiltrate was observed in the liver. Pyrogenicity testing, employing New Zealand white rabbits, revealed that parenteral glucan phosphate administration at 5 mg/kg did not significantly alter body temperature. These data indicate that the systemic administration of glucan phosphate, over a wide dose range, does not induce mortality or significant toxicity.

Browder et al. [30] have examined the therapeutic efficacy of glucan phosphate in a Phase I, randomized, placebo-controlled clinical trial *(see below)*. In this Phase I study, the primary clinical toxicities observed in trauma patients receiving intravenous glucan phosphate were chills and fever approximately 1 hour post-infusion [30]. The chills and/or febrile response to glucan phosphate appears to coincide with the peak in serum interleukin-1 levels. The febrile response is effectively blocked by pre-medication with acetaminophen or a suitable non-steroidal anti-inflammatory agents.

Pharmacokinetics

The pharmacokinetics of glucan phosphate has been evaluated in our laboratory, in male Sprague-Dawley rats, using ^{32}P-labeled glucan phosphate. The blood level time curve for ^{32}P-labeled glucan phosphate in the Sprague-Dawley rat is shown in Figure 3. One minute following IV injection 2.10 ± 0.28 % injected dose (I.D.)/ml of peripheral blood was observed. The t/2 was 17.5 ± 1.0 min for clearance of ^{32}P-glucan phosphate from the vascular compartment of Sprague-Dawley

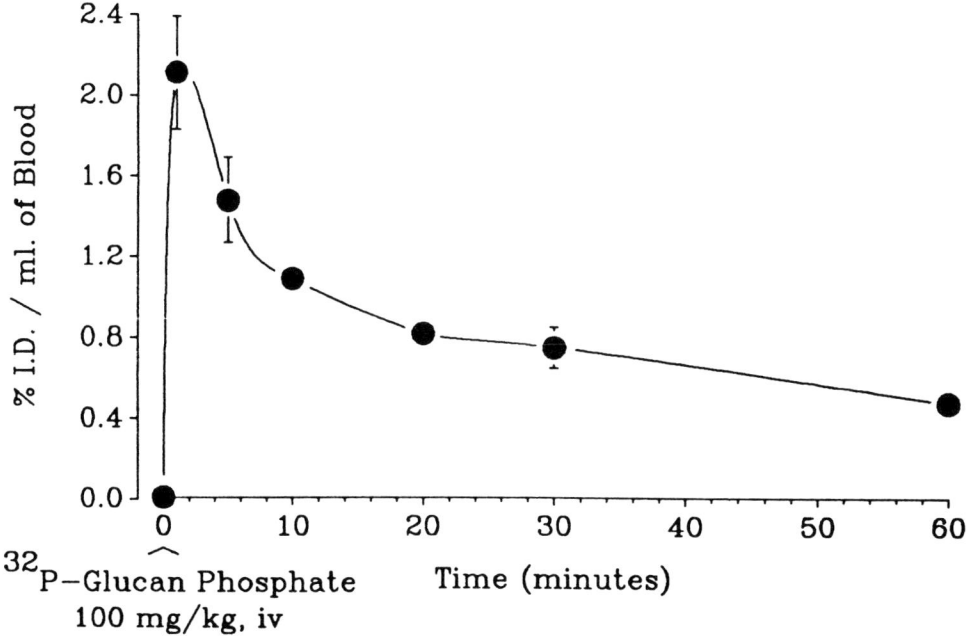

Figure 3. Blood concentration time curve of ^{32}P-labelled glucan phosphate following intravenous administration into male Sprague-Dawley rats. N = 4/group.

rats. At 60 minutes post-injection 0.47 ± 0.15 % I.D./ml of peripheral blood was observed.

Organ localization data revealed that 30 minutes following IV infusion of ^{32}P-labeled glucan phosphate <5.0 % of the injected dose was found in the liver, lung, spleen or kidneys, respectively. However, 13.12 ± 3.15 % of the injected dose was detected per 100 µl of urine 30 min post-infusion. This suggests that renal clearance mechanisms may represent an important route of elimination for glucan phosphate. By 60 minutes post-infusion, only 0.40 ± 0.01 % of the injected dose was detected per 100 µl of urine. This may indicate that lower molecular weight polymers are quickly eliminated *via* renal clearance mechanisms, while the higher molecular weight compounds are deposited at other sites in the body. In these preliminary studies it was not possible to determine the MWs (*i.e.* polymer distribution) of glucan phosphate in the urine.

Immunomodulating properties and potential mechanisms of action

Glucan phosphate has been demonstrated to enhance the functional status of macrophages [28, 30], T and B lymphocytes [5], natural killer cells [33] and neutrophils [11]. Additionally, glucan phosphate has been shown to increase synthesis and release of interleukin 1 [27], interleukin 2 [27], and colony stimulating activity [34, 35]. Previous reports from our laboratory have demonstrated that water soluble β-D-glucans stimulate various aspects of immune responsiveness in a phasic manner [31]. As an illustrative example, the effect of a single intravenous injection of glucan phosphate on bone marrow proliferation and macrophage mediated tumor cytotoxicity is presented in Figure 4. Glucan phosphate (250 mg/kg) was administered intravenously to C57Bl/6J mice on day 0. Bone marrow proliferation and macrophage mediated tumor cytotoxicity against a syngeneic tumor target were assayed as described by Pretus et al. [31]. Murine bone marrow proliferative capacity was stimulated in a biphasic manner. The first stimulatory phase peaked at 12 hours post-infusion with a return to baseline values by day 1 (Figure 4, upper panel). The second stimulatory phase was of lesser amplitude, but longer duration, with peak activity occurring on day 12 post-infusion (Figure 4, upper panel). Murine splenic macrophage cytotoxicity against a syngeneic melanoma B16 tumor target was increased on days 3, 6 and 9 following parenteral glucan phosphate administration. The first stimulatory phase was followed by a significant depression in macrophage cytotoxicity on days 15 and 21. A second stimulatory phase is observed on day 28 followed by a return to baseline values by day 35 (Figure 4, lower panel).

The precise mechanism by which β-D-glucan exerts an immunomodulatory effect is unknown. However, data suggests that β-D-glucans exert much of their activity *via* macrophage participation [10, 30]. Czop et al. [36-38] have demonstrated the presence of a β-D-glucan receptor on human monocytes. Recent studies by Czop and Kay [39] indicate the presence of two membrane proteins (160 and 180 kD) on a human myelomonocytic cell line that exhibit ligand specificity for microparticulate β-D-glucan. Goldman [40] has reported the presence of a β-D-glucan receptor on P388D1 cells, a mouse macrophage-like tumor cell line. Williams *et al.* [41] have extended these observations to demonstrate the presence of a β-D-glucan receptor on human polymorphonuclear leukocytes. Janusz *et al.* [42] have reported that the unit ligand for human monocyte β-D-glucan receptors is a heptaglucoside. Ross *et al.* [43] have reported that membrane complement receptor type three (CR_3) is the « β-glucan receptor » for particulate activation of complement. The discovery of specific β-D-glucan receptors on human immunocytes offers a tantalizing explanation for the cellular activation induced by β-D-glucans. However, the *in vivo* immunologic significance of the receptor studies is uncertain, since these experiments were largely limited to *in vitro* phagocytosis and/or phagocytosis inhibition assays. In addition, all of the receptor studies, with the possible exception of the work by Janusz *et al.* [42], employed water insoluble β-D-glucans. The precise nature of the glucan phosphate receptor has not been established. Whether the receptor for glucan phosphate is related to the receptors already identified for microparticulate β-D-glucans remains to be determined.

Singh et al. [1], Ohno *et al.* [24] and others [3, 4] have reported that the *in vivo* anti-tumor activity of β-D-glucan polymers is related to the higher structure of the polymer. Specifically, it has been suggested that β-D-glucans immunomodulatory activity is attributable to the β-1,3-interchain linkage [44, 45], the ordered (triple helical) conformation [45, 46] and/or the presence or degree of β-1,6 side chain branching [1, 24]. It may be that the molecular size, conformation and charge are important features of the β-D-glucan polymer not only for recognition by immunocyte receptors in macrophage-rich organs, but also the polymer size may facilitate retention of the polymers in the body, increasing exposure time of immunocytes to the stimulating agent.

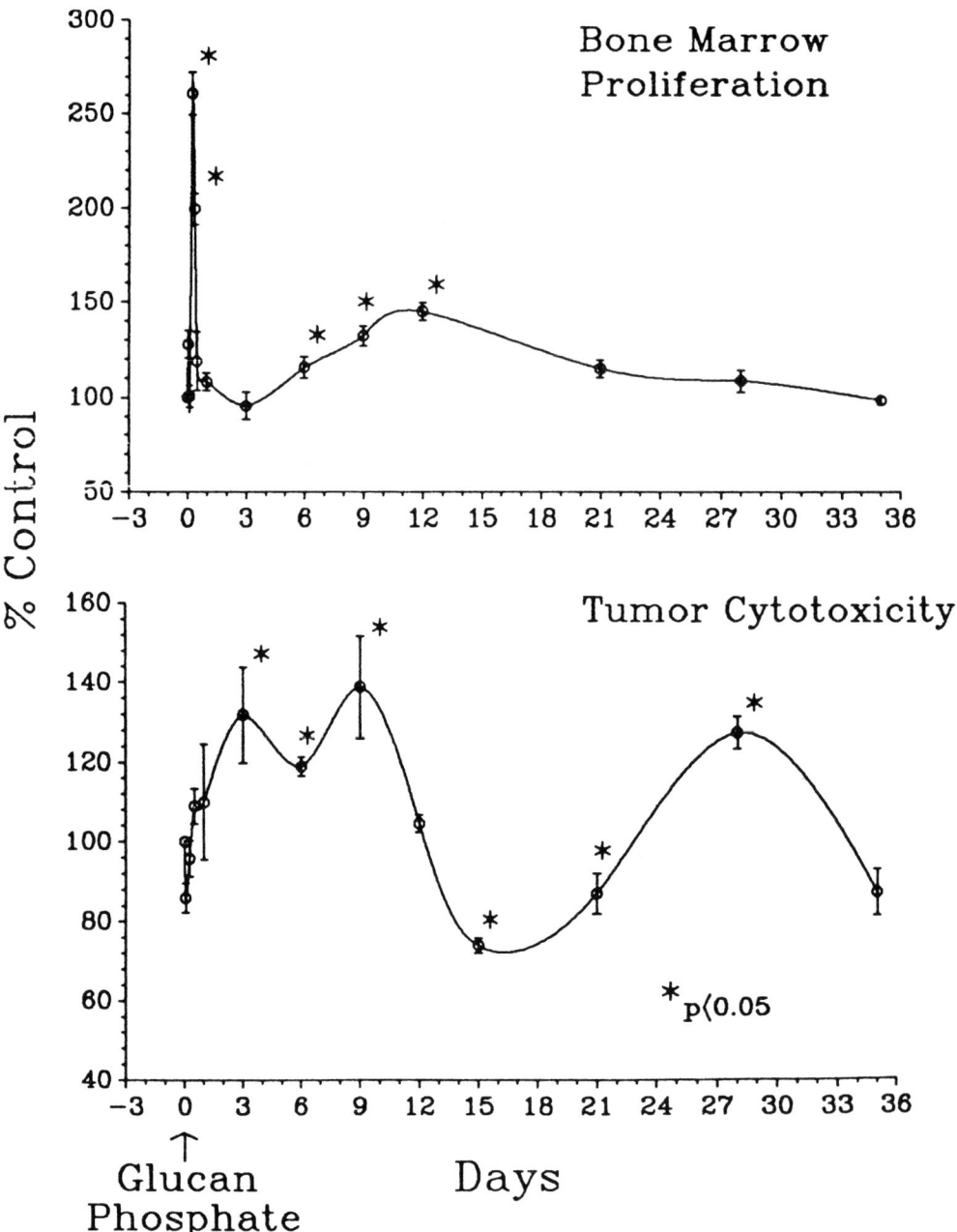

Figure 4. Temporal effect of a single intravenous injection of glucan phosphate on bone marrow proliferation (top panel) and macrophage mediated tumoricidal activity (lower panel) in male C57Bl/6J mice. Glucan phosphate was administered i.v. in the dose of 250 mg/kg. Dextrose (5 % w/v) served as control.

Therapeutic effects in animal models

• Infections

Browder et al. [29] have assessed the efficacy of glucan phosphate in a murine model of *Escherichia coli* peritonitis. More importantly, these authors have demonstrated a synergistic effect when glucan phosphate is combined with the aminoglycoside antibiotic, gentamicin, in the murine *E. coli* peritonitis model [29]. Lahnborg et al. [47] have reported similar results employing the water-insoluble form of glucan and benzylpenicillin in an ileal exclusion and devascularization model of peritonitis in the rat. In the studies by Browder et al. [29], ICR/HSD mice received glucan phosphate (4 mg/kg) 24 hours before bacterial challenge, gentamicin (0.8 mg/kg) 2 hours prior to challenge or glucan phosphate and gentamicin. Isovolumetric dextrose (5 % w/v) served as the control. While either agent is effective in this model at higher dosages [29], the doses employed for this study were below the minimally effective (*i.e.* threshold) dose. This was done in order to examine whether synergy occurred between the two drugs. All animals were challenged intraperitoneally with 1×10^8 *E. coli*. Long-term survival was significantly enhanced in the glucan phosphate-gentamicin combined therapy group (56 %, $p<0.05$) when compared with dextrose (0 %), gentamicin alone (0 %) or glucan phosphate alone (9 %) at suboptimal dosages. In addition, combined therapy significantly reduced *E. coli* bacteremia at 8 hours post-inoculation, when compared with the control groups. Combined glucan phosphate-gentamicin administration significantly enhanced bone marrow proliferation and this enhancement correlated with increased levels of circulating neutrophils. The infection model described above involved the prophylactic administration of glucan phosphate prior to microbial challenge. One might argue that prophylactic administration of an immune response modifying agent in infectious disease has limited clinical utility. However, it should be noted that antibiotics are routinely employed as prophylaxis for patients undergoing surgical procedures. It may be that an important clinical role for glucan phosphate will be prophylaxis in order to stimulate immunity and increase host resistance to infectious complications.

• Syngeneic murine tumors

Williams et al. [5] have shown that glucan phosphate, when combined with cyclophosphamide, will exert an additive and/or synergistic therapeutic effect on modification of experimental murine hepatic metastatic disease. In this study, C57Bl/6J mice were challenged subcutaneously with syngeneic reticulum cell sarcoma M5076, which preferentially metastasizes to the liver. When hepatic metastases were apparent on day 20, the mice were treated with glucan phosphate and cyclophosphamide. Treatment continued at 3 day intervals up to day 50 (a total of 11 injections). Combined therapy with glucan phosphate and cyclophosphamide resulted in a synergistic reduction of primary tumor weight and hepatic metastatic burden, when compared to either treatment alone. Survival data revealed that the combination of glucan phosphate and cyclophosphamide exerted an additive effect on extension of median survival time and the time to 100 % mortality [5]. Mechanistic studies indicated that glucan phosphate-cyclophosphamide therapy exerted anti-tumor activity by activation of Kupffer cell cytolytic activity and enhancing cell-mediated immunity. Subsequent studies by Sherwood et al. [48] have extended the work of Williams et al. [5] by demonstrating the therapeutic efficacy of glucan phosphate when combined with lymphokine activated killer (LAK) cells in the murine reticulum cell sarcoma hepatic metastases model. These data suggest the potential of glucan phosphate as prophylaxis and/or therapy for neoplastic disease. The ability of glucan phosphate to exert a synergistic effect when combined with conventional therapies, such as chemotherapy [5] and antibiotics [29], may be of practical significance. The studies of Sherwood *et al.* [48] also suggest the potential utility of combining glucan phosphate with other forms of adoptive immunotherapy. In addition, the ability of glucan phosphate to ameliorate immune suppression [30] and enhance wound healing [49] make it an appealing adjunctive agent for the therapy of human neoplasia.

- *Wound healing*

In 1978, Leibovich and Ross published a landmark paper which demonstrated that macrophage participation was essential for normal wound healing. Since that time numerous investigators [50-52] have confirmed and extended the work of Leibovich and Ross [53]. It is now well established that macrophage function is essential for effective wound debridement [53], fibroblast activity [50], angiogenesis [51], collagen synthesis [54], collagen degradation [50] and modulation of wound energy metabolism [52].

Based on the central role of the macrophage in the normal wound healing process, it is conceivable that macrophage activation might accelerate and/or improve the wound healing process. Administration of macrophage activating BRMs offers one potential approach to the therapeutic management of wounds. In addition, it may be of potentially greater benefit to administer a BRM that will augment and/or restore immune competence as well as enhance wound healing, since wounds are frequently encountered in hosts who are immunodeficient due to trauma [55], sepsis [30], surgery [56], chemotherapy [57] or a combination of these entities.

Leibovich and Danon [58] have examined the effect of glucan, levan, inulin, dextran, starch, carrageenan and talcum powder on promotion of wound healing in SWR mice with dorsal full thickness skin wounds. The authors concluded that « only glucan showed any marked beneficial effects » on wound healing [58]. Indeed, carrageenan, which is toxic to macrophages, decreased wound re-epithelialization again emphasizing the importance of macrophages in wound healing. Wolk and Danon [59] have confirmed and extended the work of Leibovich and Danon [58] by demonstrating the effectiveness of topical glucan administration in bilateral hind-limb wounds in mice, rats and guinea pigs. The authors reported that « 60-80 % of animals showed more advanced healing in the glucan-treated wound ». Kenyon *et al.* [60, 61] have investigated the effect of topical particulate glucan therapy on skin wound healing in normal mice [60], and in mice with impaired wound healing due to a genetically derived macrophage defect [61] or Sendai virus induced macrophage dysfunction [62]. These workers concluded that glucan would increase wound tensile strength in mice with normal macrophage function as well as increase wound tensile strength in mice with genetic or environmentally induced macrophage dysfunction.

All of the wound healing experiments described above employed β-D-glucan in its water insoluble, micro-particulate form. Based on the beneficial effect of particulate glucan in wound healing, it was of interest to determine the effect of glucan phosphate on experimental wound healing. Glucan phosphate is a more attractive BRM than particulate glucan because it confers the same immunologic activity and its soluble nature facilitates parenteral administration.

Browder et al. [49] have evaluated the effect of glucan phosphate on experimental wound healing. Sprague-Dawley rats (250 g) underwent 2 cm dorsal skin incisions while under pentobarbital anesthesia. Rats received normal saline (0.5 ml,IV) or glucan (20 mg,IV) 24 hours before and after incision. Other animals received glucan phosphate as a dry lyophilized powder (20 mg) in the wound site at the time of incision. All wounds were closed with sterile 9 mm autoclips, which were removed on day 3 post-incision. On post-incision days 4, 7, 10 and 14, rats were sacrificed and the skin surrounding the healing wound was excised. Wound tensile strength for fresh and formalin-fixed tissue was measured using constant speed tensiometry.

The systemic or topical administration of glucan phosphate significantly enhanced wound breaking strength on days 4 and 7 post-wounding (Table II). Measurement of wound breaking strength on days 10 and 14 following incision showed no significant difference between control and glucan phosphate groups. Subsequent analysis of wound healing at day 4 in control and intravenous glucan phosphate groups involved determination of wound breaking strength in both fresh and formalin-fixed tissue. Formalin-fixation significantly increased wound breaking strength in the control animals (Figure 5). However, formalin-fixation did not significantly enhance wound breaking strength in IV glucan phosphate treated rats. The increase in wound tensile strength after formalin-fixation in the control, but not the glucan phosphate treated animals, suggests that glucan phosphate may exert its effect, in part, by inducing maximal collagen cross-linking in the wound area.

Table II. Wound breaking strength following topical or systemic administration of glucan phosphate[1].

Group	Day 4 (gms)	Day 7 (gms)
Control	22.0 ± 2.6	29.0 ± 5.8
Intravenous glucan	49.8 ± 5.5*	49.2 ± 5.2+
Topical glucan	59.7 ± 5.6*	70.4 ± 1.2+

[1] Sprague-Dawley rats received glucan 20 mg IV or saline 0.5 ml IV 24 hours prior to and 24 hours following dorsal incision. Topical glucan animals received 20 mg glucan phosphate in the wound at the time of incision. Rats were sacrificed on days 4 and 7 following incision for measurement of wound breaking strength. Values are expressed as mean ± SEM in grams. N = 12/18/group. * $p < 0.01$, vs control. + $p < 0.05$ vs control.

To examine potential mechanisms of enhanced wound healing, glucan phosphate (100 µg/ml) was incubated in vitro with Sprague-Dawley rat splenic macrophages for 24 hours. RPMI-1640 media alone served as control. After incubation, the macrophage supernatants were aspirated, frozen, and lyophilized to dryness. Macrophage supernatant was reconstituted to 30 ml with sterile saline solution (0.9 % w/v) and divided in half ; half was used for intraperitoneal injection and the remaining 15 ml was mixed with bovine collagen for topical administration at the wound site. Supernatants were injected intraperitoneally 24 hours before and 24 hours after incision or administered topically in the rat wound model. Fresh and formalin-fixed wound breaking strengths were measured.

Intraperitoneal administration of supernatant from glucan phosphate-stimulated macrophages significantly increased wound breaking strength (258 %) when com-

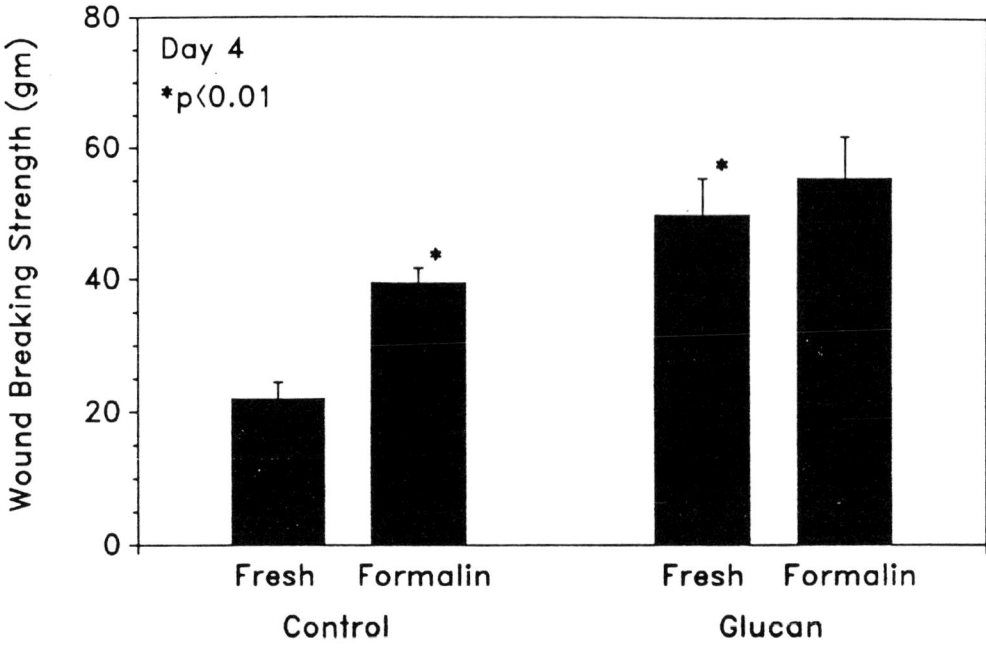

Figure 5. Wound breaking strength of fresh and formalin fixed tissues 4 days after dorsal incision. Sprague-Dawley rats were treated with saline solution or glucan phosphate 20 mg intravenously 24 hours prior to and following incision. Note that formalin fixation did not significantly increase breaking strength in the glucan phosphate treated rats. N = 6/group.

Table III. Effect of intraperitoneal administration of control or glucan-activated macrophage supernatant on wound breaking strength [1].

Group	Fresh (gms)	Formalin-fixed (gms)
Control supernatant	13.2 ± 1.5	27.0 ± 3.3*
Glucan supernatant	47.3 ± 3.3*	34.0 ± 6.8

[1] Macrophage supernatants were injected i.p. 24 hours prior to and 24 hours following incision. Supernatants were prepared as described above. Wound breaking strength was assessed on day 4. Values represent the mean ± SEM. N = 6-8/group. * $p < 0.01$ vs fresh control supernatant.

pared with intraperitoneal administration of control macrophage supernatants (Table III). Furthermore, formalin fixation did not significantly increase the breaking strength in the glucan-stimulated macrophage supernatant animals, which may indicate maximal cross-linking of collagen in these animals. In contrast, formalin fixation did significantly enhance wound breaking strength in the control supernatant animals (Table III). In subsequent studies, rats that received topical supernatants from glucan phosphate-activated macrophages showed a significant increase in wound breaking strength when compared with those receiving control supernatants. Although formalin fixation resulted in an expected increase in wound breaking strength in the control supernatant animals, wounds treated topically with glucan phosphate-activated macrophage supernatants showed no enhancement in wound breaking strength.

The practical significance of these observations are readily apparent, since increases in wound strength during the early stages of wound healing would have obvious benefits in the severely traumatized patient. In addition, the ability of soluble glucan to stimulate immune responsiveness in the immunodeficient host, who may exhibit impaired wound healing, might decrease morbidity and mortality associated with diverse injuries.

- *Amelioration of traumatic immunosuppression*

It is well established that severe injury results in suppression of diverse immune parameters [30, 55]. Extensive studies have shown that water-insoluble, microparticulate glucan will modify the course of experimental immunosuppressive disorders [13]. Pretus et al. [63] have studied the ability of glucan phosphate to ameliorate experimental post-traumatic immune suppression. Specifically, these authors examined the effect of glucan phosphate on murine splenic macrophage prostaglandin E2 release following hind-limb crush amputation injury in ICR/HSD mice. The authors noted that crush-amputation injury increased macrophage PGE2 release by 184 %. In contrast, glucan phosphate administration, prior to or following injury, reduced PGE2 levels in macrophage supernatants by 71 % and 85 %, respectively. A 52 % decrease in bone marrow proliferation was also observed 24 hours post-trauma. Glucan phosphate prophylaxis or therapy eliminated the suppression of bone marrow proliferation. These data suggest that glucan phosphate might play an important role in ameliorating post-traumatic immune suppression. Subsequent clinical studies have provided support for this concept *(see below)*.

- *Experimental pancreatitis*

In an effort to assess the impact of glucan phosphate administration on acute pancreatitis, Browder et al. [28] fed female Swiss-Webster mice a choline-deficient diet supplemented with ethionine to induce necrotizing pancreatitis. Glucan phosphate therapy resulted in improved long-term survival rates (58 % glucan phosphate vs 14 % control) and maintenance of pancreatic architecture. Glucan phosphate therapy decreased plasma and peritoneal trypsin activity as well as increased trypsin-binding activity in the peritoneum and peripheral blood. Plasma interleukin-1 and macrophage production of interleukin-1 were increased in glucan phosphate treated mice. The authors demonstrated that macrophage activation with glucan phosphate will increase interleukin-1 levels with a resultant increase in trypsin-binding activity which enzymatically inactivates trypsin released from the damaged pancreatic cells. In addition, the authors observed that α_2-macroglobulin was increased in glucan phosphate treated mice. They noted that α_2-macroglobulin is necessary for complexation of trypsin prior to removal by a hyperfunctional reticuloendothelium.

Other pharmacological properties

Hematopoietic effects

The ability of β-1,3-D-glucans, in micro-particulate or water soluble form, to stimulate hematopoiesis has been extensively investigated by Patchen et al. [34, 64, 65]. In 1986, Patchen and MacVittie examined the effect of glucan phosphate on murine hematopoiesis. They reported that a single intravenous (5 mg/mouse) injection of glucan phosphate into C3H/HeN mice increased peripheral leukocyte cellularity, bone marrow and spleen cellularity, bone marrow and splenic granulocyte/macrophage progenitor cell (GM-CFC) numbers, splenic pluripotent stem cell

(CFU-s) and erythroid progenitor cell (CFU-e) numbers. In addition, these investigators demonstrated that parenteral glucan phosphate administration increased serum granulocyte/macrophage colony stimulating activity (GM-CSA). The ability of glucan phosphate to stimulate medullary and extramedullary hematopoiesis may represent an important mechanism-of-action. Increasing the number of immunologically competent cells available to respond to neoplastic and/or infectious foci as well as repopulating the peripheral vasculature with immunocytes following a myelosuppressive event may explain, in part, the prophylactic and therapeutic activity of glucan phosphate.

- *Radioprotective effect of glucan phosphate*

Exposure of humans or animals to whole body ionizing radiation frequently results in bone marrow damage [65]. The destruction of hematopoietic progenitors by ionizing radiation results in erythrocytopenia, lymphocytopenia, granulocytopenia, immune suppression, decreased resistance to infection and, ultimately, death due to overwhelming sepsis [65]. If hematopoietic recovery following irradiation is to occur, the depression in bone marrow function must be reversed. One approach to reversing radiation induced bone marrow dysfunction is immunopharmacologic intervention [34]. Pharmacologic agents which are capable of favorably modifying the course of radiation injury are termed « radioprotectors ». Patchen *et al.* [34, 66, 67] have extensively investigated the radioprotective effects of glucan phosphate. Glucan phosphate has been shown to significantly accelerate hematopoietic recovery in sublethally and lethally irradiated mice [34]. The increased hematopoietic recovery observed in glucan-treated irradiated animals is associated with decreased opportunistic infection and increased survival [65]. Patchen *et al.* [68] have demonstrated that glucan phosphate will exert its protective effect against ionizing radiation in a therapeutic manner. More recently, these investigators have shown that glucan phosphate will exert an additive or synergistic effect on survival of irradiated animals when combined with antibiotics, recombinant hematopoietic growth factors or synthetic radioprotectors [66-68]. These composite data clearly indicate the potential of glucan phosphate as a means of inducing radioprotection.

Taken together the ability of glucan phosphate to stimulate hematopoiesis and enhance bone marrow recovery following radiation injury may have numerous practical applications in light of the myelosuppression currently encountered in patients undergoing chemotherapy or radiotherapy.

Clinical trials

Effect of glucan phosphate on interleukin 1 and 2 levels in patients with AIDS-related syndromes

Acquired immunodeficiency syndrome (AIDS) is an immunosuppressive disease predominantly observed in homosexual males and intravenous drug users [69]. AIDS is characterized by leukopenia as well as decreased *in vivo* and *in vitro* T-cell function. In view of the potent immune stimulating activity of glucan phosphate against a variety of experimentally-induced infectious disease states, immunosuppressive states and tumors, the efficacy of glucan phosphate on interleukin 1 and 2 production was evaluated in patients with AIDS.

The study was designed as an open, Phase I, dose-ranging, safety and immunologic efficacy protocol. Patient entry into the clinical protocol required that the patients : (1) belonged to one of the high risk groups for AIDS ; (2) had T-helper/inducer cells less than 750/mm^3 with a normal or elevated number of T-cytotoxic/suppressor cells ; (3) had a helper/suppressor T-cell ratio less than 0.6 ; and (4) had received no chemotherapy including steroids, radiotherapy, or immunotherapy for two weeks prior to beginning the clinical protocol. At the time of admission to the protocol, none of the patients exhibited opportunistic infections or Kaposi's sarcoma. Prior to initiating the clinical protocol all patients admitted to the study were screened and baseline evaluations of differential blood count, platelet count, serum lysozyme, serum chemistries, urinalysis, skin test for delayed hypersensitivity to the multitest battery, NK cell activity and proliferative response to mitogens stimulation were performed. Glucan phosphate diluted in sterile pyrogen free saline was administered intravenously over a 30 min period by slow i.v. drip. Patients received glucan phosphate infusions twice weekly with doses ranging from 25-150 mgm/m^2 body surface area.

Intravenous infusion of glucan phosphate (100 mgm/m^2) resulted in increased plasma IL-1 activity at 30 and 60 minutes post-injection (Figure 1). Additionally, the i.v. infusion of glucan phosphate resulted in elevation of plasma IL-2 activity 60 minutes post-injection. Interestingly, while AIDS patients are characteristically IL-2 deficient, glucan phosphate administration was capable of inducing an IL-2 response.

The systematic administration of glucan phosphate to patients with AIDS was associated with limited toxicity. Chills and fever were noted approximately 1 hour following glucan phosphate infusion. The onset of fever was associated with the peak in IL-1 activity, suggesting the pyrogenic response might be related to increased plasma IL-1. Subsequently, patients were pre-medicated with acetaminophen and diphenhydramine 1 hour prior to glucan phosphate infusion. Pre-medication eliminated the mild thermogenic response in AIDS patients. Duvic *et al.* [70] reported that 6 of 20 AIDS patients receiving glucan phosphate developed a reversible palmar and plantar keratoderma. Interestingly, this phenomenon has not been observed in any other patients receiving glucan phosphate. Duvic *et al.* [70] have speculated that this phenomenon may be limited to a specific subset of patients with AIDS.

Beneficial effect of glucan phosphate in trauma patients following laparotomy or thoracotomy

Further support for the application of glucan phosphate as an immune stimulant is provided by the clinical data of Browder *et al.* [30]. Glucan phosphate was utilized in a Phase I, randomized, double-blind, placebo controlled, perspective study of 38 trauma patients undergoing laparotomy or thoracotomy. Patients received glucan phosphate IV (50 mgm/m^2) or placebo post-operatively for 7 consecutive days. Patients who received glucan phosphate IV following trauma and surgery showed decreased ($p<0.05$) septic complications (9.5 % *vs* 47 %). Of greater importance, patients who received glucan phosphate intravenously showed increased survival (100 % *vs* 71 %), when compared to those patients who received placebo. Serum interleukin-1β levels in glucan phosphate patients increased 43 % ($p<0.05$) over the first 3 days, when compared to those patients that received placebo. Patients who were anergic on post-operative day 5 showed a higher ($p<0.01$) incidence of infection. Interestingly, glucan phosphate therapy significantly increased ($p<0.02$) skin test conversion (negative to positive, 73 % glucan vs 21 % placebo). These clinical observations indicate that : (1) systemic administration of glucan phosphate in the period immediately post-trauma resulted in decreased septic complications with a concomitant increase in survival ; (2) IL-1β levels were increased in the early post-trauma period following systemic glucan phosphate administration ; and (3) early increases in IL-1β positively correlated with skin test conversion, protection from sepsis and an increased survival.

Summary and conclusion

Glucan phosphate is a water soluble, yeast derived, -β,3-D-glucopyranose BRM that has been demonstrated to be a potent immune stimulant. Glucan phosphate administration is associated with increased resistance to a variety of experimentally-induced disease states. Phase I clinical data indicates that glucan phosphate will ameliorate immunosuppression, stimulate immunity, decrease susceptibility to infection and alter ultimate outcome in trauma patients following laparotomy or thoracotomy. These composite data suggest that glucan phosphate may be an attractive agent for immunotherapy of a variety of human and animal diseases.

References

1. Singh PP, Whistler RL, Tokuzen R, Nakahara W. Scleroglucan, an antitumor polysaccharide from *Sclerotium glucanicum*. *Carbohydr Res* 1974 ; 37 : 245-7.
2. Ohno N, Suzuki I, Yadomae T. Structure and antitumor activity of a beta-1,3-glucan isolated from the culture filtrate of *Sclerotinia sclerotiorum* IFO 9395. *Chem Pharm Bull* 1986 ; 34 : 1362-5.
3. Tabata K, Ito W, Kojima T, Kawabata S, Misaki A. Ultrasonic degradation of schizophyllan, an antitumor polysaccharide produced by Schizophyllum commune fries. *Carbohydr Res* 1981 ; 89 : 121-35.
4. Maeda YY, Watanabe ST, Chihara C, Rokutanda M. Denaturation and renaturation of a beta-1,6 : 1,3-glucan, lentinan, associated with expression of T-cell-mediated responses. *Cancer Res* 1988 ; 48 : 671-5.
5. Williams DL, Sherwood ER, McNamee RB, Jones EL, Browder IW, Di Luzio NR. Chemoimmunotherapy of experimental hepatic metastases. *Hepatology* 1987 ; 7 : 1296-304.
6. Benacerraf B, Sebestyen MM. Effect of bacterial endotoxins on the reticuloendothelial system. *Fed Proc* 1957 ; 16 : 860-7.
7. Di Luzio NR. Reticuloendothelial involvement in lipid metabolism. *Ann NY Acad Sci* 1960 ; 88 : 244-51.
8. Cutler JL. The enhancement of hemolysin production in the rat by zymosan. *J Immunol* 1960 ; 84 : 416-9.
9. Sherwood ER, Williams DL, McNamee RB, Jones EL, Browder IW, Di Luzio NR. In vitro tumoricidal activity of resting and glucan-activated Kupffer cells. *J Leukocyte Biol* 1987 ; 42 : 69-75.
10. Williams DL, Browder IW, Di Luzio NR. Immunotherapeutic modification of *Escherichia coli*-induced experimental peritonitis and bacteremia by glucan. *Surgery* 1983 ; 93 : 448-54.
11. Williams DL, Sherwood ER, Browder IW, McNamee RB, Jones EL, Rakinic J, Di Luzio NR. Effect of glucan on neutrophil dynamics and immune function in *Escherichia coli* peritonitis. *J Surg Res* 1988 ; 44 : 54-61.
12. Di Luzio NR, Williams DL. Protective effect of glucan against systemic *Staphylococcus aureus* septicemia in normal and leukemic mice. *Infect Immun* 1978 ; 20 : 804-10.
13. Di Luzio NR, Williams DL, Sherwood ER, Browder IW. Modification of diverse experimental immunosuppressive states by glucan. *Surv Immunol Res* 1985 ; 4 : 160-7.

14. Williams DL, Sherwood ER, McNamee RB, Jones EL, Di Luzio NR. Therapeutic efficacy of glucan in a murine model of hepatic metastatic disease. *Hepatology* 1985 ; 5 : 198-206.
15. Williams DL, Di Luzio NR. Glucan-induced modification of murine viral hepatitis. *Science* 1980 ; 208 : 67-9.
16. Mansell PWA, Ichinose H, Reed RJ, Krementz ET, McNamee R, Di Luzio NR. Macrophage-mediated destruction of human malignant cells *in vivo*. *J Natl Cancer Inst* 1975 ; 54(3) : 571-80.
17. Riggi SJ, Di Luzio NR. Hepatic function during reticulo-endothelial hyperfunction and hyperplasia. *Nature* 1962 ; 193 : 1292-4.
18. Bowers GJ, Patchen ML, MacVittie TJ, Hirsch EF, Fink MP. A comparative evaluation of particulate and soluble glucan in an endotoxin model. *Int J Immunopharmacol* 1986 ; 8 : 313-21.
19. Cook JA, Dougherty WJ, Holt TM. Enhanced sensitivity to endotoxin induced by the RE stimulant, glucan. *Circ Shock* 1980 ; 7 : 225-38.
20. Ohno N. Two different conformations of the antitumor B-D-glucan produced by *Sclerotinia sclerotiorum* IFO 9395. *Carbohydr Res* 1987 ; 159 : 293-302.
21. Taguchi T. *Experimental and clinical studies on Krestin*. Osaka, 1978 : 1-22.
22. Matsuo T, Arika T, Mitani M, Komatsu N. Pharmacological and toxicological studies of a new antitumor polysaccharide, schizophyllan. *Arztl Forsch Drug Res* 1982 ; 31 : 647-56.
23. Seljelid R. A water-soluble aminated beta-1,3-D-glucan derivative causes regression of solid tumors in mice. *Biosci Rep* 1986 ; 6 : 845-51.
24. Ohno N, Suzuki I, Oikawa S, Sato K, Miyazaki T, Yadomae T. Antitumor activity and structural characterization of glucans extracted from cultured fruit bodies of *Grifola frondosa*. *Chem Pharm Bull* 1984 ; 32 : 1142-51.
25. Seljelid R. Tumour regression after treatment with aminated beta 1-3D polyglucose is initiated by circulatory failure. *Scand J Immunol* 1989 ; 29 : 181-92.
26. Williams DL, Sherwood ER, Browder IW, McNamee RB, Jones EL, Di Luzio NR. Preclinical safety evaluation of soluble glucan. *Int J Immunopharmacol* 1988 ; 10(4) : 405-11.
27. Sherwood ER, Williams DL, McNamee RB, Jones EL, Browder IW, Di Luzio NR. Enhancement of interleukin-1 and interleukin-2 production by soluble glucan. *Int J Immunopharmacol* 1987 ; 9 : 261-7.
28. Browder IW, Sherwood E, Williams D, Jones E, McNamee BS, Di Luzio N. Protective effect of glucan-enhanced macrophage function in experimental pancreatitis. *Am J Surg* 1987 ; 153 : 25-32.
29. Browder W, Williams D, Sherwood E, McNamee R, Jones E, Di Luzio N. Synergistic effect of nonspecific immunostimulation and antibiotics in experimental peritonitis. *Surgery* 1987 ; 102 : 206-14.
30. Browder W, Williams D, Pretus H, Olivero G, Enrichens F, Mao P, Franchello A. Beneficial effect of enhanced macrophage function in the trauma patient. *Ann Surg* 1990 ; 211 : 605-13.
31. Pretus HA, Ensley HE, McNamee RB, Jones EL, Browder IW, Williams DL. Isolation, physicochemical characterization and preclinical efficacy evaluation of soluble scleroglucan. *J Pharmacol Exp Ther* 1991 ; 257(1) : 500-10.
32. Ogawa K, Hatano M. Circular dichroism of the complex of a (1-3)-B-D-glucan with congo red. *Carbohydr Res* 1978 ; 67 : 527-35.
33. Williams D, Jones E, Pretus H, McNamee R, Browder W. Augmentation of murine splenic natural killer (NK) cell activity following single and multiple injection regimens of soluble glucan. *J Leukocyte Biol* 1988 ; 44 : 174.
34. Patchen ML, MacVittie TJ. Hemopoietic effects of intravenous soluble glucan administration. *J Immunopharmacol* 1986 ; 8 : 407-25.
35. Patchen ML, MacVittie TJ. Comparative effects of soluble and particulate glucans on survival in irradiated mice. *J Biol Resp Modif* 1986 ; 5 : 45-60.

36. Czop JK, Austen KF. Generation of leukotrienes by human monocytes upon stimulation of their beta-glucan receptor during phagocytosis. *Proc Natl Acad Sci USA* 1985 ; 82 : 2751-5.
37. Czop JK, Austen KF. Beta-glucan inhibitable receptor on human monoyctes : its identity with the phagocytic receptor for particulate activators of the alternative complement pathway. *J Immunol* 1985 ; 134 : 2588-93.
38. Czop JK, Austen KF. Properties of glycans that activate the human alternative complement pathway and interact with the human monocyte beta-glucan receptor. *J Immunol* 1985 ; 135 : 3388-93.
39. Czop JK, Kay J. Isolation and characterization of β-glucan receptors on human mononuclear phagocytes. *J Exp Med* 1991 ; 173 : 1520-51.
40. Goldman R. Induction of a beta-1,3-D-glucan receptor in P388D1 cells treated with retinoic acid or 1,25-dihydroxyvitamin D3. *Immunology* 1988 ; 63 : 319-24.
41. Williams JD, Topley N, Alobaidi HM, Harber MJ. Activation of human polymorphonuclear leucocytes by particulate zymosan is related to both its major carbohydrate components : glucan and mannan. *Immunology* 1986 ; 58 : 117-24.
42. Janusz MJ, Austen KF, Czop JK. Isolation of a unit ligand for beta-glucan receptors of human monocytes. *Int J Immunopharmacol* 1988 ; 10(S1) : 89 (Abstract).
43. Ross GD, Cain JA, Myones BL, Newman SL, Lachmann PJ. Specificity of membrane complement receptor type three (CR3) for β-glucans. *Complement* 1987 ; 4 : 61-74.
44. Sasaki T, Takasuka N. Further study of the structure of lentinan, an anti-tumor polysaccharide from lentinus edodes. *Carbohydr Res* 1976 ; 47 : 99-104.
45. Maeda YY, Watanabe ST. Significance of the higher structure of beta-1,6 ;1,3-glucan, lentinan, for the expression of T-cell mediated responses *in vivo*. *Int J Immunopharmacol* 1988 ; 10(S1) : 87 (Abstract).
46. Yanaki T, Ito W, Tabata K, Kojima T, Norisuye T, Takano N, Fujita H. Correlation between the antitumor activity of a polysaccharide schizophyllan and its triple-helical conformation in dilute aqueous solution. *Biophys Chem* 1983 ; 17 : 337-42.
47. Lahnborg G, Hedstrom KG, Nord CE. Glucan-induced enhancement of host resistance in experimental intraabdominal sepsis. *Eur Surg Res* 1982 ; 14 : 401-8.
48. Sherwood ER, Williams DL, McNamee RB, Jones EL, Browder IW, Di Luzio NR. Soluble glucan and lymphokine-activated killer (LAK) cells in the therapy of experimental hepatic metastases. *J Biol Resp Modif* 1988 ; 7 : 185-98.
49. Browder W, Williams D, Lucore P, Pretus H, Jones E, McNamee R. Effect of enhanced macrophage function on early wound healing. *Surgery* 1988 ; 104 : 224-30.
50. Diegelmann RF, Cohen IK, Kaplan AM. The role of macrophages in wound repair : a review. *Plastic Reconstruc Surg* 1981 ; 68 : 107-13.
51. Hunt TK, Kinghton DR, Thakral KK, Goodson WH, Andrews WS. Studies on inflammation and wound healing. Angiogenesis and collagen synthesis stimulated *in vivo* by resident and activated wound macrophages. *Surgery* 1984 ; 96 : 48-54.
52. Morris A, Henry W, Shearer J, Caldwell M. Macrophage interaction with skeletal muscle : a potential role of macrophages in determining the energy state of healing wounds. *J Trauma* 1985 ; 25 : 751-7.
53. Leibovich SJ, Ross R. The role of the macrophage in wound repair. *Am J Pathol* 1975 ; 78(1) : 71-92.
54. Scott PG. Experimental wound healing : increased breaking strength and collagen synthetic activity in abdominal fasical wounds healing with secondary closure of the skin. *Br J Surg* 1985 ; 72 : 777-9.
55. Antrum RM, Solomkin JS. Monocyte dysfunction in severe trauma : evidence for the role of C5a in deactivation. *Surgery* 1986 ; 100 : 29-37.
56. Wang BS, Heacock EH, Mannick JA. Characterization of suppressor cells generated in mice after surgical trauma. *Clin Immunol Immunopathol* 1982 ; 24 : 161-70.
57. Falcone RE, Nappi JF. Chemotherapy and wound healing. In : Romm S, ed. *The surgical clinics of North America*. Philadelphia : W.B. Saunders Company, 1984 : 779-94.
58. Leibovich SJ, Danon D. Promotion of wound repair in mice by application of glucan. *J Reticuloendothel Soc* 1980 ; 27 : 1-11.

59. Wolk M, Danon D. Promotion of wound healing by yeast glucan evaluated on single animals. *Med Biol* 1985 ; 63 : 73-80.
60. Kenyon AJ, Michaels EB. Modulation of early cellular events in wound healing in mice. *Am J Vet Res* 1983 ; 44 : 340-3.
61. Kenyon AJ, Douglas DM, Hamilton SG. Defective macrophage function in wound repair of P/J mice. *Lab Anim Sci* 1985 ; 35(2) : 150-2.
62. Kenyon AJ. Delayed wound healing in mice associated with viral alteration of macrophages. *Am J Vet Res* 1983 ; 44 : 652-6.
63. Pretus HA, Browder IW, Lucore P, McNamee RB, Jones EL, Williams DL. Macrophage activation decreases macrophage prostaglandin E2 release in experimental trauma. *J Trauma* 1989 ; 29 : 1152-7.
64. Patchen ML. Immunomodulators and hemopoiesis. *Surv Immunol Res* 1983 ; 2 : 237-42.
65. Patchen ML, D'Alesandro MM, Brook I, Blakely WF, MacVittie TJ. Glucan : mechanisms involved in its « radioprotective » effect. *J Leukocyte Biol* 1987 ; 42 : 95-105.
66. Patchen ML, Chirigos MA, Brook I. Use of glucan and other immunopharmacological agents in the prevention and treatment of acute radiation injuries. *Fund Appl Toxicol* 1988 ; 11 : 573-4.
67. Patchen ML, MacVittie TJ, Wathen LM. Effects of pre- and post-irradiation glucan treatment on pluripotent stem cells, granulocyte, macrophage and erythroid progenitor cells, and hemopoietic stromal cells. *Experientia* 1984 ; 40 : 1240-4.
68. Patchen ML, MacVittie TJ, Jackson WE. Postirradiation glucan administration enhances the radioprotective effects of WR-2721. *Rad Res* 1989 ; 117 : 59-69.
69. Fauci AS, Lane HC. The acquired immunodeficiency syndrome (AIDS) : an update. *Int Archs Allergy Appl Immun* 1985 ; 77 : 81-8.
70. Duvic M, Reisman M, Finley V, Rapini R, Di Luzio N, Mansell PWA. Glucan-induced keratoderma in acquired immunodeficiency syndrome. *Arch Dermatol* 1987 ; 123 : 751-6.

5

Immunomodulators from *Nocardia opaca*

R. BAROT-CIORBARU[(1)], C. BONA[(2)]

[(1)] CNRS, URA 1116, Université Paris-Sud, Bat.432, 91405 Orsay, France.
[(2)] Department of Microbiology, Mount Sinai School of Medicine, Mount Sinai Hospital, New York, 10029, USA.

Begining with seminal work of Freund, studies of immuno stimulatory activity of substances extracted from bacteria raised a great interest.

The study of immunomodulatory activities of *Nocardia opaca*, cells walls and solubles fractions [1-3] represented an extention of studies aimed to define substances endowed with immuno stimulatory properties isolated from mycobacteria since *Nocardia* species belong to same bacterial family.

During the last twenty years, studies of *Nocardia* immunomodulatory substances were gone through three major steps. The first concerned its adjuvant activity [1-4] and the demonstration of the minimum structure concerning adjuvant activity from bacterial peptidoglycans — MDP — (N-acetyl-muramyl-L-alanyl-D-isoglutamine) is the minimal chemical structure capable of replacing mycobacteria in Freund's adjuvant [5, 6]

The second concerned the characterization of mitogen activity [7-9] of certain fractions from *Nocardia*, neoWSA — neowater soluble adjuvant [4] and, later, NWSM — nocardia water soluble mitogen [1]. Demonstration of polyclonal activation of human B cells opened the door for fruitful investigation of analysis of human B cells functions in normal and pathological conditions [3, 10-23]. It has recently been reported (Tuckova *et al.*, in preparation) that fractions of *Nocardia* are immunogenic in rabbits and mice. NWSM was used for preparation of mAbs.

The third stage covering the last years, other stimulatory functions have been discovered such as antitumoral activity [24-28], interferon release [29, 30], activation of natural killer cells [31] and of macrophages [25-27, 32], induction of interleukin-l (IL-l) [33] and other monokines [12, 33-37] and the detection and visualisation of macrophages present in the vicinity of human tumors and metastases [38]. During these studies, we found that all *Nocardia* fractions, whether soluble NWSM (nocardia water soluble mitogen), NWSMP (nocardia water soluble mitogen pellet), NSPD (nocardia soluble peptidoglycan derivative), or insoluble NDCM (nocardia delipidated cell mitogen), CW (purified cell walls), PG (peptidoglycan) and whether or not containing peptidoglycans such as NWSMP, possessed immunomodulatory properties [1, 3]. However, after purification of the *Nocardia* fractions, certain structure-activity relationships have been established [1-3]. Some fractions were found to induce only differentiation, and others proliferation of B cells [3]. We have also shown that NWSMP, a fraction devoid of PG induces interferon (INF)a/β in the mouse, whereas PG induces IFNγ [30].

The aim of the present review is to describe these fractions, various biological activities, and the different target cell populations involved.

Presentation of the fractions

Isolation of *Nocardia* water soluble mitogen (NWSM)

In early studies, we showed that a crude preparation of whole cells and hydrosoluble fractions from *N.opaca* possesses adjuvant activities [1, 2, 4]. Probably stimulated B cells and IL-l release by *Nocardia* soluble peptidoglycan fragments-activated macrophages are responsable for this effect.

In further experiments, Bona et al. [7, 8] demonstrated that these fractions are able to induce proliferation of B lymphocytes of various mamalian species.

A soluble compound containing material derived both from the cell wall peptidoglycan and the cell membrane, NWSM, was obtained after lysozyme treatment of delipidated *N.opaca* cells (NDCM) [1, 3]. This fraction which was excluded from Sephadex G75 was heterogenous, containing not only glyco- and lipoproteins but also amino sugars such as glucosamine and DAP (meso-1,6-diaminopimelic), markers of the cell wall peptidoglycans [1, 2].

The isolation of this macromolecular compound with mitogen activity was the starting point for delineating the structural requirements for the induction proliferation and differentiation of B lymphocytes. By using various bacteriolytic enzymes of known specificity, we have attempted to determine the minimal structure responsible for mitogenic activity. We have demonstrated that the minimal structure required for mitogenic activity is more complex than that required for differentiation of human lymphocytes. Figure 1 shows the scheme for preparation of mitogenic fractions from *N.opaca* [3].

Immunomodulatory activities

B cell mitogenic activity in various species

One of the most provocative and well investigated functions of NWSM is its mitogenicity [9].

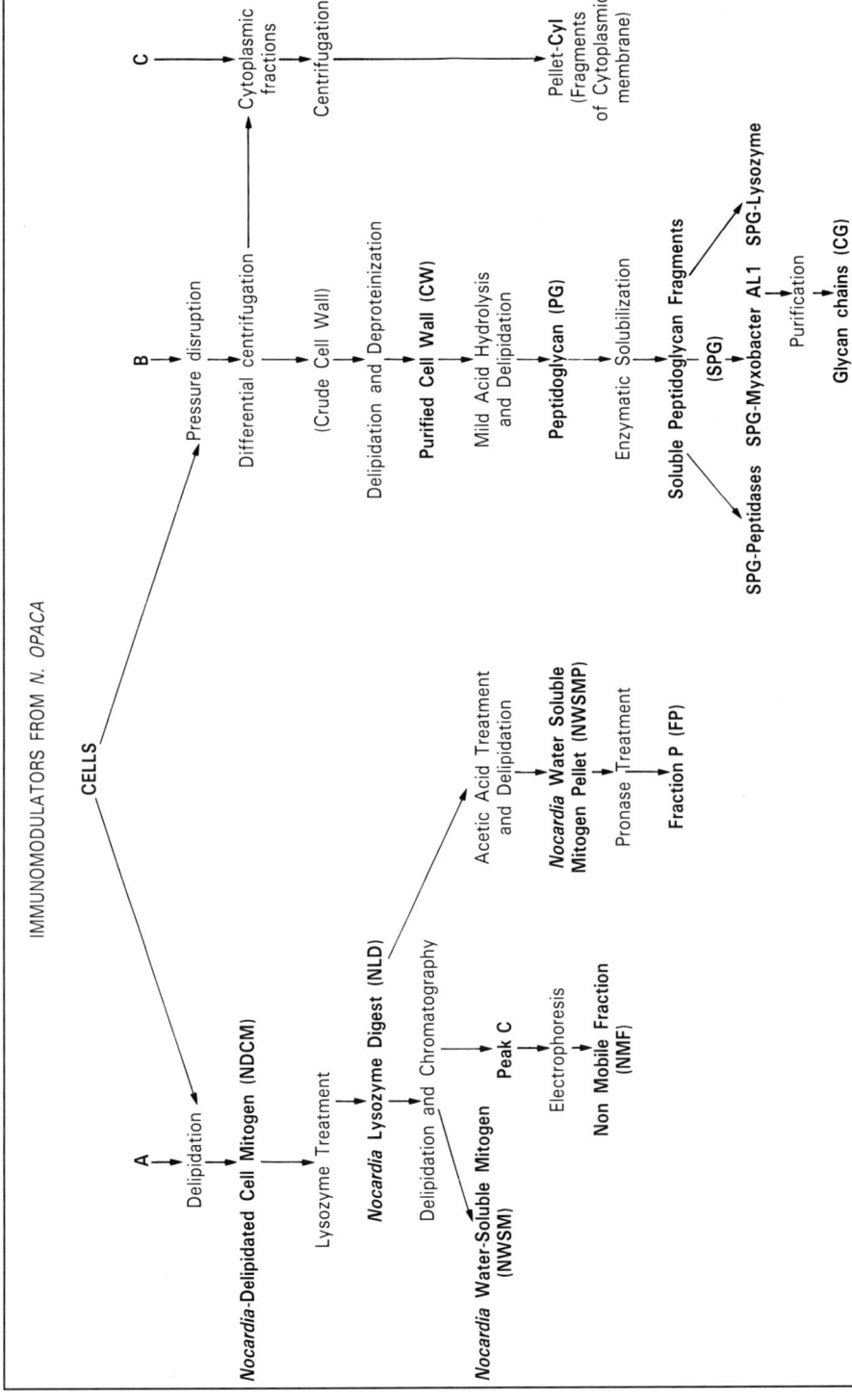

Figure 1. Scheme for preparation of mitogenic fraction from *N. opaca*. **Arrow A** indicates the products obtained by treatment of delipidated cell (NDCM) up to the obtaining of fractions devoid of C.W. constituents. **Arrow B** indicates the preparation of the C.W., PG, and SPG by using PG-degrading enzymes. **Arrow C** indicates the preparation of cytoplasmic and membrane fractions.

In contrast to the majority of B-cell mitogens such as LPS, peptidoglycan, enterotoxins, crude pneumococcal mitogens (PSIII), flagellin, dextran, levan, galactan, etc., which are powerful mitogens for murine B lymphocytes and weak or non-mitogenic for other mammalian species, NWSM is able to stimulate polyclonally the proliferation of B lymphocytes of various mammalian species : mice, rabbit and human [6-8].

In all of the above-mentioned species, it was clearly demonstrated that NWSM induced a genuine proliferation of lymphocytes evidenced by the increase of ^{3}H-thymidine incorporation as well as increase in mitosis [6]. This proliferation is also mirrored in polyclonal activation of precursors of antibody-forming cells [1, 2, 8-10, 39-41].

NWSM does not stimulate all B-cells. In mice, NWSM stimulates a subset of lymphocytes which is different from that stimulated by LPS or dextran sulfate. This subset of lymphocytes shows a low density of Ig and bears I-A but not I-E Ia antigens [9].

In the rabbit, the subset stimulated by NWSM differs from those stimulated by anti-allotype antibody or by PSIII [39, 41]. In man, it has been clearly shown that the subset stimulated by NWSM differs from that stimulated by PWM [9].

The mouse was a useful model for studying the genetic control of the response to NWSM. Two mutants of C3H/HeJ mice, which possess an autosomal dominant defect for LPS and CBA/N mice which bear an X-linked defect for various T-independent antigens, both responded to NWSM. Nonetheless, 1 :8 F_2 male progeny, originating form crosses between (CBA/N x C3H/HeJ)F_1, did not respond to NWSM or to LPS and dextran sulfate, two other B cell mitogens. Theoretically, 1 :8 of F_2 male progeny are homozygous for the autosomal defect for LPS of C3H/HeJ and also possess the X-linked defect of CBA/N. This indicates that these two defects can interact in a synergistic manner to render mice unresponsive to NWSM. Consequently, the response to NWSM is controlled by at least two genes, one located autosomally, carrying the LPS defect and the other in the X chromosome [9].

Leclerc et al. [42-44] demonstrated that NDCM, NWSMP, CW and NWSM are able to induce the proliferation of Axial organ, B-like cells of the Sea Star *Asterias rubens* at concentrations in the same range as on mammalian B lymphocytes. This activity is dependent on the presence of phagocytic cells.

Polyclonal activity and isotype (IgM, IgG, IgA)

It has also been shown that the proliferation of B cells induced by NWSM is accompanied by an increased synthesis of immunoglobulins by mice, rabbit and human B lymphocytes [7, 10, 11, 14, 16, 19]. The increased synthesis of Ig is associated with differentiation of small lymphocytes into plasma cells in response to NWSM. This conclusion is supported by several findings as follows : (a) an increased number of plasma cells in mice, rabbit and human lymphocyte cultures stimulated with NWSM ; (b) an increased number of cells which incorporate 3H-thymidine and contain Ig in rabbit lymphocyte cultures stimulated by NWSM, and (c) release from *in vivo* maternally induced allotypic suppression by *in vitro* allotypic suppression, which is due to a blockage of lymphocyte maturation [9, 41]. Release from allotype suppression obtained with NWSM can be related to its ability to break the blockage of maturation of pre B cells into Ig-secreting cells [9, 39].

The increased synthesis of Ig induced by NWSM is polyclonal [10] and affects all isotypes of Ig [11, 16]. In humans, NWSM and NDCM induces synthesis of IgA, IgM and IgG but not of IgD [3, 9, 16, 19]. Scott and Nahm [20] also studied IgG subclass expression in human lymphocyte populations (peripheral blood lymphocytes PBL, tonsils, splenocytes) stimulated with NDCM. They found that NDCM-mitogen produced all IgG subclasses excepted IgG4 : the response magnitude and pattern are similar to other T dependent mitogen.

Waldmann and Broder [16] demonstrated that total PBL cells cultured for 12 days with 100 μg of NWSM had geometric means for the synthesis and secretion of IgG, IgA and IgM of 1623, 1226 and 3016 ng per 2×10^6 lymphocytes in cultures respectively. The mean immunoglobulin stimulation ratios in the presence of NWSM as compared to culture in media and fetal calf serum alone were 9.4 for IgG, 4.7 for IgA and 27.3 for IgM, values quite comparable to those obtained for PWM. The stimulation of Ig synthesis involves a coordinate activation of all genes (i.e. V_H-V_L and C_H-C_L) which govern the synthesis of Ig molecules. Indeed, it was found that synthesis of Ig molecules induced by NWSM carried idiotypic specificities of inulin or galactan myeloma-binding proteins governed by V_H and V_L genes. Similarly, in the rabbit, NWSM is able to induce synthesis of Ig-bearing allotypes of α and β series which are located in the framework of V_H region for a series and in the CK-chain for b allotype, respectively [9, 41].

The stimulation of B lymphocytes by NWSM, which leads to duplication of DNA synthesis and mitosis, to activation of specific genes of B cells which are responsible for the synthesis of Ig and to differentiation into plasma cells, is probably associated with a widespread activation of various genes subsequent activation of B cells [9].

- *Effect of T-helper, T-suppressor and γ/δ T cells*

However, the responses to NWSM and NDCM are also regulated by signals generated by other cell types, such as T cells and monocytes-macrophages.

Waldmann and Broder [16] demonstrated that NWSM stimulated also purified B cells, to synthesize immunoglobulin but in lower quantities than in unseparated PBL cells (geometric means were 118 ng for IgG, 110 ng for IgA, and 465 for IgM). However, the quantity of immunoglobulin synthetized was increased by a factor of five when T cells were added to the cultures. Furthermore, Nagaoki et al. [14] showed that the helper function of human T cell subset, in stimulation of B cells, by NWSM, is relatively radiosensitive.

Bona et al. [9] and Revillard and Le Thi Bich Thuy [18] reported that NWSM and NDCM are not able to activate precursors of suppressor T cells. Miyawaki et al. [17] shows that the potential of human B cells to differentiate into IgM production seems to be mature at birth, but helper activity of T cells for IgM production was rather low shortly after birth and matured rapidly, during the neonatal period.

However, both B cell differentiation capacity and T cell helper function for IgG and IgA production were still immature at birth and gradually increased with age.

NWSM, NDCM and PG also activated B lymphocytes from cord and newborn infant blood [3, 14]. However, when T autologues lymphocytes were added to the culture, the capacity to generate plasma cells in the presence of these fractions was augmented. It appears that the magnitude of response of newborn infant and adult lymphocytes can be related to an ontogenic delay of Lyb5 like subset, because it is known that the newborn cannot develop an adequate response to polysaccharide vaccine (*i.e.* Streptococcus pneumoniae, or Haemophilius influenzae) as do infants or adults.

A substantial increase of γ/δ T cell was observed 7 days after i.m. injection of NDCM into pig fetuses in the middle or the end of the gestation period. Up to 70 % lymph node lymphocytes expressed γ/δ TCR (T cell receptor) after stimulation of pig fetuses with NDCM.

We suggest that γ/δ T cells might be stimulated in two possible way by this B mitogen. Either some ontogenetically early T-lymphocytes may recognize important bacterial molecules in a less subset restricted way or they may be activated secondarily as a result of the systemic reaction of the foetal immune system, *e.g.* by the secretion of interferons and other T cell stimulating substances of NK cells, macrophages and B cells [45].

- *Macrophage-monocytes independence, regulatory action of macrophages*

NWSM did not require monocytes in order to stimulate immunoglobulin production [16]. A similar monocyte independence was observed by Bona *et al.* when NWSM induced B cell proliferation was examined. In contrast, the addition of excessive numbers of monocytes (> 20 %) inhibited NWSM — induced B cell proliferation [9]. In this case, the apparent regulatory action of macrophages on B cells may be *via* T cell derived factors, or macrophage factors. The monocytes have been shown to secrete a number of products, such as prostaglandins that have been implicated in the suppressive effects of B lymphocytes proliferation by NWSM and NDCM [16, 18].

Revillard and Le Thi Bich-Thuy [18] investigated the effects of two classes of regulatory factors, which modulate Ig synthesis by B cells, stimulated by NDCM. They demonstrated the suppressor effect of aggregated IgG preparation and/or of IgFc binding factor on human B cells stimulated with NDCM.

Macrophage activation

The activation by NDCM, NWSM or CW of macrophages was evaluated by the ability of macrophages to exhibit a cytotoxic effect. Leibovici *et al.* [27] showed that, *in vitro*, peritoneal macrophages cocultured with NDCM exerted a cytotoxic effect on 3LL tumor cells. They suggested that activated macrophages must remain in contact with 3LL cell, for a sufficient length of time in order to kill them. They demonstrated that many factors affect contact, include ratio of macrophages (20 :1), macrophage density (10^6 macrophages per centimetre square minimum) and proximity of macrophages to target.

In our experiments, we showed that murine peritoneal macrophages elicited by i.p. injections of NWSM, and CW (100 µg/0.1 ml) on days 21, 8, 4 before sacrifice, exhibit cytostatic and cytotoxic activities against two tumoral targets : P815 mastocytoma cell lines and 3LL tumor cells [25, 32]. However, the acquisition of cytostatic and cytotoxic competence by activated macrophages required a supplementary transduction signal delivered by cytokines and lymphokines such as tumor necrosis factor (TNF-$\alpha\beta$), macrophage activating factor (MAF), INF-γ or by minute concentrations of LPS [25, 36]. Treatment of macrophages with these products alter surface properties of macrophages rendering sensitive to *Nocardia*. The precise mecanism by which *Nocardia* activated macrophages act to induce cytostasis and cytotoxicity is not known. It has been demonstrated that activation of macrophages is associated with a wide variety of functionnal or phenotypic changes [25, 46]. The release of cytokines such as IFN-α/β [30], IL-l and other monokines [33, 35, 36], and of TNF-α/β [12, 36, 37] has been demonstrated.

The increased secretion of lysosomal enzymes such as beta-glucuronidase, N-acetylglucosaminidase and acid phosphatase as well as oxygen metabolites, such as hydrogen peroxide [25, 32] and free oxygen radicals released by *Nocardia* activated macrophages may be involved in the cytotoxic effector mechanism.

Kozakova *et al.* (submitted) showed that NDCM exerts its effect not only on the classical immunocompetent cells but also on the enterocytes and their brush border enzymes after short-term oral treatments of germ free and normal rats. The oral treatment with NDCM changes the specific activities of enzymes such as lactase, sucrase and glucosamylase in the brush border membrane, the final localisation of these enzymes.

The activation of macrophages by *Nocardia* fractions appears to be linked to its ability to induce biochemical modification on the surface membrane and the expression of the sialylglycoproteins (sialyl and α-galactosyl residues) [47].

Release of monokines

We have also reported that adherent peritoneal cells from mice C_3H/HeJ and rats, incubated with NDCM, or NWSM or CW, release mitogenic factors acting on thymocytes from C_3H/HeJ mice. The production of IL-l and of other monokines by C_3H/HeJ macrophages was reported by Barot-Ciorbaru *et al.* [33], Moroux *et al.* [35] and Bouvet *et al.* [36, 48].

This mitogenic activity is linked to the presence of five compounds with high and low molecular weight in the 100, 45, 16, 7 and 3 kDa m.w. range. The 45 T-cell activating monokine with IL-l-like activities was characterised by chromatofocusing revealing a isoelectric point of about 4.7. Electrophoresis in SDS-PAGE, with a linear gradient 10-20 % and silver staining of gel, revealed the presence of a major peptide of 45 kDa and two minor peptides of 60 and 35 kDa. The analysis of amino acid composition showed great homology with IL-l. The high molecular weight compound (ranging from 100 to 45 kDa) activity could be related to high molecular weight precursors or intermediate forms of IL-l [35].

We have also found a novel low molecular weight monokine (NM3) with a m.w. of 3 kDa and apparent isolectric points between 4.7 and 5, which has a multiplicity of biological effects including proliferation of human B cells and thymocytes from C_3H/HeJ mice as well as differentiation of human B cells in presence of interleukin-2 (IL-2). NM3 is unable to induce the proliferation of human B-cells and of cells lines D_{10} G_H, IL-1 like dependent [36].

Finally we demonstrated that NM3 induces significant TNF-α release as detected by its cytolytic activity for L929 cells [36, 48]. This activity is probably involved in the enhanced cytotoxicity of macrophages treated with *Nocardia* fractions. In this case TNF might exert its activity by inducing the enhancement of the endogenous tumor lysosomal activities.

Induction of interferons (IFN) and other cytokines

Fractions from *Nocardia*, NWSM, NWSMP and PG have been used in experimental models to induce circulating interferon in various murine strains including C_3H/HeJ and *nude* mice [30]. The optimal effect (200-250 U/ml) was obtained after i.v. injection of 200 ug/mice of NWSM or NWSMP. The peak of α/β IFN appeared about 2 h after injection. Both IFN-α/β are produced subsequent to stimulation of macrophages by NWSM [30].

In contrast, the interferon induced by i.v. injection of PG (200 ug/mice) is a IFN-γ produced probably by activated T lymphocytes. These findings suggest that the chemical nature of *Nocardia* fraction determines the type of interferon produced by stimulated cells.

IFN-α/β can be induced by NWSM and peak B in different types of cells (peripheral blood cells, hepatocytes, lymph node cells, bone marrow cells and splenocytes), isolated from normal and *Influenza* virus infected mice.

The production of other soluble mediators by *Nocardia* stimulated lymphocytes and macrophages was also demonstrated.

In very recent investigations, Adam and Barot-Ciorbaru (unpublished data) obtained supernatant with proliferative activity for 7TD1 cells lines upon incubation of C_3H/HeJ macrophages with NWSM or CW. This effect was time and dose dependent. Interleukin-6 (IL-6) production by defective C_3H/HeB macrophages, induced by NWSM or CW, was compared with IL-1 and TNF produced in the same culture. NWSM has been reported to activated macrophages for interferon induction even in C_3H/HeJ mice [30].

Micusan *et al.* and Cavaillon *et al.* (unpublished data) have observed expression of IL-2 and IL-3 activity in stimulated murine thymocytes and splenocytes by NWSM.

Human monocytes appeared to directly produce TNF-α when incubated 12 to 24 hours in presence of NWSM and/or NLD (50 μg/1 $\times$ 106 cells). It must be noted that the maximum TNF-α level was observed after 18 h. TNF-α secretion in response to NLD and NWSM was not affected by polymyxin B, which is known to interfere with LPS. Authors also suggested that TNF-α production and regulation might be profoundly related to activation of protein kinase C (PKC). The later may act upon transcriptional and post transcriptional steps as reported for other systems. The isotype of PK involved in TNF-α secretion and the phosphoprotein induced by *Nocardia* fractions are under investigation [37].

Action on natural killer (NK) cell activity

NDCM, NWSMP and PG has been shown to increase NK cell activity in mice [35]. It was suggested that interferon was the mediator of this effect. Increased NK activity observed in mice treated i.p. with 100 ug of NDCM or NWSMP or PG was quite rapid and the peak was reached within 2 to 24 hours. Polyclonal goat antimurine IFN-α/β antiserums ablated this activity. In contrast, the activation of NK cells induced by PG was abrogated when antibodies IFN-γ were injected.

Therapeutic effects in animal models of immunological disorders

Infections

Repeated injections of NDCM and NWSM(5mg/kg) have been used in eliciting protection of Syrian hamsters inoculated with rabies virus ; their survival is slightly increased compared to normal animals. These fractions are interferon inducers and the interferon concentration in the serum reaches the peak 2 h after injection of NDCM or NWSM [29].

Tumors

The antitumor activity of *Nocardia opaca* fractions was demonstrated in various experimental tumor systems such as fibrosarcomas in rats and mice and 3LL (Lewis lung carcinoma) in mice and F6 rhabdomyosarcoma in rats.

NDCM, NWSM and CW have been reported to exhibit antitumor activity when injected intralesionally in mineral oil emulsion. They are able to diminish primary fibrosarcoma in rat and mouse : 100 % cure of rats was obtained with this treatment. Regression of treated tumors as compared with control tumors implanted contralaterally was also observed [24]. Doses of 1 mg/kg were capable to inhibiting tumor growth.

In 3LL-bearing mice we demonstrated that repeated i.p. administration of emulsified NDCM and two others compounds, NWSM and CW, resulted in a significant reduction of metastases. A combined regimen of NDCM or NWSM or CW (100 μg/ml) i.p. in 3LL-bearing mice and monokines (0.1 ml), yielded a greater antimetastatic effect than either therapy alone [25]. Monokines showed a strong synergistic effect with NWSM, CW and NDCM.

Using 3LL bearing mice, treated with NDCM, Leibovici *et al.* [26-28] examined the local cellular host response after intratumoral injection of NDCM, mg/0.2 ml/mouse. Histological analysis of the tumor site showed an increase in the mononuclear cell population around the tumor in NDCM treated mice. This population was composed, according to FACS analysis, of macrophages and Lyt-1 binding cells as well as reactive B lymphocytes [28]. Since lymphocytes were also found around non-treated tumors and they apparently did not prevent tumor development, it is possible that macrophages play a more important role in NDCM-elicited host defense against the Lewis lung carcinoma. Probably NDCM had the capacity to attract these macrophages into growing tumors in response to a tumor antigen.

A promising example of stimulation of non specific immunity is demonstrated by NDCM, which exhibits an immunotherapeutic effect. Repeated i.p. injections of NDCM (200 µg) in an oil/water emulsion (0.1 ml) were able to inhibit the appearance of lymph node and lung metastases after surgical removal of a grafted F6 rhabdomyosarcoma in Wistar AG rats. Ten days after the death of the last untreated animal all the treated rats were alive and 6 rats out of 10 were completely free from lung nodules. The median number of metastases was 0 as shown in Table I. NDCM was very effective in reducing metastases, when associated with surgical removal of primary tumor [25].

Table I. Effect of NDCM on the dissemination of the F6 transplanted rhabdomyosarcoma in the Wistar AG rat.

Treatment of rats[1]	Number of rats with invasion of local lymph nodes[2]	Individual count of lung tumor nodules	Median
Oil water emulsion	7	7, 10, 19, 31, 36, 45, 51, 66, 107, 155	40
NDCM in oil water emulsion	1	0, 0, 0, 0, 0, 0, 1, 4, 18, 69	0

[1] Rats were treated by i.p. administration of 200 µg/0.1 ml *Nocardia* delipidated mitogen (NDCM), twice weekly until sacrificed (see *Materials and methods*).
[2] Tumor invasion reached the axillary or inguinal lymph node areas.

In summary, these experiments suggest that *Nocardia* fractions activate a series of processes resulting in the inhibition of metastases. We are far from being able to indicate which mechanism is directly responsible for the reduction of established metastases. Even if macrophages are considered to be the principal responding cells for these stimulating agents, helper effects of other cells cannot be excluded. For example, these findings could be the results of IFN-γ stimulation, which we have shown can be induced by the cell wall peptidoglycan derivative [30]. Stimulation of the NK lymphocyte system which occurs after injection of *N.opaca* fractions [31] could play a role in the inhibition of metastatic spread.

Recently the induction of NO⁻ synthase in a macrophage cell line J 774 cells by fractions from *Nocardiae* was investigated (McCall and Barot, in preparation). NLD induce NO synthase in these cells in a concentration dependent manner with maximum induction observed at 100 µg/ml (382 ± 33 pmoles NO/min/mg/protein) after 12 h incubation. This delay may reflect the need for NLD-mediated cytotoxicity production by the cells prior to induction of NO synthase.

Regardless of the mechanism involved, the main goal of these studies remains the effective prevention of metastasis.

Immunology disorders

Concerning the use of NWSM to define disorders of regulatory monocytes, Waldmann and Broder [16] observed that lymphocytes from patients with aplasic anemia (monocytopenia, *i.e.* 0-1 %) have a markedly deficient responses to NWSM.

Gugliemi *et al.* [15] demonstrated that NDCM is a T cell independent activator of CLL (chronic lymphocytic leukemia) B lymphocytes, when the B cells are in an advanced state of differentiation. Bernheim *et al.* [12] developed an assay in order to investigate the presence of SIg and Ph¹ (Philadelphia chromosome) in mitotic cells obtained by stimulation of blood mononuclear cells PBL in chronic myelocytic leukemia (CML) by NDCM.

In untreated patients with Hodgkin's disease (HD), B cell enriched populations from PBL were unresponsive to NDCM, which is able to induce Ig synthesis in normal B cells, even in the absence of T cells [49].

Visualisation of submacroscopic metastases

In preliminary experiments it had been observed that an immunomodulator isolated from *N.opaca* NSPD (nocardia soluble peptidoglycan derivative) [3] selectively bound to a model of activated macrophages [38]. A hypothesis has been put forward that the enhanced detection of macrophages that are usually present in the vicinity or inside tumors should represent a polyspecific test for scintigraphy of a variety of metastases.

NSPD radiolabelled with ^{99m}Technetium cannot be injected intravenously due to its physicochemical properties. It has therefore been encapsulated into liposomes (phosphatidylcholine, phosphatidylserine and cholesterol in the molar ratio 8 :2 :10), then administered *via* the respiratory tract as an aerosol. Amphiphilic properties, as well as its low molecular weight, allow a rapid diffusion of NSPD in blood. Scintigraphy of metastases was possible from 1.5 to 6 h after inhalation [38].

The first stage of the study was carried out on 5 patients bearing known metastases (skin, lymph nodes, bone) from malignant melanoma that all were imaged with ^{99m}Tc-NSPD. The test was then applied to patients with a high risk of recurrent cancers (melanoma : 6, breast tumor : 7) based on the detection in their plasmas of high lipid associated sialic acid (LASA), (sensitive marker for many forms of neoplasia) concentrations. The association of these two sensitive techniques has resulted in the detection of very small metastases that were not seen using conventional scintigraphy : they were then confirmed histologically (Table II) [38].

The results obtained demonstrate that NSPD is able to concentrate in the metastases of two very different types of tumor, melanoma and breast carcinoma, with such an affinity that it allows the scintigraphic detection of submacroscopic or even microscopic lesions.

As far as the mechanism of action is concerned, we now believe that metastases can only be visualised when the macrophages have reached a certain level of activation, as a result of signals received from the tumor cells and from NSPD. The synergy between the two signals allows the detection of certain types of tumor but not of others (Barot-Ciorbaru et al., unpublished data).

Recently, Le Pape et al. (unpublished data) using the same type of experiment investigated another type of pathological feature characterized by an important recruitment of inflammatory macrophages, i.e. sarcoidosis such as *Berylliosis*. Promising results have been obtained for the evaluation of inflammatory lesions of lung granulomatosis.

Table II. Clinical data on patients investigated from residual minimal disease of breast cancer or melanoma. + symbol is used for indicating pathological values 17.1 µg/100 ml for LASA and to express the observation of a fixing area in scintigraphy. The observations on patients 2 and 9 have been more extensively documented in the text.

No.	Patient	Sex	Age	Type of initial tumor and duration from first treatment	LASA	99m Tc-NSPD scintigraphic localization : and relative ratio	Histological confirmation of tumor cells
1	La...	F	49	Breast : 3 yr T2N+	+	+ Breast (1.18)	+
2*	Mo...	F	41	Breast : 1 yr	+	+ Breast (1.22)	+
				T1N0		+ Sternum skin (1.28)	+
3	Pa...	F	65	Breast : 4 yr T1N+	−	+ Lung (1.15)	ND
4	Si...	F	63	Breast : 8 yr T1N+	+	+ Arm (1.30)	−
5	Fo...	F	40	Breast : 4 yr T2N+	+	+ Breast (1.26)	±
6	Gr...	F	50	Breast : 4 yr T3N+	+	−	ND
7	Ju...	F	46	Breast : 3 yr T2N+	+	+ Sternum skin (1.23)	−
8	Ca...	M	56	Melanoma : 2 yr	+	+ Neck (1.19)	+
9*	Be...	M	54	Melanoma : 5 yr	+	+ Scarpa area (1.40)	+
						+ Buttock (1.35)	+
10	St...	F	65	Melanoma : 1 yr	+	+ Axillary area (1.20)	ND
11	Ni...	M	41	Melanoma : 3 yr	+	−	ND
12	Gi...	M	47	Melanoma : 8 yr	+	−	ND
13	Lo...	F	62	Melanoma : 10 yr	+	−	ND
14	Bl...	F	32	Melanoma : 2 yr	−	−	ND
15	Ra...	M	35	Melanoma : 1 yr	−	−	ND

Conclusion

The demonstration of the mitogenic activity of *N.opaca* fractions and the studies carried out in the area have allowed the role of the B lymphocyte to be elucidated.

The activation of macrophages and the secretion of active mediators, with a role in the control of tumor growth and in the visualisation of metastases, represents a more spectacular field and promises well for future advances.

The potential of these fractions and of the mediators which they are able of releasing permits us to advance in the study of the anti-tumoral and anti-infectious effect for which we already have promising results.

In memory of Professor Edgar Lederer.

References

1. Ciorbaru P, Adam A, Petit JF, Lederer E, Bona C, Chedid L. Isolation of mitogenic and adjuvant active fractions from various species of *Nocardiae*. Infect Immun 1975 ; 11 : 257-64.
2. Ciorbaru R, Petit JF, Lederer E, Zissman E, Bona C, Chedid L. Presence and subcellular localization of two distinct mitogenic fractions in the cells of *Nocardia rubra* and *Nocardia opaca* : preparation of soluble mitogenic peptidoglycan fractions. Infect Immun 1976 ; 13 : 1084-90.
3. Barot-Ciorbaru R, Brochier J, Miyawaki T, Preud'homme JL, Petit JF, Bona C, Taniguchi N, Revillard JP. Stimulation of murine, rabbit and human B lymphocytes by NDCM (Nocardia delipidated cell mitogen) from *N. opaca* and derived fractions structure activity-relationship. J Immunol 1985 ; 135 : 3277-83.
4. Adam A, Ciorbaru R, Petit JF, Lederer E. Isolation and properties of a macromolecular, water-soluble, immuno-adjuvant fraction from the cell wall of *Mycobacterium smegmatis*. Proc Natl Acad Sci USA 1972 ; 69 : 851-4.
5. Ellouz F, Adam A, Ciorbaru R, Lederer E. Minimal structural requirements for adjuvant activity of bacterial peptidoglycan. Biochem Biophys Res Commun 1974 ; 59 : 1317-25.
6. Lederer E. Synthetic muramyl peptides. Science 1982 ; 218 : 330.
7. Bona C, Damais C, Dimitriu A, Chedid L, Ciorbaru R, Adam A, Petit JF, Lederer E, Rosselet JP. Mitogenic effect of water-soluble extract of *Nocardia opaca* : a comparative study with some bacterial adjuvants on spleen and peripheral lymphocytes of four mammalian species. J Immunol 1974 ; 112 : 2028-35.
8. Bona C, Chedid L, Damais C, Ciorbaru R, Shek PN, Dubiski S, Cinader B. Blast transformation of rabbit B-derived lymphocytes by a mitogen extracted from Nocardia. J Immunol 1975 ; 114 : 348-53.
9. Bona C, Broder S, Dimitriu A, Waldmann TA. Polyclonal activation of human B lymphocytes by Nocardia water soluble mitogen (NWSM). Immunol Rev 1979 ; 45 : 69-92.
10. Brochier J, Bona C, Ciorbaru R, Revillard JP, Chedid L. A human T-independent B lymphocyte mitogen extracted from *Nocardia opaca*. J Immunol 1976 ; 117 : 1434-40.
11. Le Thi Bich-Thuy, Ciorbaru R, Brochier J. Human B cell differentiation immunoglobulin synthesis induced by Nocardia mitogen. Eur J Immunol 1978 ; 8 : 119-23.
12. Prieur AM, Pham Huu T. Lymphotoxin and chemotactic factor produced *in vitro* by human lymphocytes during their proliferative response in the presence of phytohaemagglutinin and Nocardia soluble mitogen. Ann Immunol (Paris) 1980 ; 131D : 223-32.

13. Bernheim A, Berger R, Preud'homme JL, Labaume S, Bussel A, Barot-Ciorbaru R. Philadelphia chromosome positive blood B lymphocytes in chronic myelocytic leukemia. *Leukemia Res* 1981 ; 5 : 331-8.
14. Nagaoki T, Miyawaki T, Ciorbaru R, Yachie A, Uwadana N, Moriya N, Taniguchi N. Maturation of B-cell differentiation ability and T-cell regulatory function during child-growth assessed in a *Nocardia* water-soluble mitogen driven system. *J Immunol* 1981 ; 126 : 2015-9.
15. Guglielmi P, Preud'homme JL, Ciorbaru-Barot R, Seligmann M. Mitogen-induced maturation of chronic lymphocytic leukemia B lymphocytes. *J Clin Immunol* 1982 ; 2 : 186-96.
16. Waldmann TA, Broder S. Polyclonal B-cell activators in the study of the regulation of immunoglobulin synthesis in the human system. *Adv Immunol* 1982 ; 32 : 1-63.
17. Miyawaki T, Nagaoki T, Yokoi T, Yachie A, Uwadana N, Taniguchi N. Cellular interactions of human T cell subsets defined by monoclonal antibodies in regulating B cell differentiation : a comparative study in Nocardia water soluble mitogen and pokeweed mitogen-stimulated culture systems. *J Immunol* 1982 ; 128 : 899-905.
18. Revillard JP, Le Thi Bich-Thuy. Ig-G binding factors and polyclonal activation of human B cells. *Clin Immunol News Letter* 1983 ; 4 : 116-20.
19. Le Thi Bich-Thuy, Revillard JB. Modulation of polyclonally activated human peripheral B cells by aggregated IgG and IgG subclass synthesis. *J Immunol* 1984 ; 133 : 544-9.
20. Scott MG, Nahm MH. Mitogen-induced human IgG subclass expression. *J Immunol* 1984 ; 135 : 2454-60.
21. Tlaskalova-Hogenova H, Bartova J, Mrklas L, Mancal P, Broukal Z, Barot-Ciorbaru R, Novak M, Hanykova M. Stimulation of human blood lymphocytes by different polyclonal B cell activators of bacterial and plant origin : production of IgM, IgG and IgA estimated by Elisa method. *Folia Microbiol* 1985 ; 30 : 258-66.
22. Tlaskalova-Hogenova H, Mandel L, Stepankova R, Bartova J, Barot R, Leclerc M, Kovaru F, Trebichavsky I. Autoimmunity : from physiology to pathology. Natural antibodies, mucosal immunity and development of B cell repertoire. *Folia Biologica* 1992 ; 38 : 202-15.
23. Emilie D, Crevon MC, Chicheportiche R, Auffredou MT, Barot-Ciorbaru R, Lenoir G, Dayer JM, Galanaud P. Cystic fibrosis patients B lymphocyte response is resistant to the *in vitro* enhancing effect of corticosteroids. *Eur J Clin Invest* 1990 ; 20 : 620-6.
24. Barot-Ciorbaru R, Petit JF, Chassoux D, Salomon JC. Antitumoral activity of intralesionally administered *Nocardia opaca* preparations in rat and mouse tumors : a comparison with BCG and *Corynebacterium parvum*. *J Immunopharmacol* 1980 ; 3 : 115-22.
25. Barot-Ciorbaru R, Cornil J, Grand-Perret T, Poupon MF. Antimetastatic activity of immunomodulators from *N.opaca* in mice and rats. Activation of peritoneal macrophages in mice by these fractions. *Cancer Immunol Immunother* 1987 ; 25 : 111-8.
26. Leibovici J, Hoenig S, Horodniceanu E, Barot-Ciorbaru R. Local cellular host response induced by Nocardia delipidated cell mitogen in Lewis lung carcinoma bearing mice. *In vivo* 1990 ; 4 : 299-308.
27. Leibovici J, Hoenig S, Pinchassov A, Barot-Ciorbaru R. Macrophage involvement in the antitumoral effect of Nocardia-delipidated cell mitogen (NDCM). *In vivo* 1991 ; 5 : 365-74.
28. Leibovici J, Hoenig S, Pinchassov A, Horodniceanu E, Barot-Ciorbaru R. Mechanism of the antitumoral effect of two *Nocardia opaca* immunomodulatory fractions in Lewis lung carcinoma. In : Wegmann RJ, Wegmann MA, eds. *Recent advances in cellular and molecular biology, immunology, autoantibodies, lymphomas, infectious diseases, tumors.* Vol. 1. Leuven, Belgium : Peeters Press, 1992 : 231-9.
29. Barot-Ciorbaru R, Yokota Y, Petit JF, Chedid L, Atanasiu P. Induction de la synthèse d'interféron chez le hamster par des fractions de *Nocardia :* essais de protection contre la rage par le NWSM. *Ann Microbiol (Inst.Pasteur)* 1979 ; 130B : 263-9.
30. Barot-Ciorbaru R, Catinot L, Wietzerbin J, Petit JF, Chedid L, Falcoff E. Involvement of a radioresistant cell in the production of circulating interferon induced by *Nocardia* fractions in mice. *J Reticuloendothel* 1981 ; 30 : 247-57.

31. Barot-Ciorbaru R, Linna TJ, Patel MR, Altman J, Carnaud C. Enhancement of natural killer cell activity by *Nocardia opaca* fractions. *Scand J Immunol* 1989 ; 29 : 133-41.
32. Bravo-Cuellar A, Barot-Ciorbaru R, Homo-Delarche F, Cabannes J, Nowacki W, Orbach-Arbouys S. When adjuvants are sequentially administered, inhibition may take place : preliminary results. *Int J Immunother* 1989 ; V(1) : 21-4.
33. Barot-Ciorbaru R, Boschetti E, Petit JF. Sécrétion par des macrophages péritoneaux stimulés par les parois de *Nocardia opaca* de plusieurs facteurs mitogènes, pour des thymocytes murins. *CR Acad Sci Paris* 1984 ; tome 298, série III, n° 17 : 483-6.
34. Moroux Y, Boschetti E, Barot-Ciorbaru R, Plassat JL, Egly JM. Synthetis of Trisacryl sorbents for metal chelate chromatography. Application to monokine separation. In : Chaiken JM, Wilchek M, Parikh I, eds. *Affinity chromatography and biological recognition.* Orlando, San Diego, New York, London, Toronto, Montreal, Sydney, Tokyo, Sao Polo : Academic Press, Inc., 1983 : 275-8.
35. Moroux Y, Boschetti E, Bouvet JP, Barot-Ciorbaru R. Application of chromatographic methods to the analysis of macrophages factors induced by *Nocardia opaca* cell walls. *J Chromatogr* 1988 ; 440 : 113-30.
36. Bouvet JP, Souvannavong V, Lasfargues A, Adam A, Mysiakine E, Crevon C, Boschetti E, Barot R. IL-l-release and biological properties of low molecular weight monokines by C3H/HeJ macrophages, treated with cell wall from *N.opaca*. The macrophage, annual conference of the Upper Rhine Universities, Freiburg. Basel, Munchen : Karger, 1990 : 4-5.
37. Mege JL, Sangueldoce MV, Jacob T, Bongrand P, Capo C, Myssiakine EB, Barot-Ciorbaru R. *Nocardia* fractions, NLD and NWSM, induce tumor necrosis factor-α secretion in human monocytes : role of protein kinase C. *Eur J Immunol* 1993 ; 23 : 1582-7.
38. Le Pape A, Barot-Ciorbaru R, Musset M, Baulieu J, Jubault C, Lemarie E, Pourcelot L, Besnard JC, Nicolau C, Mathe G. An original method for submacroscopic metastases visualization in case of cancer minimal residual disease. *Biomed Pharmacother* 1986 ; 40 : 392-8.
39. Cazenave PA, Juy D, Bona C. Ontogeny of lymphocyte functions during embryonic life of rabbit. *J Immunol* 1978 ; 121 : 444-55.
40. Cavaillon JM, Udupa TNS, Chou CT, Cinader B, Haeffner-Cavaillon N, Dubiski S. Rabbit B spleen lymphocytes and T helper cells.I. Responsiveness to mitogens of B cell subpopulations of different sedimentation velocities and subpopulations bearing or lacking FC receptors. *J Immunol* 1979 ; 123 : 2231-8.
41. Primi D, Mami F, Le Guern C, Cazenave PA. Mitogen-reactive B cell subpopulations selectively express different sets of V regions. *J Exp Med* 1982 ; 156 : 181-6.
42. Leclerc M, Brillouet C, Barot-Ciorbaru R. Evidence for a B-like cells stimulatory factor in *Asterias rubens*. *Med Sci Res* 1987 ; 15 : 211-2.
43. Leclerc L, Bahamaoud T, Brillouet C, Tlaskalova-Hogenova H, Petit JF, Barot-Ciorbaru R. Stimulation of Sea Star *Asterias rubens* axial organ B-like cells by Nocardia-delipidated cell mitogen and derived fractions. *Folia Biologica* 1988 ; 34 : 182-90.
44. Leclerc M, Bajelan M, Barot R, Tlaskalova-Hogenova H. Effect of silica on the spontaneous cytotoxicity of Axial organ cells from *Asterias rubens*. *Cell Biol Int* 1993 ; 17 : 787-8.
45. Pospisil R, Trebichavsky I, Rehakova Z, Rejnek J, Tuckova L, Tlaskalova H, Kovaru F, Barot R. The expression of $\tau\delta$ T cell receptor and proliferation of $\tau\delta$ cells during T cell ontogeny in pig. *Immunology* (in press).
46. Lemaire G, Tenu JP, Petit JF, Lederer E. Effects of microbially derived products on mononuclear phagocytes. In : Hadden JW, Szentivanyi A, eds. *The reticuloendothelial system*, Vol. 8. New York and London : Plenum Press, 1985 : 181-245.
47. Hoenig S, Skutelsky E, Leibovici J, Barot-Ciorbaru R. Changes in distribution of lectin receptors in macrophages activated by Nocardia water soluble molecules. *Cell Mol Biol* 1993 ; V : 39 (in press).
48. Bouvet JP, Souvannavong V, Boschetti E, Adam A, Barot-Ciorbaru R. Release and characterization of monokines induced by murine macrophages treated with cell walls from *Nocardia opaca*. *Exp Cell Biol* 1989 ; 57 : 87-90.
49. Griesinger F, Bergmann L, Barot-Ciorbaru R, Mitrou PS. Intrinsic B lymphocyte defect in untreated patients with Hodgkin's disease. *Cancer Immunol Immunother* 1990 ; 32 : 256-60.

6

Lentinan

R. BOMFORD

Unité d'Épidémiologie des Virus Oncogènes, Institut Pasteur, 28, rue du Docteur-Roux, 75724 Paris Cedex 15, France.

Product

Historical background

Lentinan is a fungal polysaccharide, a β-1,3-glucan, extracted from the Japanese edible mushroom, *Lentinus edodes*, which was shown to possess anti-tumor activity by Chihara *et al.* in 1969, who has recently reviewed its immunopharmacology and therapeutic effects [1]. It is being developed by Ajimoto jointly with Morishita and Yamaouchi as an immunostimulant and anti-neoplastic agent, and was launched in Japan for the treatment of stomach cancer in 1986. It is not to be confused with lentinacin (eritadenine), which is also isolated from *Lentinus edodes*, and is a (2R,3R)-dihydroxy-4-(9-adenyl) butyric acid used as a hypocholesterolemic.

Chemical and physico-chemical properties

The molecular weight of lentinan is between 300,000 and 800,000 dalton as measured by gel permeation chromatography and quasielastic light scattering, and the β-1,3-glucan has two β-1,6-glucopyranoside branches for every five β-1,3-glucopyranoside linear linkages [2, 3].

The anti-tumor activity of lentinan is dependent on its higher structure, being decreased after denaturation with urea or dimethyl sulfoxide, but recovered after the removal of the denaturants [3].

Experimental and preclinical studies

Toxicology

After intravenous (i.v.) injection into mice, rats, dogs or monkeys, the LD_{50} of lentinan is greater that 50 mg/kg. However in chronic toxicity studies in rhesus monkeys, it was found that daily intravenous treatment at any dose above 0.5 mg/kg produced a variety of clinical and histological changes such as skin rashes, bleedings, foam cells in the liver, spleen and lymph nodes, renal granulomata and vasculitis, etc. [4].

Pharmacokinetics

The i.v. administration of lentinan to rats revealed that it has a plasma half-life of about eight hours and is thereafter gradually removed from the circulation, probably by phagocytosis by Kupffer cells in the liver, and persists for up to seven days [5].

Immunomodulating properties and mechanisms of action

• **In vivo *and* ex vivo *studies***

The immunomodulating effect of lentinan is expressed through the promotion of non-specific effector functions of macrophages and natural killer cells, and also of specific T-cell mediated immunity. In rodents lentinan functions as an immunological adjuvant for T cells [6, 7] and augments alloreeactive cytotoxic T lymphocytes [8]. It stimulates helper T cells in the peripheral blood of rats after oral administration [9] and, in mice which are low-responders to the antigens of tumors induced by the Rous sarcoma virus, it activates specific anti-tumor immunity when given intraperitoneally (i.p.) after the subcutaneous injection of mitomycin-C-inactivated tumor cells [10]. The peritoneal macrophages of mice become activated to inhibit the incorporation of 3H-TdR by tumor cells *in vitro* after i.v. injection of lentinan [11]. In certain cancer patients an elevation of the NK cell activity of peripheral mononuclear cells was observed during lentinan treatment [12]. Enhanced production of interleukin-1 and tumor necrosis factor by peripheral monocytes has been observed after lentinan treatment in gastric cancer patients [13], and the same effect was observed for induction of lymphokine-activated killer activity [14]. Administration of 2 mg of lentanin twice to patients with gastric cancer (3-9 days before surgery and the day before surgery) did not change lymphocyte subsets in the periperal blood, but there was an increase in the ratio of CD4 cells in the lymph nodes, and in the tumor infiltrating lymphocytes the number of CD4, Leu11 and LeuM3 cells increased [15].

• **In vitro *studies***

— **Animal cells** : The phagocytic activity of mouse peritoneal macrophages is raised by *in vitro* exposure to lentinan and this is mediated through a specific cell-surface β-glucan receptor [16]. Lentinan also raises the cytostatic activity of mouse peritoneal macrophages against metastatic target cells, although a highly metastatic variant of the Lewis lung carcinoma was found to be resistant [17].

— **Human cells** : Lentinan increases the ^{3}H-TdR incorporation of peripheral blood lymphocytes from healthy volunteers or cancer patients [18], stimulates interleukin-1 production by human monocytes [19] and promotes the cytotoxic function (NK cells and antibody dependent cellular cytotoxicity) of lymphocytes from patients with chronic lymphoïd leukemia [20].

• *Molecular activity mechanims*

As mentioned above, lentinan binds to specific β-glucan receptors on the surface of monocytic cells, which causes their activation [16], and this in turn could cause the stimulation of specific T-cell mediated immunity through the induction of T-cell growth factors such as interleukin-1 [19]. In addition, lentinan activates the complement system by the alternative pathway [21], which could also contribute to macrophage activation [11]. The intracellular messengers involved in the activation of cells by lentinan do not yet seem to have been investigated.

Therapeutic effects in animal models of immunological disorders

- *Infections*

Lentinan has predominantly been studied as an anti-tumor agent, and little work has been reported on its effects on infectious disease. However, it does limit post-chemotherapeutic relapse in experimental mouse tuberculosis [22] and it increases resistance to a cestode parasite in mice [23]. Intranasal administration of lentinan conferred significant protection against aerosol influenza virus infection in mice, and activated broncho-alveolar macrophages as measured by chemiluminescence [24]. The anti-microbial activity of lentinan and related polysaccharides has recently been reviewed [25].

- *Tumors*

Since the original observations by Chihara *et al.* in 1969 [26], the anti-tumor activity of lentinan has been demonstrated with a variety of tumors in mice, both allogeneic, syngeneic and autochthonous [27, 28]; reviewed in [29]. In typical experiments, the tumor cells are injected subcutaneously, and lentinan treatment is commenced 24 hours later with daily i.p .doses of one or a few mg/kg, leading to a retardation of tumor growth. Recently lentinan has been shown to act synergistically with interleukin- 2 in a model of spontaneous metastasis in the mouse [30] and this anti-metastic effect was correlated with the induction of lymphokine-activated killer (LAK) activity in the spleen.

Clinical studies

Pharmacokinetics and tolerance in healthy human volunteers

The administration of 1 mg of lentinan predissolved in 2 ml of distilled water containing 2 mg dextran-40 and 100 mg mannitol, mixed with a drip infusion solution (glucose or saline) and then slowly infused i.v. caused no ill effects in volunteers or patients [31].

Pharmacokinetics on patients

The discovery that lentinan levels can be measured by the limulus test usually used for endotoxin made it possible to study the pharmacokinetics of lentinan in man [5]. Lentinan was stable when incubated *in vitro* in human plasma at 37 °C for an hour. The pharmacokinetics of lentinan in the blood of ten healthy volunteers and three patients with advanced gastric cancer was measured. During the i.v. administration of 1 mg of lentinan over a two hour period, the plasma concentration peaked at 50-80 ng/1 ml at the end of the infusion period and decreased gradually thereafter.

Clinical trials phase I

Clinical trials with lentinan against colon, rectal, lung, gynaecological and breast cancers, and against AIDS, are underway in Japan (16th International Congress Chemotherapy (Jerusalem), 1989, 17), and in the USA in phase I-II trials against AIDS, a total of 16/44 patients receiving 2-10 mg/1 week of lentinan showed rises in CD4 cell counts (6th International Conference AIDS on (San Fransisco), 1990, Abs. SB487).

Lentinan has been used in conjunction with another immunopotentiator, OK-432, with the object of inducing the secretion of cytokines such as tumor necrosis factor-α or interferon-gamma into the serum (tumor necrosis factor serum) post-operatively in cancer patients [32]. Eighteen cancer patients received pre-operative priming treatment with lentinan (4-10 mg, total dose), with OK-432 being given i.v. or i.p. immediately after their operation. Plasma TNF-α levels were elevated 2-3 hours following treatment, and IFN-γ after one day. The adverse effects were a high fever, as well as mild hypotension not requiring any supportive therapy. Intra-abdominal and intrapleural injection of lentinan at a dosage of 4mg/week for four weeks has been used to treat malignant ascites and pleural effusion, and 16/20 patients showed a clinical response [33].

Lentinan treatment in two Japanese patients with antibodies against human T leukemia virus I and III caused the disappearance of the antibodies and of $HTLV_p24$ antigen [31].

Clinical trials phase II-III

The original reports on a phase III trial of lentinan in gastric cancer are in Japanese [34] but an overview in English is available [29]. A randomised controlled study was conducted of lentinan in combination with the chemotherapeutic agent tegafur for the treatment of inoperable and recurrent gastric cancer. Tegafur (600 mg per day, orally) was given alone to 68 patients, or together with lentinan (1 mg twice a week or 2 mg once a week) to 77 patients. The inclusion of lentinan in the treatment regimen prolonged lifespan significantly ($p = <0.01$) and this remained the case when the patients were divided according to Zubrod's performance status, histology, tumor spread and Borrmann type. Toxicity was observed in 6.8 % of the 469 patients who entered phase I, II or III studies of lentinan, and included eruption and redness (1.9 %), headache and a feeling of heaviness in the head (0.6 %), hot sensation (0.6 %), sweating (0.6 %), and fever (0.4 %), etc. Lentinan treatment was discontinued in only two patients.

Conclusion

Until recently Lentinan and related polysaccharide immunomodulators of fungal origin such as Krestin have been principally studied in Japan, and have only received licences for clinical application in Japan, where they are very widely used, principally for gastric cancer. Interest in these agents is now developing outside Japan, particularly in the possibility that they may be useful for the immunotherapy of AIDS, and the results from further clinical studies can be expected in the not too distant future.

References

1. Chihara G. Recent progress in immunopharmacology and therapeutic effects of polysaccharides. *Dev Biol Stand* 1992 ; 77 : 191-7.
2. Chihara G, Hamuro J, Maeda YY, Arai I, Kukuoka F. Fractionation and purification of the polysaccharides with marked antitumor activity, expecially lentinan, from Lentinus edodes (Berk.) Sing., (an edible mushroom). *Cancer Res* 1970 ; 30 : 2776-81.
3. Maeda YY, Watanabe ST, Chihara C, Rokutanda M. Denaturation and renaturation of a β-1, 6 ; 1, 3 -glucan, lentinan, associated with expression of T-cell-mediated responses. *Cancer Res* 1988 ; 48 : 671-5.
4. Aoki T, Miyakoshi H, Horikawa Y, Usuda Y. Staphage lysate and lentinan as immunomodulators and I or immunopotentiators in clinical and experimental systems. In : Hersh EM, Chirigos MA, Mastrangelo JM, eds. *Augmenting agents in cancer therapy* New York : Raven Press, 1981 : 101-12.
5. Yajima Y, Satoh J, Fukuda I, Kikuchi T, Toyota T. Quantitative assay of lentinan in human blood with the limulus colorimetric test. *Tohoku J Exp Med* 1989 ; 157 : 145-51.
6. Dennert DW, Tucker D. Antitumor polysaccharide lentinan : a T-cell adjuvant. *J Natl Cancer Inst* 1973 ; 51 : 1727-9.
7. Dresser DW, Phillips JM. The orientation of the adjuvant activities of Salmonella typhosa lipopolysaccharides and lentinan. *Immunology* 1974 ; 27 : 895-902.
8. Hamuro J, Rollinghof M, Wagner H. β(1-3) glucan-mediated augmentation of alloreactive murine cytotoxic T-lymphocytes *in vivo*. *Cancer Res* 1978 ; 38 : 3080-5.
9. Hanaue H, Tokuda Y, Machimura T, Kamijoh A, Kondo Y, Ogoshi K, Makuuchi H, Nakasaki H, Tajima T, Mitomi T, Kurosawa T. Effects of oral lentinan on T-cell subsets in peripheral venous blood. *Clin Ther* 1989 ; 11 : 614-22.
10. Toko T, Fujimoto S. Augmentation of anti-tumor immunity in low-responder mice by various biological response modifiers : analysis of effector mechanism. *Jpn J Cancer Res* 1989 ; 80 : 1212-9.
11. Bomford R, Moreno C. Mechanisms of the anti-tumor effect of glucans and fructosans : a comparison with *C. parvum*. *Br J Cancer* 1977 ; 36 : 41-8.
12. Miyakoshi H, Aoki T, Mizukoshi M. Acting mechanism of lentinan in human. II. Enhancement of non-specific cell-mediated cytotoxicity as an interferon inducer. *Int J Immunopharmacol* 1984 ; 6 : 373-9.
13. Arinaga S, Karimine N, Takamuku K, Nanbara S, Nagamatsu M, Ueo H, Akiyoshi T. Enhanced production of interleukin 1 and tumor necrosis factor by peripheral monocytes after lentinan administration in patients with gastric carcinoma. *Int J Immunopharmacol* 1992 ; 14 : 43-47.
14. Arinaga S, Karimane N, Takamuku K, Nanbara S, Inoue H, Nagamatsu M, Ueo H. Enhanced induction of lymphokine-activated killer activity after lentanin administration in patients with gastric cancer. *Int J Immunopharmacol* 1992 ; 14 : 535-9.
15. Takeshita K, Watanuki S, Iida M, Saito N, Maruyama M, Sunagawa M, Habu H, Endo M. Effect of lentinan on lymphocyte subsets of peripheral blood, lymph nodes, and tumor tissues in patients with gastric cancer. *Surg Today* 1993 ; 23 : 125-9.
16. Abel G, Szollosi J, Chihara G, Fachet J. Effect of lentinan and mannan on phagocytosis of fluorescent latex microbeads by mouse peritoneal macrophages : a flow cytometric study. *Int J Immunopharmacol* 1989 ; 11 : 615-21.
17. Ladanyi A, Timar J, Lapis K. Effect of lentinan on macrophage cytotoxicity against metastatic tumor cells. *Cancer Immunol Immunother* 1993 ; 36 : 123-6.
18. Miyakoshi H, Aoki T. Acting mechanisms of lentinan in human. I. Augmentation of DNA synthesis and immunoglobulin production of peripheral mononuclear cells. *Int J Immunopharmacol* 1984 ; 6 : 365-71.
19. Fruehauf JP, Bonnard GD, Herberman RB. The effect of lentinan on production of interleukin-1 by human monocytes. *Immunopharmacol* 1982 ; 5 : 65-74.
20. Peter G, Karoly U, Imre B, Janos F, Kaneko Y. Effects of lentinan on cytotoxic functions of human lymphocytes. *Immunopharmacol Immunotoxicol* 1988 ; 10 : 157-63.

21. Okuda T, Yoshioka T, Ikekawa G, Chihara G, Nishioka K. Anti-complementary activity of anti-tumor polysaccharides. *Nature, New Biol* 1972 ; 238 : 59.
22. Kanai K, Kondo E, Jacques PJ, Chihara G. Immunopotentiating effect of fungal glucans as revealed by frequency limitation of post chemotherapy relapse in experimental mouse tuberculosis. *Jpn J Med Sci Biol* 1980 ; 33 : 283-93.
23. White TR, Thompson RC, Penhale WJ, Chihara G. The effect of lentinan on the resistance of mice to *Mesocestoides corti*. *Parasitol Res* 1988 ; 74 : 563-8.
24. Irinoda K, Masihi KN, Chihara G, Kaneko Y, Katori T. Stimulation of microbicidal host defence mechanisms against aerosol influenza virus infection by lentinan. *Int J Immunopharmacol* 1992 ; 14 : 971-7.
25. Kaneko Y, Chihara G. Potentiation of host resistance against microbial infections by lentinan and its related polysaccharides. *Adv Exp Med Biol* 1992 ; 319 : 201-15.
26. Chihara G, Maeda YY, Hamuro J, Sasaki T, Fukuoka F. Inhibition of mouse sarcoma 180 by polysaccharides from Lentinus edodes (Berk.) Sing. *Nature* 1969 ; 222 : 687-8.
27. Zakany J, Chihara G, Fachet J. Effect of lentinan on tumor growth in murine allogeneic and syngeneic hosts. *Int J Cancer* 1980 ; 25 : 371-6.
28. Suga T, Shiio T, Maeda YY, Chihara G. Antitumor activity of lentinan in murine syngeneic and autochthonous hosts and its suppressive effect on 3-methylcholanthrene-induced carcinogenesis. *Cancer Res* 1984 ; 44 : 5132-7.
29. Taguchi T, Kaneko Y. Lentinan : an overview of experimental and clinical studies of its action against cancer. In : Urushizaki I, Aoki T, Tsubura E, eds. *Host defence mechanisms against cancer*. Asmterdam : Excerpta Medica, 1986 : 221-8.
30. Yamasaki K, Sone S, Yamashita T, Ogura T. Synergistic induction of lymphokine (IL-2)-activated killer activity by IL-2 and the polysaccharide lentinan, and therapy of spontaneous pulmonary metastasis. *Cancer Immunol Immunother* 1989 ; 29 : 87-92.
31. Aoki T, Miyakoshi H, Usuda Y, Chermann JC, Barre-Sinoussi F, Ting RC, Gallo RC. Antibodies to HTLV I and III in sera from two Japanese patients, one with possible pre-AIDS. *Lancet* 1984 ; (ii) : 936-7.
32. Abe Y, Miyake M, Miyazaki T, Horiuchi A, Kimura S. The endogenous induction of tumor necrosis factor serum (TNS) for the adjuvant postoperative immunotherapy of cancer — Changes in immunological markers of the blood. *Jpn J Surg* 1990 ; 20 : 19-26.
33. Oka M, Yoshino S, Hazama S, Shimoda K, Suzuki T. Immunological analysis and clinical effects of intraabdominal and intrapleural injection of lentinan for malignant ascites and pleural effusion. *Biotherapy* 1972 ; 5 : 107-12.
34. Taguchi T, Furve H, Kimura T, Kondo T, Hattori T, Itoh I, Ogawa N. Late results of the phase III study of a random comparison test in cases of cancer of the digestive organs (stomach and colon). *Jpn J Cancer Chemother* 1985 ; 12 : 366-78 (in Japanese).

7

RU 41740 (Biostim), an immunomodulating agent from bacterial origin

C. BLOY[1], M. MORALES[1], M. GUENOUNOU[2]

[1] Laboratoire Cassenne, 17, rue Pontoise, 95520 Osny, France.
[2] Laboratoire d'Immunologie, Faculté de Pharmacie, 31, rue Cognacq-Jay, 51100 Reims, France.

RU 41740 (trade name : Biostim) is a glycoprotein complex extracted from *Klebsiella pneumoniae* 01 : K2. It acts as an immunomodulating agent which has been shown to reduce the number and length of infectious episodes in chronic bronchitis patients [1-3]. Experimental studies have shown that RU 41740 enhances both humoral and cell-mediated immune responses and protects against bacterial, fungal and viral infections [4-6].

Biochemical studies have shown that the treatment of RU 41740 with cetyltrimethylammonium bromide led to the isolation of two distinct macromolecular fractions : the F1 fraction (RU 41821), with an LPS-like structure associated with protein [7] and the P1 fraction (RU 41825), which has a proteoglycanic structure, and is most likely from capsular origin [8]. Extensive studies have been performed both in murine and human systems. Taking into consideration the numerous interactions and regulatory mechanisms operating within the immune system, experiments have been carried out on isolated cell populations to determine the target cells of RU 41740. These studies indicated that phagocytic cells and B lymphocytes are selective targets for RU 41740, in LPS responder and LPS non-responder cells. Cytokine network is also highly improved. In view of its bacterial origin, the possible involvement of LPS-like and LPS- non related molecules was also studied. Data showed that both molecules were active on immuno-competent cells, most likely, *via* different cellular receptors.

Immunomodulating properties and mechanisms of action

Activation of phagocytic cells

Macrophages play a major role in antigen presentation, cytokine-dependent activation of T and B lymphocytes, phagocytosis and bactericidy. RU 41740 is active throughout the major stages of phagocytosis. Macrophage stimulation is evidenced by the enhancement of glucosamine incorporation [5], the production of superoxide anions and the release of lysosomal enzymes [9, 10]. The production of free radicals by rat peritoneal macrophages is notably increased by RU 41740 *in vitro* and to a lesser extent *in vivo*. Oral administration of RU 41740 increases phagocytosis and generation of superoxide anions by alveolar macrophages and polymorphonuclear cells in pigs [11]. Similar results were found in murine models [12, 13]. The mechanism involved in increased polymorphonuclear cell attraction has been partially clarified by the observation that macrophages incubated with RU 41740 secrete a chemotactic factor for human neutrophils. In addition, in hairless rats, RU 41740 restores the migratory capacity of polymorphonuclear neutrophils initially depressed by niflumic acid treatment. Oral administration of RU 41740 stimulated the phagocytic function of polymorphonuclear cells in elderly subjects [14].

Studies using rat neutrophils showed that RU 41740 has different effects on polyphosphoinositide metabolism in PMNs, according to the patho-physiological state of the animals. Indeed, RU 41740 modulates fMLP and zymosan receptor-mediated signal transduction, inducing an attenuation of the phosphatidylinositol hydrolysis response. Treatment by RU 41740 also reduced intracellular multiplication of *Legionella pneumophila* in human monocytes-macrophages [15], and enhanced cytotoxic activity of human monocytes [16]. Incubation of human blood with RU 41740 induced an enhancement of receptors complement receptors (CR-1, CR-3) expression [17].

Blood monocyte functions were also investigated in chronic bronchitis patients, treated by RU 41740. Data showed that RU 41740 administered *per os* (at 2 or 8 mg/day) enhanced phagocytosis and intra-cellular killing capacity of peripheral blood monocytes in treated patients as compared to the placebo group, as evidenced by yeasts engulfement and candidacidal activity [18].

Activation of B cells

It is well established that RU 41740 acts as a polyclonal B cell activator either in murine [19-21] or human systems [22], inducing differentiation which results in increased antibody synthesis. RU 41740 was found mitogenic for spleen cells from both normal and athymic mice. The effect on B cells seems independent of T cell intervention. Indeed, purified B lymphocytes do respond to RU 41740 stimulation, in the virtual absence of T cells or macrophages.

RU 41740 is isolated from Gram-negative bacteria, since the possibility that endotoxin-like components could be involved in its biological activities has been raised. It was therefore necessary to determine the respective involvement of the LPS non-related molecule (P1 fraction) and the LPS-like structure (F1 fraction) in the activation of B cells and macrophages by RU 41740. The P1 fraction was found mitogenic for B lymphocytes from LPS non-responder C3H/Hej mice. Besides, using Polymyxin B, which interacts with the lipid A moiety of the endotoxin molecule, we found that P1 fraction, as well as RU 41740, were not sensitive to Polymyxin B. This antibiotic inhibited B cell proliferation induced by LPS or by the F1 fraction [23]. Oral or parenteral administration of RU 41740 to mice immunized with SRBC induced an increase of the number of anti-SRBC plaque-forming cells, particularly of the IgG type [4]. *In vitro*, immunization also showed that RU 41740 enhanced anti-SRBC plaque forming cells [24].

Finally, another study [25] has established the potentializing effect of Biostim with anti-IgM stimulation of B cells, in the presence or absence of cytokines. This result clearly demonstrates that RU 41740 amplifies the humoral immune response, even when B cells are activated *via* their physiological receptor (membrane Ig), as does antigen *in vivo*.

T lymphocytes and NK cells

The effect of RU 41740 on T lymphocytes is not so clear-cut. *In vitro*, RU 41740 potentiates the proliferative response to T cell mitogens [4, 26]. However, RU 41740 alone did not induce cell proliferation in T cells enriched population.

T cell activation is dependent on macrophages (monocytes) help and, as it appears that the concentration of these cells is a critical factor, the observed effects may be simply associated to macrophage activation. The effect of RU 41740 on the proliferative response in mixed lymphocyte culture [4] also seems to be mediated by macrophages since RU 41740 stimulates the production of interleukin-1 (IL-1) in human and murine phagocytic cells [21, 27, 28]. It should be noted that the incubation of human prothymocytes with RU 41740 stimulates the expression of surface differentiation markers, particularly CD 4 (J.L. Touraine, personal communication).

RU 41740 also enhances, albeit to a limited extent, the cytotoxicity of natural killer cells [4, 28, 29].

In vivo, RU 41740 potentiates the delayed hypersensibility reactions (DTH) to ovalbumin in the guinea pig [4, 5] and to DNCB in the pig. Oral administration of RU 41740 to mice stimulates T helper cell function to the extent that it potentiates the graft *versus* host reaction (GvH).

Parenteral and oral treatment with RU 41740 induced an enhancement of NK cell activity, particularly in the lungs [12]. *In vivo*, RU 41740 potentiates IL-2 induced generation of NK activity [30].

Production of cytokines

RU 41740 has been shown to affect multiple cells, either directly and/or through the secretion of various cytokines leading to an amplification of the initial stimulatory process. Early results have demonstrated the enhancing effect of RU 41740 on the production of IL-1 by human monocytes and murine macrophages [21, 27], as well as NK cells [28]. In monkey, IL-1 activity was detected in serum following oral administration of RU 41740 [31]. Because IL-1 plays a central role in a wide range of biological phenomenons, some of the properties of RU 41740 can be partially explained by its capacity to increase IL-1 production. No direct evidence for the modulation of IL-2 or interferon γ production by T cells was provided (unpublished data).

Hemopoietic growth factors are produced by a number of cells including monocytes/macrophages. These cells produce TNF and IL-1 which can in turn stimulate growth factor production by endothelial cells. Apart from its effects on phagocytic cells described above, RU 41740 has also an effect on hematopoieis. Parenteral administration to mice increases the number of circulating polymorphonuclear neutrophils as well as that of the myeloid cells and the granulo-monocyte stem cells (GM-CFU) in the bone marrow and spleen. The parenteral or oral administration of RU 41740 to mice increased the serum levels of GM-CSF and facilitated hemopoietic reconstitution in irradiated mice [32, 33]. Production of cytotoxic factors was found in murine and human macrophages [34, 35]. RU 41740 also induced a rapid increase in TNF release by NK cells [16].

Low amounts of the drug produced a rapid increase in IL-1, IL-6 and TNFα production by human blood cells. In the same conditions, higher concentrations were needed with LPS from the same strain. Northern blot analysis showed that in quiescent macrophage populations, both IL-1α and IL-1β mRNA levels were dramatically increased in response to RU 41740. In parallel experiments, LPS was effective only at higher concentrations [36]. Using F1 and P1 fractions, we showed that both molecules were able to induce IL-1, TNFα and IL-6 production by murine macrophages and human monocytes. F1 activity was abolished by Polymyxin B and was not found using macrophages from LPS non-responder mice [23].

The cytokine network is a highly sophisticated system, with positive and negative signals ; acting on one site of this network may influence all the immune system. It is well established that CD4 T cells play a pivotal role in the induction and regulation of the immune response and that macrophages are important element in T cells activation. Recently, it has become clear that different CD4 + T cell subsets can be distinguished (TH1 and TH2 cells). These subsets exhibit distinct immunological functions and different cytokine pattern : TH1 cells produce IL-2 and IFNγ and are involved in delayed type hypersensitivity and macrophage activation, whether TH2 cells produce IL-4, IL-5 and IL-10, and are involved in help for IgE production. TH1 and TH2 cells develop from a TH0 state. Cell environment is crucial for the balance between TH1 and TH2. Cytokines produced by TH1 and TH2 cells reciprocally regulate the functions of each other. IFNγ antagonizes a number of biological functions of IL-4, which in turn, as well as IL-10, inhibits the production of IFNγ and other cytokines by TH1 cells. IFNγ, in association with TNF and GM-CSF, is a potent activator of macrophage functions, resulting in an enhancement of resistance towards infections and cancer. Recently, it has been shown that RU 41740 inhibits IL-4 activity on different target cells (unpublished data) and potentiates IL-2 induced activities. This may favour the TH1 response, resulting in an improvement of resistance to infections. By regulating cytokine levels before and during encounter with infectious agents, RU 41740 may constitute a potent agent for the prevention of recurrent infections.

- *Intracellular mechanism of action*

A recent study [37] on the effect of RU 41740 on a second intercellular IP3 messenger, common to all immune cells, has provided us with more detailed information about the product's intracellular mechanism of action.

In rat polynuclear cells subjected to preliminary immunosuppression by burning, RU 41740 restores the polymorphonuclear intracellular level of IP3 with respect to the basal state.

These studies are important as IP3 is a second messenger involved in intracellular variations in Ca^{2+} levels and its production passes through the phospholipase C activation route. This route involved a membrane receptor, a G protein and other enzymatic effectors. We believe that future work will enable us to understand at which point RU 41740 intervenes in this activation route.

- *Effect of RU 41740 on experimental infections*

Experimental infections represent adapted models for the study of the anti-infectious effect of immunostimulants. The process consists in producing a lethal infection in two mice populations, one treated by RU 41740, the other by placebo. The anti-infectious capacity of RU 41740 is assessed by comparing the survival rate of animals in each of the two groups.

This method is advantageous because it makes possible to test the product with chosen germs thus prompting different lines in the anti-infection defence system.

RU 41740 was tested by oral, intraperitoneal and aerosol routes and was found to have an anti-infective activity [4, 6, 38] against numerous germs such as :
— bacteria with extracellular development *(Staphylococcus aureus, Escherichia coli, Pseudomonas aeruginosa, Streptococcus pneumoniae, Klebsiella pneumoniae, Proteus)*,
— bacteria with intracellular development *(Listeria monocytogenes, Salmonella typhimurium)*,
— viruses *(Influenza*, encephalomyocarditis virus),
— *Candida albicans.*

This protective effect was demonstrated by the statistically significant increase in the survival rate of groups of mice treated with RU 41740 compared to placebo.

All these pharmacological studies, both *in vivo* and *in vitro*, demonstrate the effect of RU 41740 on the immunocompetent cells and on the principal messenger of the immunological process. The stimulation of various elements of the anti-infectious defence mechanism means that RU 41740 is effective whatever the type of germ encountered.

- *Other studies*

Two *in vitro* studies on different cell populations were carried out on RU 41740 with the aim of obtaining a pre-requisite in a pathology involving immunosuppression : AIDS.

A first study was carried to test the possible effect of RU 41740 on HIV replication. The protocol was based on :
— examining the effect of RU 41740 on the proliferative response of T lymphocytes, to non-specific (PHA) or to specific (mixed lymphocyte reaction model = MLR) stimulation ;
— studying HIV replication under standard conditions in mononucleated blood cells infected *in vitro* and kept in culture, in the absence or presence of RU 41740.

This protocol showed that RU 41740 had no effect on the capacity for HIV infection or on viral replication. Addition or maintenance of RU 41740 in culture did not lead to any increase in the amount of virus produced by infected cells and did not accelerate the occurrence of cytopathogenic effects.

A second study was carried to investigate any possible effect of RU 41740 on the production of HIV virus in monocyte and macrophage cell lines. The cells used were human monocytes / macrophages U937 and TPH1 line cells.

The results of this study are as follows :
— With monocytic cells (U937), no significant effect was found, whatever the route and concentrations studied, on infectivity, viral infection, cytopathogenic effect and cell proliferation.
— With macrophagic cells (TPH1), treatment with RU 41740 in the course of marked infectivity (2500 TCID50) did not inhibit infectivity and viral replication in the long term. On the other hand, with limited infectivity (250 TCID50) or after elimination of residual viruses and slow replication, treatment or pre-treatment with RU 41740 inhibited HIV replication and its infectivity in this cell type.

Clinical pharmacology

Clinical pharmacology trials verified the effect of RU 41740 on the components of the immune system, thus confirming the immunological points of impact, predetermined *in vitro* and *in vivo* in animals.

Double-blind studies *versus* placebo tested various dosages and, in most cases, concerned populations with a defect in one compartment of the immune reaction.

Effect of RU 41740 on phagocytic function

The effect of RU 41740 on phagocytosis function was carried out on a group of 29 patients with chronic bronchitis [39]. Administration of RU 41740 was accompanied by a significant increase in the phagocytic index of these cells and in the candidacidic activity of monocytes compared to the placebo group ($p < 0.01$).

An identical study [19] tested two different RU 41740 dosages (2 mg/day every second week or 8 mg/day every second week for 3 months) *versus* placebo. The phagocytic and candidacide capacity of circulating monocytes was evaluated in 20 patients with chronic bronchitis before and after treatment. A significant increase in phagocytosis ($p < 0.05$) and candidacidy ($p < 0.05$) was found with the two RU 41740 dosages whereas the placebo group showed no change.

Effect of RU 41740 on immunity by cellular transmission

In studies on cellular immunity, the effect of RU 41740 on delayed hypersensitivity was evaluated in 70 hypoergic or anergic patients presenting lymphoma in remission [40]. Several dosing schedules were tested in double-blind trials *versus* placebo (8 mg/day for 7 days ; 2, 8 and 32 mg/day for 14 days). In these two trials, cutaneous hypersensitivity was measured by the Merieux Multitest (7 antigens tested) before and after treatment. The results showed a significant increase in the mean score for skin tests and number of positive reactions to antigens for the RU 41740 group compared to the placebo group.

Effect of RU 41740 on immunity by humoral transmission

The effect of RU 41740 on humoral immunity was evaluated in the course of 2 trials in patients receiving anti-influenza vaccination in addition to the treatment [41]. In the study of Profeta et al., 42 patients aged over 65 years received either 4 mg of RU 41740 or placebo for 14 days starting on the day of vaccination. At the 2nd, 3rd and 4th week, the level of anti-*Influenza* antibodies and the number of patients responding to treatment were much higher in the group treated with RU 41740 ($p < 0.05$).

Effect of RU 41740 in a model for the study of chronic respiratory infection : cystic fibrosis

Cystic fibrosis is a disease characterized by abnormalities in ion transport in different glands in the organism, particularly in the bronchial epithelium glands. This leads to abnormalities of the bronchial mucous membrane (increase in viscosity due to dehydration), and chronic bacterial colonization. ORL infection, often viral at the begining of the disease, plays an important role in the occurrence of acute exacerbation and secondary bacterial infections of the lower respiratory tract.

This pathology, in which viral and bacterial infections are extremely common, constitutes an interesting model for the study of the anti-infectious preventive effect of an immunostimulant.

For this reason, studies have been carried out and constitute an interesting prerequisite for development of Biostim further :
— The first trial, a multicentre double-blind trial *versus* placebo, included 50 children [42]. Monitoring was carried out over a 12-month period. The usual dosage regimen was multiplied by 4 and repeated during 6 months. The results showed that a significant reduction occurred at the 6th and 12 month in ORL infections ($p = 0.04$ and $p = 0.05$ respectively) and the duration of antibiotherapy ($p < 0.05$) with respect to the placebo group.
— A second study, including 60 patients, was carried out with pairing (= control group consisting of close relatives free of the disease). This study, based on the same therapeutic programme as the previous one trial, monitored 56 patients with cystic fibrosis and 54 controls (not treated) for 6 months. It showed a reduced probability of contracting ORL and/or bronchopulmonary infections during treatment with RU 41740 when compared to the period without treatment ($p = 0.002$).

Similarly, length of infectious episodes, duration of antibiotherapy, frequency of hospitalization and number of antibiotic courses required were reduced during the treatment period when compared to the period without treatment ($p = 0.002$).

Finally, a single-centre open study [43] on the oxidative metabolism of phagocytic cells in 17 children with cystic fibrosis before and after treatment with RU 41740, at a dose rate of 8 mg/day for 8 days, showed that :
— before treatment, children with cystic fibrosis had hypersecretion of chloramines (oxidizing radicals with a long half-life) after cell stimulation (by PHA and Zymosan) ($p = 0.001$) ;

— 30 days after the completion of treatment, a statistically significant reduction in chloramine levels produced by phagocyte cells in children with cystic fibrosis was obtained (p = 0.002).

This study demonstrates Biostim's ability to regulate production of chloramines by phagocyte cells in children with cystic fibrosis.

Clinical efficacy in the preventive treatment of recurrent respiratory infections

Several immunological abnormalities have been identified in patients presenting with recurrent respiratory infections, patients with chronic bronchitis and in fragile elderly patients and children with recurrent infections. These abnormalities preferentially affect one or more of the elements of anti-infectious defence [44].

RU 41740, with its *in vitro* and *in vivo* proven effects in humans and in animals on the three elements of anti-infectious defence, can be used to attenuate or normalize the various immune disorders associated with recurring respiratory infections.

The clinical efficacy of RU 41740 as a mean of preventing infection has been established by double-blind *versus* placebo trials.

RU 41740 in chronic bronchitis

In patients with chronic bronchitis, recurrent respiratory infections contribute probably to the aggravation of obstructive ventilatory disorders and may also be the source of acute failure of the disease. The immune defects identified in these patients essentially affect phagocytosis with a reduction in the functional capacity of monocytes and polymorphonuclear cells [44].

Five trials [1-3, 39, 45] were carried out on different stages of this disease — I and II : simple or purulent chronic bronchitis, III and IV : obstructive chronic bronchitis with or without chronic respiratory insufficiency. For all these clinical studies :
— the study design was a double-blind randomized, parallel, trial *versus* placebo ;
— RU 41740 (or the placebo) was administered at a regimen of 8 days per month for 3 months, 2 tablets per day for the 1st course of treatment and 1 tablet per day for the 2nd and 3rd courses ;
— patients were vaccinated against influenza and received neither anti-bacterial vaccination nor any systematic antibiotherapy.

• *Non-obstructive chronic bronchitis (stages I and II)*

One study [1] included 73 patients suffering from simple chronic bronchitis (38 in the RU 41740 group and 35 in the placebo group). Patients were seen at the 3rd, 6th and 9th month. Several points emerge from this study :
— RU 41740 significantly increases the number of patients with no infectious episodes during the 3-month trial period (78 % for the RU 41740 group *versus* 53 % for the placebo group) (p < 0.05) ;
— RU 41740 significantly reduces the average duration of infectious episodes as

compared to placebo : 13 ± 5.8 days *versus* 33 ± 5.8 days, that is to say 20 days less of infectious episodes in 9 months ($p < 0.05$) ;
— RU 41740 reduces antibiotic consumption after 9 months of observation in the RU 41740 group, that is 30 days less of antibiotics over a period of 9 months : 11.5 ± 1.4 days *versus* 41 ± 9.8 days in the placebo group ($p < 0.01$).

- *Obstructive chronic bronchitis (stages III and IV)*

In another study [45], RU 41740 was tested in subjects suffering from chronic bronchitis at the respiratory insufficiency stage, compensated or not, in which the occurrence of infectious episodes might compromise vital prognosis. Thirty-five patients were divided, by randomization, between the RU 41740 group (exactly the same dosage as the previous study) or to placebo group. Patients were examined at the 3rd, 6th and 9th month. A third of patients in each group underwent tracheotomy and were on home mechanical ventilation. By the 9 month of observation, RU 41740 had significantly reduced the number of patients with infectious episodes ($p = 0.002$). No respiratory infection was observed in 41 % of patients in the RU 41740 group *versus* 12 % in the placebo group ($p < 0.04$) after 9 months of observation.

The anti-infectious prevention of RU 41740, observed whatever the degree of severity of chronic bronchitis, is seen from its effects on the immune system. This close immuno-clinical correlation was established by a trial conducted by Fietta [39] which showed the link between an improvement in phagocytic capacity of monocytes due to RU 41740 and the reduction of bronchial infections.

Meta analysis was carried out of the Bonde, Boutin, Carles, Chrétien and Fietta trials. The results showed that the relative risk for the placebo group to catch at least one infection over the 0-6 month period is equal to 1,43. That means that the risk to catch at least one infection during this period is upper to 43 % in the placebo group than in the RU 41740 group ($p = 0.0009$) (decreased to 30 % for the RU 41740 group). We also calculated that the relative risk for the placebo group during the 3-6 month period is equal to 2.36 ($p = 0.001$).

Overall, the efficacy of RU 41740 in preventing respiratory infections in patients with chronic bronchitis has been demonstrated. RU 41740 leads to a significant reduction in the frequency and duration of infectious episodes. In the long term, an improvement in the prognosis of the disease with a reduction in acute decompensation risks and degradation in respiratory function can be hypothetized. Furthermore, RU 41740 is the only one oral immunostimulant with a Marketing Authorization in this indication.

RU 41740 in elderly patients

In addition to patients with chronic bronchitis, other fragile subjects can develop recurrent bronchial or bronchopulmonary infections, particularly true of elderly subjects. In fragile elderly persons, it is mainly immunity by cellular transmission and by humoral transmission which seems to be defective.

A study coordinated by Hugonot *et al.* (1988) focused on 1-year follow-up of Biostim's efficacy in this type of population with a high risk of respiratory infections as the subjects were in long-stay institutions and already suffering from subjacent pathologies (chronic bronchitis, cardiovascular disease, metabolic diseases,...).

Three hundred and fourteen patients were included in this double-blind study. Half of them received RU 41740 according to the usual programme while the other half received the placebo. After 12 months, the group treated with RU 41740 was still significantly protected against respiratory infection with :
— a larger number of patients without pulmonary infection in the RU 41740 group than in the placebo group (75 out 140 in the RU 41740 group *versus* 89 out of 140 in the placebo group, p = 0.045) ;
— the average number of pulmonary infections was significantly lower than in the placebo group (0.77 episode *versus* 1.1, p = 0.02) ;
— a shorter antibiotherapy period (p = 0.03).

RU 41740 in children

Respiratory infections in children are characterized by their frequency, great diversity of clinical symptoms, ranging from straightforward rhinopharyngitis to serious bronchopneumopathy and, finally, in their tendency to recurrent episodes thus exposing the child to various complications.

Although the aetiology of these recurrent infections is multifactorial (allergic regions, group life, passive smoking,...), the physiological immaturity of the immune system is also an important factor. Various immunological abnormalities occur which can affect one or more of the 3 lines of defence against infection : functional defects of the T lymphocytes, abnormal antibody production, ineffective phagocytosis.

The tablet form of RU 41740 was studied in the first instance in children suffering from repetitive respiratory infection, both upper and lower, in either an allergic or non-allergic region. Four multicentre double-blind trials *versus* placebo were thus carried out. A total of 240 children, from 1 to 14 years of age were included. Of these, 119 received RU 41740 and 121 received placebo ; all were monitored over a period of 6 months. All the children presented with infections — rhinopharyngitis, otitis, laryngitis, angina, rhinobronchitis — for at least a year. In one of the trials, children also underwent adenoidectomy associated or not with amygdalectomy about one month before inclusion.

The dosage programme retained was the same for all the studies : one course per month for 3 months with a 3-week period between each course at the following dosage :
— 1st course : 2 mg/day for 8 days,
— 2nd course : 1 mg/day for 8 days,
— 3rd course : 1 mg/per for 8 days.

A clinical examination was carried out before treatment and after the 1st, 2nd, 3rd and 6th month.

The clinical efficacy of RU 41740 was proven in each trial. This was seen from a reduction in the frequency and duration of infectious episodes and associated antibiotherapy as compared to the placebo group :
— significantly greater number of children without infection after 6 months (8 out of 38 *versus* 0 out of 40, p = 0.02, 11 out of 39 *versus* 5 out of 39, p = 0.05) ;
— a significantly reduced average number of infections per patient (1.9 angina

over 6 months *versus* 3.2 in the placebo group, p < 0.0005, 0.23 rhinopharyngitis per month *versus* 0.37, p < 0.01) ;
— a significantly reduced duration of infection (during the 6-month follow-up period, 10.9 days *versus* 19.9 days, p < 0.001 and 10 days *versus* 34 days, p < 0.05) ;
— a significantly reduced number of antibiotherapy courses (0.86 courses per patient *versus* 1.51, p < 0.03) ;
— a significantly reduced duration of antibiotherapy (5.79 days *versus* 11.48 days, p < 0.005, 10 days *versus* 20 days, p < 0.05).

At a later date, two other trials were carried out which demonstrated the efficacy and ease of use of a new pharmaceutical form of RU 41740 adapted to younger children (capsule) [43].

Meta-analysis was carried out of the Paupe, Pech and Piquet trials. It included 165 children. The results showed there were :
— a statistically significant reduction in the number of infections in the RU 41740 group as compared to the placebo group (p = 0.05) at the end of 6 months (1,9 placebo *versus* 1,3 RU 41740) ;
— the relative risk for the placebo group to catch at least one infection over a 3-6 month period is equal to 1,78. Finally, the risk to catch one infection during this period is upper of 78 % in the placebo group than in the RU 41740 group (p = 0,024). That also means that the risk to catch at least one infection over a 3-6 month period decreases for 44 % (= 1-1/1.78) in the RU 41740 group.

In conclusion, the efficacy of RU 41740 in children is demonstrated by the reduction in the number and duration of infectious episodes as well as by the reduced severity of such episodes, evaluated from the decrease in the number and duration of antibiotic courses. This efficacy has been demonstrated for the two pharmaceutical forms of RU 41740, the capsule form adapted to young children, as it can be taken with food, and the tablet form for older children.

Co-prescription of RU 41740 with an antibiotherapy

The efficacy of RU 41740 in preventing respiratory infections was also verified in the case of treatment at the beginning of an acute infectious episode, in combination with antibiotherapy.

Three double-blind trials *versus* placebo were carried out on a population of elderly patients or patients with chronic bronchitis presenting acute bronchitis or an acute bronchopulmonary episode. Each patient received either RU 41740 or the placebo, at the same time antibiotherapy was started (Amoxycillin, Ampicillin, Macrolide or Tetracyclin). The three studies found a significantly faster improvement in symptoms in the RU 41740 group accompanied by a shorter recovery time. The tolerance of the association was excellent. These results confirm the possibility of starting preventive RU 41740 treatment in association with antibiotherapy during an acute respiratory episode.

Biostim tolerance

In parallel to the evaluation of the beneficial effects of RU 41740, other studies focused on investigation of any adverse events linked to the product's mechanism of action on the immune response. Particular attention was paid to auto-immune risk and atopical risk.

Clinical tolerance

Clinical tolerance was assessed in adults and children in the group of patients having received RU 41740 during one of the trials.

— **In adults** : 2 open studies including 3 110 patients and 8 double-blind studies *versus* placebo including 751 patients [1, 2] were carried out. No serious iatrogenic complication was found in any of these patients. In the double-blind *versus* placebo studies, tolerance was identical in the RU 41740 and placebo groups (7.9 % of side effects with RU 41740 *versus* 6.7 % with the placebo). The side effects are also superimposable in the two groups with a predominance of minor digestive disorders (nausea, vomiting, swelling, diarrhea,...).

— **In children** : 4 open studies including 4 687 children (aged between 1 and 15 years) and 4 double-blind studies *versus* placebo including 751 patients were carried out. Out of the groups of children receiving RU 41740, 57 (1.2 %) presented intolerance, mainly of the digestive type. Confirmation of good clinical tolerance was supported by double-blind studies *versus* placebo in which intolerance was reported in 7 out of 122 children treated with RU 41740 (5.7 %) *versus* 2 out of 121 children receiving only the placebo (1.65 %). In the same way as for adults, these side effects are benign, temporary (or quickly reversible on discontinuance of treatment) and mainly digestive in nature.

In conclusion, clinical tolerance of RU 41740 verified in the course of 18 trials on 8791 patients is excellent in both children and adults. French drug monitoring data, collected since the product was put on the market (1982), confirmed that it is well tolerated [46]. Apart from minor digestive disorders, a few cases of exacerbation of infectious symptoms at the start of the course of treatment have been reported. These temporary symptoms (rhinorrhea, coughing,...) might be due to RU 41740 although the possibility of coincidence cannot be ignored. These symptoms regress spontaneously within the space of a few days and do not require treatment to be stopped.

Immunological tolerance

It was verified in animals then in humans in the course of two specific immunotolerance trials carried out on adults and on children. These trials focused on two particularly important points regarding tolerance of an immunostimulating product, namely the auto-immune risk and the risk to allergic patients.

• *Effect of Biostim on auto-immunity*

— **In animals** : the effects of long-term treatment with RU 41740 (10 mg/kg/day) were evaluated in NZB/NZW mice with a spontaneous disorder similar to human lupus disease. Two parameters were selected to monitor the disease : survival rate after 11 months (animals aged between 3 and 4 weeks at the beginning of treatment) and proteinuria values at different times between 6 and 19 weeks. None of the two parameters studied were worsened by RU 41740. Rather, a significant increase in the survival rate at 11 months was found (p < 0.05 — 62.5 % *versus* 25 % in the control group).

— **In adults** : a specific double-blind immunotolerance trial *versus* placebo was carried out on 21 patients with chronic bronchitis having received RU 41740 according to the usual dosage regimen. Quantitative determination of the principal parameters made it possible to evaluate auto-immunity (anti-nuclear, native anti-DNA and anti-erythrocyte antibodies, rheumatoid factors, circulating immune complexes, complement fractions C3 and C4, proetinuria, HLM). There was no significant difference between the RU 41740 group and the placebo group 2 9 months later.

— **In children** : the same specific investigation was carried out on a population of 65 children with plasma determination of anti-nuclear antibodies and native anti-DNA antibodies, determination of total haemolytic complement and investigation of rheumatoid factor and anomalous agglutinins. This showed there was no significant difference between the various parameters analyzed for values before and after 3 months of RU 41740 treatment (usual dosage regimen). Examination of individual values did not reveal any pathological change.

The auto-immune risks of RU 41740 were thus evaluated in detail. The different studies carried out do not provide any evidence in favour of an increased risk of auto-immune pathology or aggravation of pre-existing auto-immunity. However, as a precautionary measure, the product is contraindicated in the case of known auto-immune disease.

• *Effect of Biostim in allergic patients*

Allergy represents one of the multifactorial causes of recurring respiratory infection, particularly in children. Allergic patients presenting recurrent ORL or bronchial infections justify administration of an immunostimulant, providing the product is well-tolerated.

In the course of therapeutic or specific tolerance trials on RU 41740, a large number of allergic patients (rhinitis, conjunctivitis, asthma) received the product without this leading to any particular clinical symptoms.

Moreover, a retrospective open study was aimed at evaluating tolerance in a population of atopic adults. Out of the 113 patients studied, 94 % were being desensitized and 63 % were asthmatic. Six of these patients (5.3 %) presented disorders possibly related to the treatment (2 cases of rhinitis, 2 cases of purulent rhinitis and 2 cases of bronchitis). The frequency of adverse reactions did not seem to be higher in allergic patients than in non-allergic patients.

From the biological point of view, quantitative determination of total IgE in the serum was carried out before and after treatment (usual 3-month dosage programme) in an open trial on 65 children [46] (14 of whom were true allergics). This study showed that changes in total IgE were independent of RU 41740 treatment. This was confirmed by 4 double-blind studies *versus* placebo including 85 children (35 % of these were allergic) and on 50 cases of chronic bronchitis [1]. In these trials, no significant increase in total IgE was found in the RU 41740 group compared to the placebo groups.

In conclusion

Biostim constitutes an interesting approach to the preventive treatment of these infections,
— by the reproducibility of biological and clinical effects, good understanding of the pathways and distribution of the product, a well-elucidated mechanism of action and particularly the potentializing effect of biostim on the prestimulated B cells,
— by an excellent continuity of results throughout the developmental phase, proven clinical efficacy, with an excellent tolerance.

Biostim, with all this properties, offers a good way to minimize infections and should constitute part of the physician's therapeutic arsenal.

References

1. Viallat JR, Costantini D, Boutin C, Farnisse P. Étude en double aveugle d'un immunomodulateur d'origine bactérienne (RU 41740) dans la prévention des épisodes infectieux chez le bronchitique chronique. *Poumon Coeur* 1983 ; 39 : 53-7.
2. Anthoine D, Blaive G, Cabanieu G, Chrétien J. Étude en double aveugle du Biostim dans la prévention des surinfections des patients atteints de bronchopathie chronique. *Rev Pneumol Clin* 1985 ; 41 : 213-7.
3. Bonde J, Dahl R, Edelstein R, Kok-Jensen A, Lazer L, Punakivi L, Seppala A, Soes-Petersen U, Viskum K. The effect of Biostim, an immune modulating compound in the prevention of acute exacerbations in patients with chronic bronchitis. *Eur J Respir Dis* 1986 ; 69 : 235-41.
4. Griscelli C, Grospierre B, Montreuil J, Fournet B, Bruvier C, Lang JM, Marchiani C, Zalisz R, Edelstein R. Immunomodulation by glycoprotein fraction isolated from *K. pneumoniae*. In : Yamamura Y, Kotani SK, eds. *Immunomodulation by microbial products and related synthetic compounds*. Amsterdam : Excerpta Medica, 1982 : 261-5.
5. Takada H, Tsujimoto M, Ogawa T, Ishihara Y, Kawasaki A, Konati S, Tanaka A, Nagao S, Kushima K, Fujiki TF, Kato A. Immunomodulating activities of Biostim. In : Yamamura Y, Konati S, eds. *Immunomodulation by microbial products and related synthetic compounds*. Amsterdam : Excerpta Medica, 1982 : 266-9.
6. Rudent A, Zalisz R, Quero AM, Smets P. Enhance resistance of mice against influenza virus infection after local administration of glycoprotein extracts from *K. pneumoniae*. *Int J Immunopharmacol* 1985 ; 7 : 525-31.
7. Kol O, Montreuil J, Fournet B, Smets P, Zalisz R. Purification of lipopolysaccharide from *K. pneumoniae* 01 : K2 by high performance liquid chromatography. *J Chromatogr* 1987 ; 396 : 281-6.
8. Kol O, Montreuil J, Fournet B, Zalisz R, Smets P. Separation by high performance liquid chromatography of oligosaccharides obtained after mild acid hydrolysis of *Klebsiella pneumoniae* 01 :K2 (NCTC 5055) lypopolysaccharides. *J Chromatogr* 1989 ; 474 : 452-6.
9. Roch-Arveiller M, El Abbouyi A, Paul JL, Smets P, Raichvarg D, Giroud JP. Effects exerted by Biostim on oxidative metabolism and migration of rat polymorphonuclear leukocytes collected after induction of one acute non specific inflammatory reaction. *Int J Immunopharmacol* 1987 ; 9 : 417-24.
10. Fiszer Safarz B, Rommain M, Brossard C, Smets P. Hyaluronic acid-degrading enzymes in rat alveolar macrophages and in alveolar fluid : stimulation of enzyme activity after oral treatment with the immunomodulator Biostim. *Biol Cell* 1988 ; 63 : 355-60.
11. Laval A, Rommain M, Fortier M, Zalisz R, Dahan R, Smets P. Immunomodulating

effects of orally administered Biostim (Biostim) in the swine. In : Proceedings of the International Symposium Immunomodulators and non-specific host defence mechanisms against microbial infections, Berlin, 6-8 May 87, Pergamon Press. *Adv Biosci* 1988 ; 68 : 103.

12. Sozzani S, Luini W, Brascheschi L, Spreafico F. The effect of Biostim (Biostim) on natural killer activity in different mouse organs. *Int J Immunopharmacol* 1986 ; 8 : 845-53.
13. Radermecker M, Rommain M, Maldague MP, Bury T, Smets P. Increase in the number and the phagocytic function of guinea pig pulmonary and peritoneal macrophages following oral administration of Biostim, a glycoprotein extract from *Klebsiella pneumoniae*. *Int J Immunopharmacol* 1988 ; 8 : 913-7.
14. Minonzio F, Ongari AM, Palmieri R, Bochicchio D, Guidi G, Capsoni F. Immunostimulation of neutrophil phagocytic function by Biostim (Biostim) in elderly subjects. *Immunol Clin* 1989 ; 2 : 87-95.
15. Rajagopalan P, Dournon E, Vilde JL, Pocidalo JJ. Direct activation of human monocytes delivered macrophages by a bacterial glycoprotein extract inhibits the intracellular multiplication of virulent *Legionella pneumophila* serogroup 1. *Infect Immun* 1987 ; 55 ; 9 : 2234-9.
16. Sozzani S, d'Alessandro F, Capsoni F, Luini W, Barcellini W, Guidi G, Spreafico F. *In vitro* modulation of human monocytes functions by Biostim (Biostim). *Int J Immunopharmacol* 1988 ; 10 : 93-102.
17. Capsoni F, Minonzio F, Ongari AM, Bonara P, Guidi G, Zanussi C. Increased expression of C3b and C3bi receptors on human neutrophils and monocytes induced by a glycoprotein extract from *Klebsiella pneumoniae* (Biostim). *Int J Immunopharmacol* 1991 ; 13 : 227-33.
18. Nielsen H, Bonde J. Immunostimulation of blood monocyte function by Biostim (Biostim) in patients with chronic bronchitis. *Int J Immunopharmacol* 1986 ; 8, 6 : 589-92.
19. Guenounou M, Smets P, Agneray J. Activation des lymphocytes B de souris par le Biostim, un extrait glycoprotéique de *K. pneumoniae*. *CR Acad Sci, Paris* 1984 ; 298, série III : 135-8.
20. Wood CD, Moller G. Influence of Biostim, a glycoprotein extract from *K. pneumoniae*, in the murine immune system. I. T-independant polyclonal B cells activation. *J Immunol* 1984 ; 132 : 616-21.
21. Guenounou M, Vacheron F, Zalisz R, Smets P, Agneray J. Immunological activities of Biostim, a glycoprotein extract from *K. pneumoniae*. I. Activation of murine B cells and induction of interleukin-1 production by macrophages. *Ann Inst Pasteur Immunol* 1985 ; 135D : 59-69.
22. Martinez-Maza O, Wood C, Britton S. IgM and IgG secretion by human B cells exposed to Biostim, a glycoprotein extract from *K. pneumoniae*. *Cell Immunol* 1985 ; 90 : 569-76.
23. Vacheron F, Perin S, Kodari E, Smets P, Zalisz R, Guenounou M. Immunological activities of Biostim, a glyco-proteic complex extracted from *Klebsiella pneumoniae*. III. Role of LPS-like and LPS-non-related molecules. *Res Immunol* 1989 ; 140 : 159.
24. Guenounou M, Smets P, Agneray J. Immunomodulating activity of Biostim, a glycoprotein extract from *Klebsiella pneumoniae*. *Farm Ter* 1985 ; 1 : 28-32.
25. Bloy C, Sautes C, Fridman WH. RU 41740 (Biostim) increases the proliferation and the immunoglobulin M and G secretion of preactivated murine B lymphocytes. *Fundam Clinic Pharmacol* 1994 ; (sous presse).
26. Wood CD, Moller G. Influence of Biostim, a glycoprotein extract from *K. pneumoniae*, in the murine immune system. II. RU41740 facilitates the response to Con A in otherwise unresponsive T-enriched cells. *J Immunol* 1985 ; 135 : 131-6.
27. Guenounou M, Vacheron F, Nauciel C, Agneray J. Induction of interleukin-1 secretion by murine macrophages and human monocytes after stimulation by Biostim, a bacterial immunomodulator. *Int J Immunopharmacol* 1985 ; 7, 2 : 287-90.
28. Herman J, Kew MC, Rabson AR. The effect of Biostim (Biostim) on the production of interleulin-1 by monocytes and enriched large granular lymphocytes in normals and patients with hepatocellular carcinoma. *Cancer Immunol Immunother* 1986 ; 21 : 26-30.

29. Viland H, Blomgren H. Augmentation of spontaneous cytotoxicity of human lymphocytes by Biostim, a glycoprotein extract from *K. pneumoniae*. *Anticancer Res* 1987 ; 7 : 17-22.
30. Migliorati G, Guidi G, Cannarile L, Riccardi C. Effect of Biostim (Biostim) on natural killer cell generation from bone marrow precursors. *Int J Immunopharmacol* 1989 ; 11 : 77-82.
31. Guenounou M, Perin S, Vacheron F, Smets P. Induction of circulation interleukin-1 (IL-1) activity after oral administration of Biostim, a bacterial immunomodulator, in monkeys. In : Proceedings of the International Symposium Immunomodulators and non-specific host defence mechanisms against microbial infections, Berlin, 6-8 May 87. Pergamon Press, *Adv Biosci* 1988 ; 68 : 245-50.
32. Andreux JP, Renard MH, Andreux MH, Smets P. Modulation of murine hemopoiesis by repeated injections of a glycoprotein extract from *K. pneumoniae*. *Int J Immunopharmacol* 1986 ; 8, 2 : 147-54.
33. Rezzoug F, Touraine JL, Zalisz R, Smets P. Effect of Biostim on autologous hemopoietic reconstitution of sublethally irradiated mice. *Int J Immunopharmacol* 1990 ; 12 : 491-6.
34. Vacheron F, Smets P, Nauciel C, Guenounou M. Immunological activities of Biostim, a glycoprotein extract from *Klebsiella pneumoniae*. II. Activation of macrophages cytotoxicity against tumor cells and production of a cytotoxic factor. *Ann Inst Pasteur Immunol* 1987 ; 138 : 571-80.
35. Viland H, Blomgren H. Augmentation of spontaneous cytotoxicity of human lymphocytes by Biostim is due to monocytes derived factors distinct from interleukin-2, interferon alpha and gamma. *Anticancer Res* 1987 ; 7 : 23-8.
36. Meredith C, Scott MP, Pekelharing II, Miller K. The effect of Biostim (Biostim) on the expression of cytokine mRNA in murine peritoneal macrophages *in vitro*. *Toxicol Lett* 1990 ; 53 : 327-37.
37. Tissot M, Mathieu J, Mirossay L, Thuret A, Giroud JP. Polyphosphoinositide metabolism in polymorphonuclear cells from healthy and thermally injured rats : effect of the immunomodulator Biostim. *J Leuko Biol* 1991 ; 50 : 607-14.
38. Rudent A, Zalisz R, Quero AM, Smets P. Enhancement of resistance to experimental infections by purified immune modulator of bacterial origin. *Int J Immunopharmacol* 1982 ; 4 : 256-9.
39. Fietta A, Bersani C, De Rose V, Mangiarotti P, Merlini C, Uccelli M, Guildi G, Gialdroni-Grassi G. Double-blind trial RU 41740 *vs* placebo : immunological and clinical effects in a group of patients with chronic bronchitis. *Respiration* 1988 ; 54 : 145-52.
40. Lang JM, Gastaut JA, Sotto JJ, Troncy J, Marchiami C. Enhancement of delayed cutaneous hypersensitivity by oral administration of RU 41740 in lymphoma patients : a randomized double-blind multicentric trial. *Int J Immunopharmacol* 1986 ; 8 : 687-90.
41. Profeta ML, Guidi G, Meroni PL, Palmieri R, Palladino F, Cantone V, Zanussi C. Influenza vaccination with adjuvant RU 41740 in the elderly. *Lancet* 1987 ; 1, 8539 : 973.
42. Lenoir G, Sommelet Olive D, Derelle L, Chazalette JP, Douchain F, Loeuil M, Ounis I. A double-blind comparison of RU 41740 (Biostim) and placebo in recurrent upper respiratory tract infections in children with cystic fibrosis. *Drug Invest* 1991 ; 3 : 76-81.
43. Duhamel JF. Utilisation du Biostim dans les infections respiratoires récidivantes de l'enfant. Étude en double insu de deux formes galéniques orales. *Rev Int Ped* 1990 ; 198 : 67-72.
44. Nielsen H. Inflammatory indices in chronic bronchitis. Monocyte-macrophage microbicidal activity. *Agents Actions* 1990 ; 30 : 213-8.
45. Carles P, Fournials F, Bollinelli R. Intérêt du RU 41740 dans la prévention des épisodes de surinfection des insuffisants respiratoires par bronchite chronique ou dilatation des bronches. *Gaz Med France* 1981 ; 88 : 1-3.
46. Testud F. Toxicologie clinique et effets secondaires des médicaments immunostimulants. *J Toxicol Clin Exp* 1990 ; 37 : 535-40.

8

Immunostimulating lipopeptides

Danièle MIGLIORE-SAMOUR, Pierre JOLLÈS

Laboratoire des Protéines, Université René-Descartes, CNRS, Paris-V, 45, rue des Saints-Pères, 75270 Paris Cedex 06, France.

Among chemically defined immunostimulants of relatively low molecular weight which are already in clinical use or at the stage of advanced preclinical or clinical testing, the molecules of prokaryotic origin keep up an important place. These substances are used in an effort to enhance immune functions such as antibody production, resistance to infection, rejection of malignant cells in immunologically normal subjects or to restore them to a normal level in immunocompromised patients.

This review deals with natural or synthetic lipopeptides and acyl-peptides, excluding desmuramylpeptidolipid derivatives which will be described in another chapter. In 1979, our group in close collaboration with the Research Laboratories of Rhône-Poulenc Santé (Vitry/Seine, France) described the first lipopeptide, the lauroyltetrapeptide (LTP), which was as effective as the muramyldipeptide (MDP), in spite of the absence of the sugar moiety, for stimulation of host against bacterial infection [1]. LTP is the representative of a new family of immunostimulants the activities of which are directed towards cellular immunity illustrated by the models of delayed-type hypersensitivity (DTH) and of resistance to infection to *Listeria monocytogenes* in mice. In the same line of compounds, a research group of Fujisawa Pharmaceutical Co (1981, Osaka, Japan) reported that a lactoyltetrapeptide, FK-156, showed protective activity against bacterial infection [2]. Another family of lipopeptides pertaining to derivatives of the lipoprotein of the outer membrane of *Escherichia coli* was described by Cybulla *et al.* as a potent mitogen for B-lymphocytes [3].

Lauroyl peptides

Presentation of the compounds (Figure 1)

- *History of the discovery*

In the course of researches devoted to the determination of the smallest active part of Mycobacteria implicated in Freund's complete adjuvant (FCA), we isolated a short peptidoglycan from mycobacterial peptidoglycolipids (waxes D), structurally related to the bacterial cell wall peptidoglycan [4], which was able to replace whole Mycobacteria in FCA for an adjuvant effect on DTH in guinea-pig [5]. As for N-acetyl-muramyl-L-alanyl-γ-D-isoglutamine (MDP), the minimal adjuvant active structure of cell wall bacteria [6], presence of mineral oil was required to obtain the adjuvant effect on DTH. Nevertheless, the use of such preparations for human immunization would only be possible after elimination of the mineral oil responsible for undesirable side effects. Following the observation that selective induction of DTH may be obtained by acylation of proteins [7], we coupled lauric or palmitic acid to water-soluble peptidoglycans from Mycobacteria. The compounds became adjuvant active on DTH in guinea-pig in absence of mineral oil [8]. At that time, the Rhône-Poulenc laboratories were interested in a *Streptomyces* strain (NRLL 76) called *Streptomyces stimulosus*. We isolated and purified from the water-soluble extracts a tetrapeptide (L-Ala-D-Glu [(LL-A_{2pm}-Gly)] NH_2 which, after coupling to lauric anhydride, acquired immunostimulating activity. This semi-synthetic lipopeptide, *in vitro*, stimulated thymidine incorporation by mouse spleen cells and enhanced phagocytosis of sheep red blood cells (SRBC) by mouse peritoneal macrophages and, *in vivo*, increased the number of anti-SRBC plaque forming cells in mouse spleen and the resistance of mice against *Listeria monocytogenes* [1]. For the first time it was proved that the presence of the sugar moiety in the minimal adjuvant structure of the bacterial peptidoglycan was not a prerequisite for immunopotentiating activities and may be advantageously replaced by a lipidic moiety.

These potent biological activities prompted Rhône-Poulenc Santé to perform the total synthesis of a close lauroyltetrapeptide analog, RP 40639 (pimelautide), which was a mixture of two stereo-isomers where the diaminopimelic acid (A_{2pm}) was present under two forms: LL-A_{2pm} and DD-A_{2pm}. This compound exhibited the same adjuvant activities as those of the semi-synthetic lipopeptide [9]. The total synthesis of each stereo-isomer led to the conclusion that only the LL-A_{2pm} stereo-isomer (RP 44102) was active, the DD-A_{2pm} form (RP 53204) being totally devoid of any *in vivo* activities. Among the intermediates of the active lauroyltetrapeptide, the direct precursor lauroyltripeptide, RP 56142, exhibited potent immunological activities quite similar to the relevant lipotetrapeptide, RP 44102 [10].

Thus, after a biological assessment of a great number of synthetic analogs [11] the following molecules were selected (Figure 1):

— RP 40639 (pimelautide) which is a mixture of 2 stereo-isomers of lauroyltetrapeptides,
— RP 44102, the active forme (LL-A_{2pm}) of RP 40639,
— RP 56142, the active tripeptide.

• *Chemistry and physicochemical properties*

Synthesis of these compounds was performed by conventional methods used in peptide synthesis [12].

Structural formulae (Figure 1)

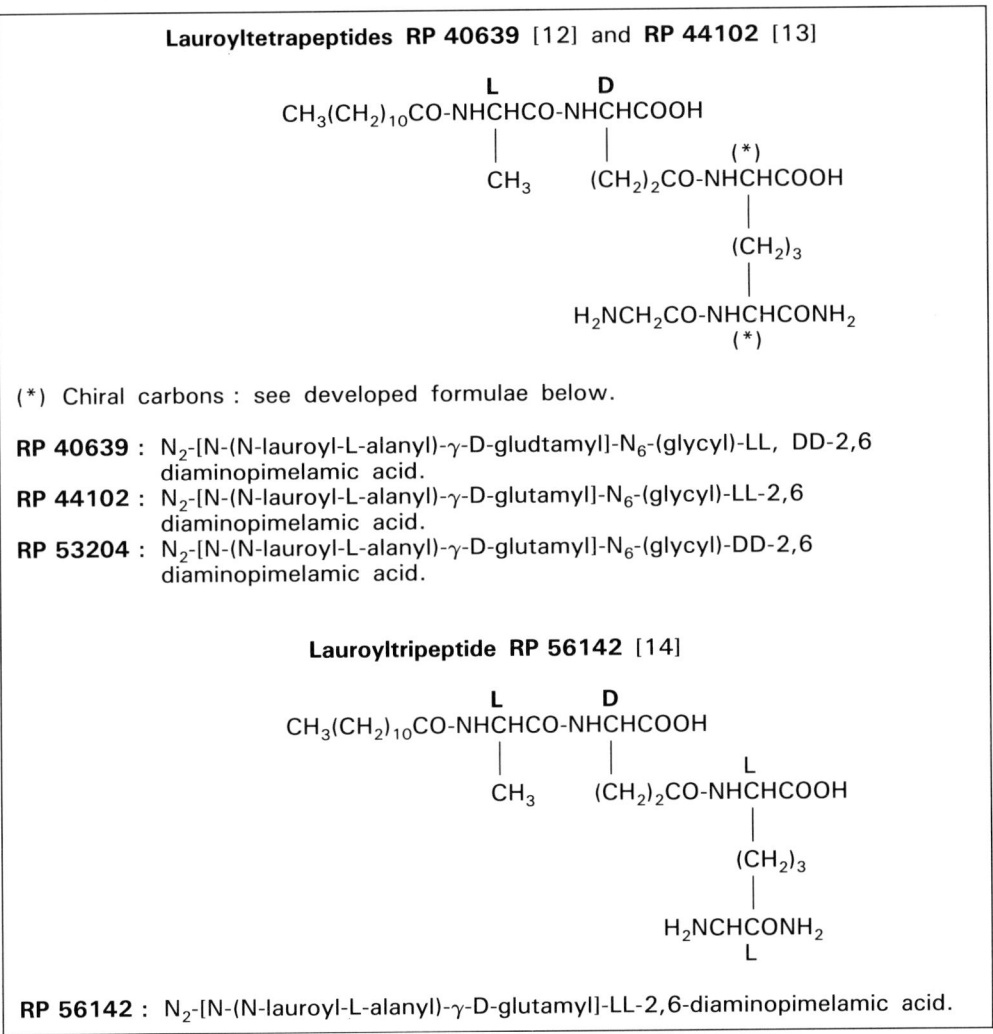

Figure 1. Chemical structure of lauroylpeptides.

Physicochemical properties

Lauroyltetrapeptides (M.W. 628.77 ; m.p.180-184°C) and lauroyltripeptide (M.W. 571.72) are white powders, which can be solubilized in aqueous solutions either as hydrochlorides or as sodium salts. Formation of micelles (diameter ranging between 3.500 and 10.000 Å) is observed when lipotetrapeptides are suspended at 90 μg/ml in phosphate buffer or in saline, a fact which is in accordance with the amphipathic character of this molecule [12].

The lauroyltetrapeptide has been shown to interact with Cu(II) to form chelated complexes dependent on pH [15].

Experimental immunopharmacology

- *Toxicological data* [12]

The acute LD_{50} of the lipotetrapeptide RP 40639, in adult mice by the intravenous route, is 410 mg/kg ; as in all immunostimulating *in vivo* tests, the active doses never exceed 3 mg/kg by parental routes, the margin of safety of this compound appears quite important. The lipopeptides caused hyperthermia in the rabbit at doses higher than 0.4 mg/kg i.v. At this dose, the compounds were devoid of histaminoid activity in the cat. Lack of anaphylactogenic activity was demonstrated in guinea-pigs treated for 3 consecutive days with 1 mg/kg s.c. RP 40639 and challenge intravenously at 1 mg/kg 16 days after the last s.c. injection.

A one-month toxicity study was performed in dogs which received three times a week subcutaneous injections of 0.2 and 1 mg/kg RP 40639 : clinical, ophthalmological, hematological, biochemical and histopathological examinations showed that the compound was very well tolerated.

In the pentobarbital-anesthetized dog, RP 40639 injected i.v. at 0.4 mg/kg did not exert any activity on the cardiovascular, respiratory and neurovegetative systems.

Similar toxicological results were obtained with the lauroyltripeptide, in accordance with the fact that metabolic studies, based on a perfused liver assay, revealed that RP 44102 was rapidly metabolized into RP 56142, the lauroyltetrapeptide could thus be considered as a prodrug of the lauroyltripeptide [10].

- *Immunomodulating properties, target cells and mechanisms of action*
  In vivo *and* ex vivo *studies*

Effects of RP 40639 on DTH reactions : In experimental DTH reactions to SRBC in mice, an enhancing effect was consistently observed at doses ranging between 0.3 and 10 mg/kg. DTH reactions were also demonstrated in guinea-pigs immunized with bovine gamma-globulins (BGG) and boostered with DNP-BGG in presence or not of RP 40639. Guinea-pigs which have received lipopeptide showed an enhanced reactivity to DNP-BGG compared to the control animals.

In these experiments and various others performed in mice and guinea-pigs, the simultaneous injection of Freund incomplete adjuvant (FIA) was not required to obtain enhancement of DTH by RP 40639, in contrast of muramyldipeptide (MDP) [16].

Adjuvant effect on antibody production [12, 16] : In the above mentioned experimental systems, used to determine the effects of RP 40639 on DTH reactions, the lipopeptide also potentiated antibody production. Adjuvant effect of lipotetrapeptide on antibody production, in absence of FIA, was proved in mice immunized against the A/Texas (H3N2) strain of human influenza virus or with type C meningococcal polysaccharide.

The lipotetrapeptide has been shown, by various experimental procedures, to exert a significant adjuvant activity on the production of antibodies against a number of antigens, even in absence of FIA. Furthermore, it is reasonable to assume from some results that this compound should be injected at very low doses for optimal adjuvant activity on humoral immunity.

Stimulation of the clearing activity of the reticuloendothelial system (RES) : Efficiency of the mononuclear-phagocyte system was measured by the rate of clearance of a colloidal suspension of carbon particles injected i.v. in blood of mice. RP 40639 administrated i.p. at doses of 2 and 10 mg/kg doubled the clearance speed of the reticuloendothelial system. The same clearance activity was observed in mice treated orally with 30 mg/kg of RP 56142, and infected 18 h later with 1.5×10^7 *Salmonella typhimurium* showing an activation of the first line of non-specific immune defences [10].

Effect on the induction of cytolytic T lymphocytes (CTL) in mice immunized against allogenic tumor cells : Significant increase in CTL activity in the spleen of mice immunized with P 815 cells was observed after a single administration of RP 40639 (1-3 mg/kg) on day 4 or after three successive administrations at days 4, 6 and 8 after immunization, doses ranging between 0.001 to 0.1 mg/kg. The treatment with the compound enhanced the migration of CTL from the spleen to the peritoneal cavity, which is the site of multiplication of allogeneic cells [16].

Effect on the recruitment of pre-thymic lymphocytes : RP 40639 was administered (3 mg/kg) to CBA mice 6 weeks after thymectomy. The number of autologous rosette-forming cells from the spleen removed 1 or 5 days after treatment was increased by a factor of 1.4 or 1.5 compared with that of untreated mice.

Effect on natural killer (NK) cells : RP 40639 was able to stimulate, *in vivo*, spleen and peripheral blood NK cells in 5-weeks-old C57BL/6 mice in a highly significant manner and to restore spleen NK activity in aged mice (23 months). The lipotripeptide RP 56142 was able to enhance, *in vivo*, spleen NK activity whatever routes of administration : subcutaneous, oral, intravaenous, intranasal or intramuscular. Only the optimal doses differed from one route to another. Fractionated doses or repeated injections remained quite active. RP 56142 was directly active on peripheral blood NK cells (even in splenectomized mice), the optimal dose was 1 mg/kg [14].

In vitro studies on target cells
In the *in vitro* assays, activities of the lauroylpeptides were observed with concentrations ranging between 10^{-5} to 10^{-7} M.

Activities on animal cells : (a) Lauroylpeptides stimulated the phagocytic activity of murine peritoneal macrophages against SRBC and the phagocytic and bactericidal activities against *Listeria monocytogenes* [12] ; (b) RP 40639 [12] and RP 56142 [14] highly enhanced the cytostatic activity of murine peritoneal macrophages against P 815 tumor cells after 24 h incubation ; (c) RP 40639 exerted a mitogen-like activity on murine thymus cells increasing 4-5 fold the DNA synthesis. By contrast, this compound manifested only a slight activity (stimulating index : 1.5 – 2.5 at 10^{-6} M) on murine spleen cells cultured *in vitro* containing a large number of cells from B-lymphocyte subset [16] ; (d) RP 40639 increased secretion of anti-SRBC antibodies by spleen cells of mice pre-immunized 4 days before with SRBC.

RP 40639 would act on B cells through T cell and/or macrophage cooperation, since its effect was markedly diminished after depletion of adherent cells from the suspension and abolished on non-adherent cells after anti-Thy serum treatment [16].

Activities on human cells: (a) RP 40639 *in vitro* enhanced the phagocytic (130-170 %) and the bactericidal (40-80 %) activities of human monocytes (from cirrhotic ascites) compared to controls. Similar results were obtained with cells of HL-60 line differentiated in macrophages with phorbol myristate acetate (PMA) [16]. The lipotripeptide RP 56142 stimulated the phagocytic activity of human blood monocytes-macrophages for senescent human red blood cells [17]. *In vitro*, RP 40639 (10^{-6}M) incubated with human PMNL was unable to stimulate by itself the reduction of nitroblue tetrazolium test (NBT) by those cells. However, when the compound was incubated with PMNL which were subsequently stimulated with a suboptimal dose of LPS (1 µg/ml), the enhancing effect of LPS was significantly boosted ; (b) RP 40639 *in vitro* increased the helper activity of human blood T-lymphocytes for the differentiation of B-lymphocytes into plasmocytes.

Mechanisms of action of the lauroylpeptides

Stimulation of O^{2-} production by macrophages: The superoxide anion O^{2-} production is involved in the bactericidal and also the tumoricidal activities of stimulated macrophages. At concentrations ranging between 1 and 30 µg/ml RP 40639, *in vitro*, increased the production of O^{2-} by resident peritoneal macrophages stimulated with PMA [16].

Stimulation of interleukin 1 (IL-1) and tumor necrosis factor (TNF) production by macrophages: At concentrations between 10^{-5} and 3×10^{-7} M, RP 40639 enhanced the IL-1 intracellular and extracellular content of macrophages [16]. RP 56142 induced the mRNA expression for IL-1α, IL-1β and TNF-α in murine peritoneal macrophages [18].

Enhancement of the interleukin-2 (IL-2) production by human lymphocytes: The addition of RP 40639 (10^{-5} and 10^{-6} M), *in vitro*, enhanced the IL-2 production of human peripheral blood leukocytes stimulated with PHA in presence of ketoprofen to block production of prostaglandins [16].

Production of serum colony stimulating factor (CSF) in the mouse: The serum of mice treated, *in vivo*, with RP 40639 (0.5 or 1 mg/kg i.v.) and collected 4 h later, exerted, *in vitro*, CSF-like activity on murine bone marrow cells. The CSF level reached a peak 6-8 h after the injection [16]. This activity is mainly due to M-CSF [18]. Similar results were obtained with RP 56142 delivered by oral route at 10 and 100 mg/kg. This compound also induced CSF production in athymic and 5-fluorouracil (5-FU)-immunocompromised mice treated with 1 mg/kg s.c. [10, 19].

- *Therapeutic effects in animal models*

Anti-infectious activities

Enhancing effect on resistance to bacterial infections [10, 16] : (a) *Klebsiella pneumoniae* infection : The lauroylpeptides are active against *K. pneumoniæ* septicaemia whatever the route of administration. RP 56142 was active at doses as low as 0.03 mg/kg (s.c., i.p., i.v., i.m.) and 10 mg/kg by the oral route in a single administration were able to protect the treated animals. High doses up to 100 mg/kg (i.m.) still exerted a strong protective effect ; (b) *Listeria monocytogenes* infection : The lauroylpeptides exerted a potent protection against mortality of animals at doses ranging between 0.1 and 10 mg/kg i.p., i.v. or s.c. The protection was also observed after *per os* treatment (50 mg/kg) and when the compound was administered intranasally : a single low dose (1 mg/kg) of RP 56142 protected the animals ; (c) the protective effect conferred by lauroylpeptides is also observed in models using other bacteria such as *Escherichia coli* and *Salmonella typhimurium*.

Protective effects against bacterial infections in murine models relevant to human therapy : In combined treatment protocols, suboptimal doses of RP 56142 given preventively (day - 1) or curatively (day + 4) significantly protected mice receiving antibiotics at doses which were ineffective when administered alone. Given s.c. 1 or 2 days before infectious challenge, RP 56142 was able to normalize and even enhance significantly the resistance of mice previously immunocompromised by lomustine, 5-FU or hydrocortisone [10].

Anti-tumoral activities

The lipopeptides alone have no effect on survival of mice bearing tumors or on metastatic growth. But administered in association with suboptimal doses of cyclophosphamide, RP 40639 enhanced the activity of this anticancer drug on L 1210 leukemia and Lewis lung carcinoma [16] and RP 56142, in combination with surgery or suboptimal doses of cisplatin, exerted synergistic prophylactic and therapeutic effects on spontaneous liver metastases of M 5076 histiocytosarcoma [14].

- *Other pharmacological properties*

The immunostimulating lauroylpeptides RP 44102 and RP 56142 exerted, *in vivo*, in mice, a protective effect against lethal lipidic peroxidation induced by paracetamol and depressed some of the liver microsomal cytochromes P-450 [13].

Radioprotective effects were obtained with these compounds on lethal γ-ray irradiation of mice [18].

Clinical trials, phase I [16]

- *Activities of RP 40639 on human polymorphonuclear leukocytes (PMNL)*

In vivo, in healthy volunteers, at doses of 0.1-0.3 and 1 mg/individual s.c., RP 40639 exerted a direct effect on respiratory burst of PMNL detected with nitroblue tetrazolium (NBT) reduction. Capacity of phagocytosis itroblue tetrazolium (NBT) reduction. Capacity of phagocytosis of these cells was enhanced as shown by the increase of the PMNL chimioluminescence index of the volunteers receiving 1 mg of RP40639.

These results were confirmed by a study performed with PMNL obtained from a family suffering from chronic granulomatosis (congenital enzymatic deficiency of PMNL). *In vivo,* RP 40639 stimulated PMNL of the heterozygotes whereas it was inefficacious on PMNL of homozygotes (total enzymatic defection).

Ex vivo, RP 40639 stimulated bactericidal activities of human PMNL evaluated in two different models using either *E. coli* or *S. aureus*

• *RP 40639 as an adjuvant for vaccines*

In double blind clinical trial performed in collaboration with the Mérieux Institute, the adjuvant activity of RP 40639 was studied in 159 elderly people receiving an anti-influenza vaccine (« VAXIGRIP ») at the same time. Three weeks after vaccination, the group which had received 0.1 mg of RP 40639 and the vaccine had higher antibody titers than the controls receiving vaccine alone.

Conclusion

At the present time, in spite of extensive experimental and preclinical studies performed with RP 40639, the lauroyltripeptide RP 56142 is the only compound proposed for clinical development. The new steps for the physicians will consist in assessing the potency of this lauroylpeptide in immunocompromised patients as well as its therapeutic effectiveness in cancer, in combination with surgery, radiotherapy and conventional chemotherapy, and in infectious diseases. Construction of vaccines after coupling to viral peptide segments would be a new research field for their development.

Japanese acylpeptides

Presentation of the compounds (Figure 2)

• *History of the discovery*

In 1981, in their studies devoted to novel antibiotics, the Fujisawa research Laboratories in Osaka characterized, in fermentation broths of *Streptomyces* strains, substances which manifested discrepancy between their *in vivo* efficiency and their *in vitro* antibacterial activity. An effective compound found in crude extracts of *Streptomyces olivaceogriseus* was extracted, purified and named FK-156 [2]. Its structure was proposed as D-lactyl-L-alanyl-γ-D-glutamyl-(L) meso-diaminopimelyl (L)-glycine. FK-156 showed a stimulatory activity on the reticuloendothelial system (RES) and protective efficiency against experimental infections in animals. A subsequent synthetic program yielded a series of structurally related lipopeptides. The D-configuration of Glu and the L-configuration of the carbon of A_{2pm} combined with Glu and Gly are essential, while the configuration of lactic acid and Ala are of lesser importance. Compounds which differed by the acyl part and/or were lacking the L-Ala displayed potent anti-infectious and anti-neoplastic activity. Replacement of D-lactyl acid by n-heptanoic acid gave a compound with an enhanced anti-infectious activity and the stearoyl analog showed a tumor-supressive activity which was lacking in FK-156. Particularly, FK-565, heptanoyl-γ-D-glutamyl-(L)-meso-diaminopimelyl-(L)-D-alanine, was found to be more active for bacterial infections, increase of NK cell activity and prevention of tumor metastasis. Some more intensively studied analogs of these two peptides are described in Table I.

• *Chemistry and physicochemical properties*

Synthesis of these compounds was performed by conventional methods using a novel copper chelate amino-protection [20, 21].

Structural formulae (Figure 2)

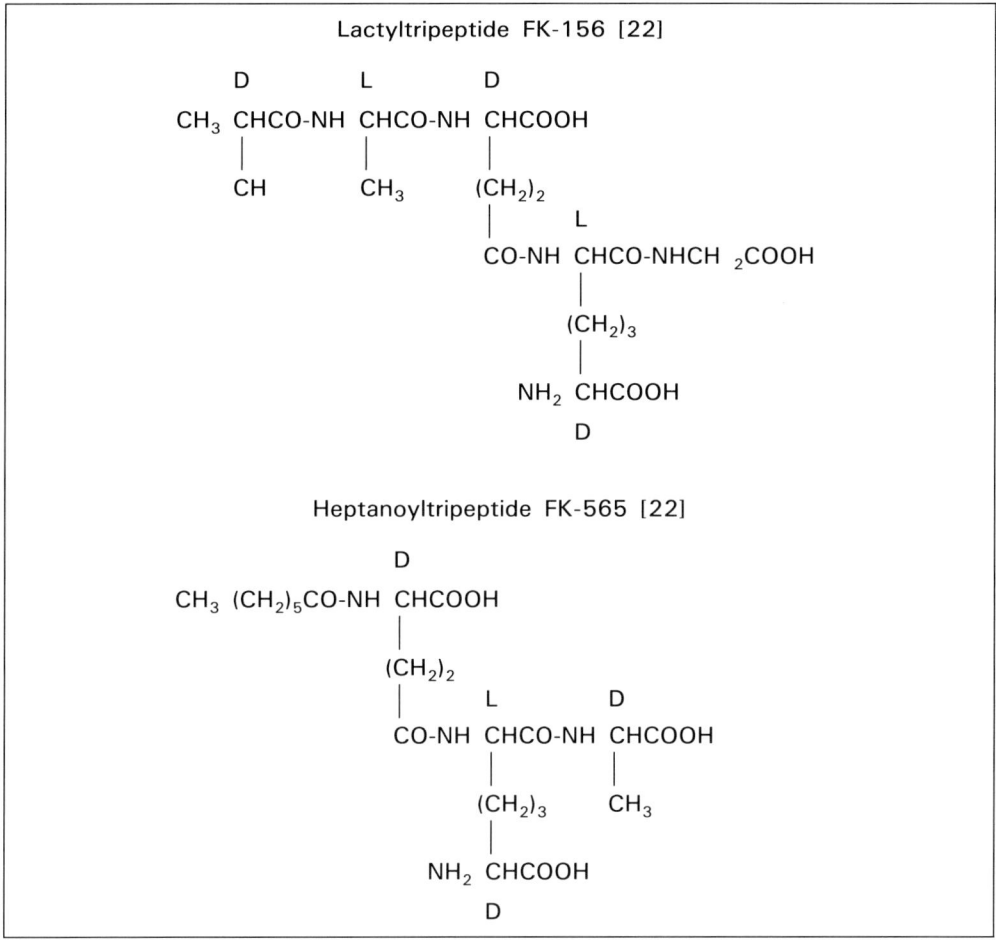

Figure 2. Chemical structure of Japanese acylpeptides.

Table I. Synthetic acyltripeptides and some related compounds [23].

Name	Chemical structure
FK-156	Lactyl-L-Ala-γ-D-Glu-(L)meso-α,ε-A_2pm(L)-Gly
FR-42148	Stearoyl-L-Ala-γ-D-Glu-(L)meso-α,ε-A_2pm(L)-D-Ala
FR-48217	Behenoyl-L-Ala-γ-D-Glu-(L)meso-α,ε-A_2pm(L)-D-Ala
FK-565	Heptanoyl-γ-D-Glu-(L)meso-α,ε-A_2pm(L)-D-Ala
FK-42149	Stearoyl-γ-D-Glu-(L)meso-α,ε-A_2pm(L)-D-Ala

Recently, a new convenient synthesis of FK-156 and FK-565 was described [24].

Physicochemical properties
FK-156 (M.W. 447, m.p.143-148°C) is a white powder which is water soluble with pKa' values 4.3, 5.8, 6.3 and 10.9. Measurement of optical rotation gave $[\alpha]$ D -30.0° (c 0.5, water). It is slightly soluble in methanol and almost insoluble in other organic solvents [25]. FK-565 (M.W. 503) is a powder with a $[\alpha]$ D -15.7° (c 0.5, methanol). Both acylpeptides are soluble in physiological saline.

Experimental immunopharmacology

- *Toxicological data*

FK-156 exhibited low toxicity in mice. The LD_{50} value is greater than 1 g/kg when administered i.v. to ICR mice (male and female, 6 weeks old).

- *Immunomodulating properties, target cells and mechanisms of action*

In vivo *and* ex vivo *studies*

Effect of FK-156 and FK-565 on DTH reactions and antibody production : The two compounds strongly enhanced DTH reaction against antigens in presence of ACF [25, 26].

Stimulation of the clearing activity of RES : The carbon clearance in mice 24 h after i.p. injection of FK-156 increased dose-dependently (0.01 to 1 mg/kg) and, at doses of 1 and 10 mg/kg, was three times higher than in non-treated control mice [25].

Mitogenic activities on murine splenic lymphocytes : FK-156 significantly increased the incorporation of labeled thymidine in mouse spleen cell culture. The maximal response was observed at a concentration of 100 µg/kg [25]. FK-565 also exerted mitogenic activity on peripheral blood and splenic lymphocytes [26].

Stimulation of phagocytic cells : FK-156 and FK-565 subcutaneously injected at 1 mg/kg to normal mice significantly increased counts of peripheral and peritoneal PMNL and monocytes. These compounds at 1 mg/kg s.c. and i.p. enhanced the *in vitro* chemotactic, phagocytic and killing activities of peritoneal macrophages and PMNL [27].

Effect on NK cells : In C57BL/6 mice low doses of FK-565 (0.1-100 µg/kg, s.c.) selectively activated splenic and peripheral blood NK cells. Increase of peripheral NK activity occured about one day after subcutaneous injection of FK-565 and the elevated level declined to baseline in 2 to 3 days after maximal augmentation [26]. In all experiments, activation of NK cell activity by FK-565 was significantly greater in peripheral blood than in splenic cells.

In vitro *studies on target cells*

Activities on animal cells : Murine alveolar and peritoneal macrophages can be rendered tumoricidal by incubation with FK-565 and its analogs [28].

FK-565 encapsulated in liposomes, composed of phosphatidylcholine and phosphatidylserine, was more effective than the free compound in rendering rat alveolar macrophages tumoricidal [29]

Activities on human cells : Human blood monocytes were activated to tumoricidal state by incubation *in vitro* with FK-565 (0.5 to 100 µg/ml) ; this activity was dependent on the concentration of acylpeptide and on the ratio of monocytes to target tumor cells. Several analogs were more potent activators than FK-565, among them FR-42148 and FR-42149 which were found as effective as LPS. rIFN-γ at subthreshold concentrations had a synergic effect with acylpeptides in activating human monocytes, whereas rIFN-α and rIFN-β had additive effects [23].

A strong stimulatory effect on superoxide generation by resting human monocytes and granulocytes was observed over a wide range of FK-565 concentrations [30].

Mechanisms of action of acylpeptides
FK-156 and FK-565 were able to induce colony-stimulating factor in murine serum [31] and to release IL-1 from murine macrophages [32].

- *Therapeutic effects in animal models*
Anti-infectious activities
Enhancement of host resistance to microbial infection in mice : In the course of seeking new antibiotics, the development of these acylpeptides started with the observation that some microbial metabolites showed higher *in vivo* antibacterial activities compared to those based on their *in vitro* MIC (maximal inhibiting concentration) values. FK-156 and related compounds exerted protective efficiency against experimental infections in animals.

FK-156 and FK-565 enhanced significantly the defence of mice against extracellular bacteria such as *Pseudomonas aeruginosa, Escherichia coli* and *Serratia marcescens* as well as a fungus, *Candida albicans,* and against facultative intracellular bacteria such as *Listeria monocytogenes* and *Salmonella enteritidis*. The two drugs were also effective against local infection such as subcutaneous abscess by *Staphylococcus aureus*. The protective effect of these compounds depended on the route, time and doses. FK-565 was more potent than FK-156 and was most active through oral and parenteral administration, whereas FK-156 was most active through intravenous or subcutaneous routes [22].

Restoration of host resistance to microbial infection in immunocompromised mice : FK-156 and FK-565 were given to immuno depressed mice (with cyclophosphamide, carrageenan, mitomycin C, hydrocortisone or implantation with sarcoma 180) before infectious challenge. Subcutaneous injection of FK-156 (0.1 and 1 mg/kg) increased host resistance to systemic infections with extracellular and facultative intracellular parasites in immunosuppressed mice. A similar effect was obtained with the same administered orally doses of FK-565 [33].

The therapeutic effect of ticarcillin or gentamicin alone against *Pseudomonas* infection in cyclophosphamide- and hydrocortisone-treated mice and tumor-bearing mice was much lower than in normal mice. The protective efficiency of the antibiotics was markedly enhanced (and restored to nearly normal level for ticarcillin) by combined therapy with FK-156. Acylpeptides restored depressed defence mechanisms in immunocompromised mice by (a) increasing PMNL, macrophages and lymphocytes counts, (b) stimulating exudate response and the chemotactic, phagocytic and killing activities of macrophages and PMNL, (c) enhancing RES fonctions [33]. The synergism of ticarcillin and acylpeptides against infection is thought to be induced by synergistic effect of antibacterial ticarcillin and activated phagocytes.

Protection against viral infections : FK-156 and FK-565 were active in protecting animals against viral infections, especially with Herpes virus and showed therein therapeutic as well as prophylactic activities [26].

FR-48217 (Table I) was investigated in mice vaccinated with inactivated influenza virus. It exerted a strong adjuvant effect on the survival rate of mice infected with influenza virus A/PR/8/34 28 days after vaccination. The titers of virus-specific IgA and IgG antibodies were higher in mice treated with the acylpeptide than in control mice. Whereas there was a temporary decrease of antibodies titer in the serum just after the viral infection, the free IgA and IgG antibody levels in the pulmonary lavage fluid of vaccinated mice increased after day 4, suggesting that the serum antibodies were transported to the lung epithelial tissues and consumed to neutralize the virus upon infection [34].

FK-565 alone and in combination with zidovudine (AZT) inhibited retroviral infections by Friend leukemia virus in mice [35].

Antitumoral activities
FK-156, FK-565, FR-48217 and other derivatives as FR-46758, an alcoholic analog of FK-565, substantially suppressed solid tumor growth when directly injected into a tumor mass (P 388 cells, injected subcutaneously into the flank of DBA/2 mice) or into a site far from the tumor. The mechanisms of growth inhibition were strongly suggested to be host-mediated because these peptides had remarkably low cytotoxicity against P 388 cells *in vitro* [36].

Low doses of FK-565 (0.1-100 µg/kg) reduced the pulmonary metastases of NK-sensitive B 16 and 3 LL tumor cells ; these results might be correlated with the activation of peripheral blood NK cells, probably based on the induction of CSF in the serum. The activity of FK-565 in the therapy model of metastasis was also confirmed by the Biological Response Modifying Program (BRMP) in the National Cancer Institute [37]. Optimal therapeutic activity was observed at approximately 25-50 mg/kg administered i.v. three times per week for 4 weeks [38].

FK-565 at 0.05 µg/kg enhanced host resistance to syngeneic X 5563 plasmacytoma and MH 134 hepatoma, augmented by immunization with vaccinia virus-modified tumors. FK-565 also enhanced cytotoxic T-lymphocyte response to X 5563 tumor cells and suppression of the growth of both tumors in Winn assay [39].

Conclusion

Acylpeptides increase protection against bacterial and viral infections in animals with either compromised or competent immune systems. The chemotherapeutic activity of antibiotics is enhanced and antimetastatic activity of FK-565 based on the activation of NK cells in experimental animals suggests that this compound and/or some analogs have potential efficiency for the management of cancer metastases. Phase I clinical trials are in progress.

Lipopeptides from N-terminus of *Escherichia coli* lipoprotein

Presentation of the compounds (Figure 3)

• *History of the discovery*

In 1969 Braun *et al.* demonstrated the presence in the outer membrane of *Escherichia coli* of a lipoprotein covalently attached to the murein of the cell wall. At the N-terminal end the polypeptide chain contains 2 ester-linked and 1 amide-linked fatty acids bound to glyceryl-cysteine and is covalently bound by the C-terminal lysine to the carboxyl group of a diaminopimelate residue of the murein. The lipoprotein is a potent mitogen of B-lymphocytes and this specific response was independent on T-lymphocytes and did not need serum factors of adherent cells. The lipoprotein also stimulated B-lymphocytes from C3H/HeJ mice (low responders to mitogenic stimulation by LPS) indicating two distinct stimulation sites for lipoprotein and lipopolysaccharide on B-lymphocytes [40]. This lipoprotein is also a potent mitogen for lymphocytes of several species [41]. The molecular structure responsible for the mitogenicity resides in its N-terminal fatty-acid containing part; removal of the ester-linked fatty acids from the lipoprotein by weak alkali hydrolysis abolished its mitogenic activity. Lipopeptide fragments prepared by enzymatic digestion, which carried three fatty acids bound to glyceryl-cysteine attached to an oligopeptide chain of 3-5 aminoacids, were fully active. Fragments carrying only one fatty acid still exhibited reduced mitogenicity [42]. Analogs carrying one fatty acid bound to cysteine (N-terminal amino acid of the lipoprotein) or to glutamic acid were synthesized and exhibited mitogenic activity towards B-lymphocytes comparable to the effect of lipoprotein [3]. Ciba-Geigy laboratories (Basel, Switzerland) have been involved in lipoprotein research since 1977; the potent mitogenic action of the *E.coli* lipoprotein on mice B cells prompted them to study its effect on antibody synthesis *in vivo*. The compound proved highly active and was considered worthy of further chemical and medical investigations. They have also been engaged in synthesis of lipopeptide analogs [43].

• *Chemistry and physicochemical properties*

Synthesis of analogs of N-terminal part of *E. coli* lipoprotein, carrying one fatty acid bound to cysteine (Pam-Cys-OMe) or to glutamic acid (Pam-Glu-OMe), was first described by Cybulla *et al.* [3]. Synthesis of three fatty acid (palmitoyl) derivatives [44] was the key to produce various lipopeptides from the N-terminal end of the *E. coli* lipoprotein, among them a lipopentapeptide containing the five N-terminal amino acids (Cys-Ser-Ser-Asn-Ala) of the native lipoprotein [45] or several other peptidic analogs [46].

Structural formulae : [3, 44, 45, 47] (Figure 3)

Physicochemical properties

All these compounds are insolule in water and almost insoluble in most solvents including dimethylsulfoxide, dimethylformamide, alcohols and chlorinated solvents. From diluted warm solutions in chloroform, Pam_3-pentapeptide precipitated as a gel and forms opalescent multilamellar sheets on the glass wall upon slow evaporation of the solvent [45]. The lipopentapeptide seemed to be a suitable and interesting additive for the preparation of lipid bilayers and vesicles [45].

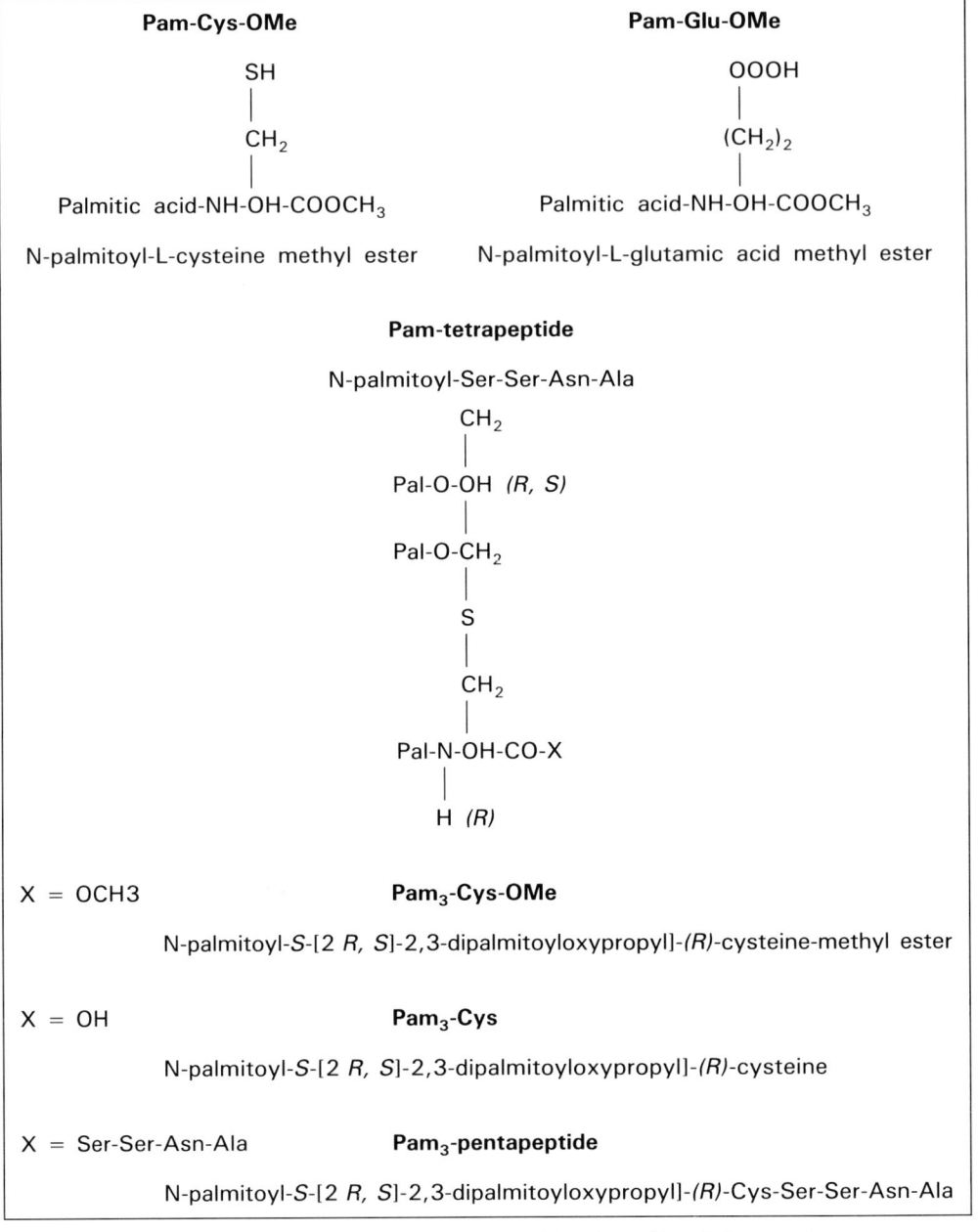

Figure 3. Chemical structure of lipopeptides from *E. coli* lipoprotein.

Monolayer experiments with Pam_3-peptide derivatives, dissolved in chloroform or mixed with cholesterol and dipalmitoylphosphatidylcholine, were performed to obtain the surface areas for the lipopeptides in isotherms and hysteresis isotherms, in view to estimate their ability to form liposomes as well as to get some informations about the interactions of the lipopeptides with membrane forming lipids [46].

All biological assays were carried out after sonication of the lipopeptides in culture medium.

Experimental immunopharmacology

- ### Immunomodulating properties, target cells and mechanisms of action
  In vivo *and* ex vivo *studies*

In regard to their *in vitro* mitogenic activity on murine spleen cells, *in vivo* effects of Pam_3-pentapeptide and Pam_3-Cys were determined in Balb/c mice. A marked enlargement of the spleen was apparent 3 days after i. v. administration of 35 µg lipopeptides, comparable to that induced by either lipoprotein or LPS. Splenocytes of treated mice were polyclonally stimulated into immunoglobulin secretion, as the plaque-forming cells against trinitrophenylated erythrocytes increased markedly ; compared to control mice, Pam_3-Cys had a significant but less pronounced effect than Pam_3-pentapeptide [48].

In vitro *studies on target cells*

Effects of Pam-peptides on B-cell mitogenicity : Lipoprotein of *E. coli* was known to be a potent mitogen for lymphocytes of several species. Thus, the first investigations with the synthetic derivatives were orientated towards this activity. Analogs carrying one fatty acid bound to one amino acid such as cysteine or glutamic acid [3], or bound to a longer peptide [47] exhibited stimulatory activity on B-lymphocytes, as measured by ^{3}H-thymidine incorporation and by hemolytic plaque assays, for several inbred mice strains, particularly for the C3H/HeJ strain, genetically no-responder to LPS. However, the stimulating action of these compounds was less pronounced than the effect of the native lipoprotein [41] or of the synthetic tripalmitoyl-pentapeptide (Pam_3-pentapeptide) [49]. The increased hydrophobicity due to three fatty acid residues was likely to favour mitogen-cell interactions and to further increase the stimulatory effect. *In vitro*, Pam_3-pentapeptide was a potent immune adjuvant : in the presence of 0.33 to 33 µg/ml, antibody response towards SRBC or trinitrophenylated (TNP)-SRBC was markedly enhanced as measured by hemolytic plaque assay ; IgM and IgG response were increased as shown by ELISA. In the secondary *in vitro* response to TNP-SRBC, enhancement of the antibody titer was obtained with the lipopeptide. The application of Pam_3-pentapeptide and antigen had to occur concurrently in order to achieve a strong adjuvant effect [50]. Lipopeptides also enhance the growth of the BCL1 cell line, which exhibits the phenotype of immature B-lymphocytes [47].

If lipopeptides constitute potent immunoadjuvants in combination with antigens, this activity is conserved after covalent linkage to low molecular-mass compounds like peptides [51]. The conjugates were capable of inducing anti-hapten-specific IgM and IgG without further adjuvants or carriers [52]. Conjugation of Pam_3-Cys-Ser with the extracytoplasmic domain of epidermal growth factor receptor (residues 516-529) lead to a non-toxic synthetic peptide-adjuvant conjugate capable of inducing specific antibodies when injected i.p. into Balb/c mice [53].

Stimulation of human and murine adherent cells and neutrophils : The ability of two synthetic compounds, Pam_3-pentapeptide and Pam_3-Cys-Ser, to directly activate primary adherent cells or macrophages was tested.

The two lipopeptides were able to stimulate the proliferation of the P388D1 murine macrophage cell line. At concentrations of 10-100 µg/ml they induced IL-1 secretion by these cells and by murine peritoneal macrophages and human mononuclear cells. Moreover, murine peritoneal exudate cells were stimulated to secrete prostaglandins E_2 (PG_{E2}) and F_{2a} (PGF_{2a}). The stimulation of murine B cells by Pam_3-pentapeptide was strongly impeded if macrophages were depleted, though a significant residual B-cell activation could still be observed in all performed experiments [54].

Two more soluble lipopeptide analogs, Pam_3-Cys-Ala-Gly and Pam_3-Cys-Ser-(Lys)4, were able to induce tumor cytotoxicity in murine bone-marrow-derived macrophages (BMDM) tested against the tumor cell line L929 ; the optimal concentration for cytotoxicity was around 100 µg/ml for both lipopeptides. The effects were comparable or superior to those exerted by LPS [55]. Pam_3-Cys-Ala-Gly induced the secretion of IL-1, IL-6 and TNFα in BMDM [56] and was a potent activator of the oxidative L-arginine pathway leading to the formation of nitric oxide (NO) and nitrite (NO_2-) [57] ; Pam_3-Cys-Ser-(Lys)4 activated superoxide formation and lysozyme release in human neutrophils [58].

Mechanisms of action
The proteinkinase C (PKC) activation by lipopeptide induced B cell stimulation was investigated. Pam_3-Cys-Ala-Gly failed to induce phosphoinositide degradation and the generation of the two second messengers cAMP and cGMP.

Thus B cell activation bypasses phosphatidyl metabolism and PKC translocation [59]. Similar results were obtained on BMDM where the lipopeptide induced a rapid rise in cytosolic Ca^{2+}, which was due to an influx of extracellular calcium as well as to a redistribution of intracellular calcium [60].

Lipopeptides were effective stimulators of tyrosine phosphorylation in human myeloid cells and human neutrophils [61].

Lipoprotein and derived lipopeptides were demonstrated to bind to defined membrane proteins of murine spleen cells or macrophages, including proteins of the major histocompatibility complex. In order to follow the routes and to determine the distribution of the lipopeptide analogs within macrophages after stimulation, the novel method of electron energy loss spectroscopy was used. The lipopeptide Pam_3-Cys-Ser was present in different compartments of the cell. The major amount was located within the cytoplasm and the plasma membrane and minor quantities were detected within the nuclear membranes and the nucleus [62, 63].

- *Therapeutic effects in animal models*
  Anti-infectious activities
  Enhancement of host resistance to microbial infections : Enhancement of protection against *Salmonella typhimurium* infection in NMRI mice was obtained with Pam_3-pentapeptide associated with acetone-killed *S. typhimurium* vaccines. Con-

sidering the LD_{50}, a great percentage of the S. *typhimurium* vaccine could be replaced by the adjuvant lipopeptide without a recognizable decrease in protective immunizing capacity. However the lipopeptide alone was not effective in protecting mice from infection [64].

An analog synthezised by Ciba-Geigy, CGP-31, where the peptide moiety was modified with taurine [43], displayed a marked anti-infectious activity (60-70 % survival) when administrated prophylactically or simultaneously with infectious organisms, whatever the route of administration, the best results being observed when the route of infection and the one of administration of lipopeptide were the same.

Synthetic peptide vaccines : The potentiality of these immunoadjuvants to stimulate the antibody response, even when they are covalently coupled to peptide antigens [52, 53], lead to production of low-molecular-weight synthetic vaccines for viral infections.

(a) The synthetic antigenic determinant VPI (135-154) of foot-and-mouth disease (FMD) virus strain O_1K was coupled to Pam_3-Cys-Ser-Ser [65]. The immunization of cattle with synthetic antigenic peptide free of any carrier induced only limited protection and the antibody response to such a peptide was very low. Guinea-pig vaccination has proved to be a useful model for the evaluation of FMD vaccines. No local reactions of the animals were observed after s.c., i.p. or i.m. injection of this novel vaccine (emulsified in egg lecithin by sonication). The animals were challenged by intradermal inoculation of virulent O_1K FMD virus 25 days after priming. The protection (estimated by absence of any lesions for 10 days) and antibody titers were strongly increased compared to a mixture of the lipopeptide with the antigenic peptide or to the lipopeptide alone. The protection rate was 100 % after 3 weeks, 75 % after 4 and 12 weeks and 50 % after 6 weeks.

(b) Cytotoxic T-lymphocytes (CTL) constituted an essential part of the immune response against viral infections. They recognized peptides derived from viral proteins associated with major histocompatibility complex (MHC) class I molecules on the surface of infected cells and usually required *in vivo* priming with infectious virus. An influenza nucleoprotein epitope [NP147-158 (R-)], the most efficient peptide to be recognized by $H-2^d$-restricted CTL specific for influenza nucleoprotein, was coupled with Pam_3-Cys-Ser-Ser. When BALB/C ($H-2^d$) mice were immunized with the epitope alone or with the lipopeptide alone, after 6 days, *in vitro* stimulated spleen cells failed to kill peptide-incubated or virus infected P 815 ($H-2^d$) target cells. By contrast, mice immunized with Pam_3-Cys-Ser-Ser-NP147-158 (R-) conjugate produced a virus specific CTL response as strong as that induced by priming with infectious virus. The lipopeptide-conjugate priming is MHC class I restricted [66].

Experiments with lipopeptide-HIV-peptide-conjugates to induce a cellular immune response involving helper T lymphocytes and cytotoxic T cells recognizing HIV infected targets are in progress [67].

Antitumor activities

Though some Pam_3-peptides were able to strongly stimulate *in vitro* tumor cytotoxicity of BMDM [55], a most important modification of the peptide moiety is needed to obtain an *in vivo* response. CGP 31 362, from Ciba-Geigy laboratories, induced mesurable rejection of pulmonary metastases after not only i.v. but also p.o. administration [43].

Conclusion

Except on the non-pyrogenicity of these lipopeptides, there are so far no data on the toxicity of these compounds. These lipopeptides are strong B cell mitogens, partly due to their stimulating activity on macrophages. Interesting results obtained by conjugating Pam_3-Cys-Ser-Ser to viral epitopes seem to indicate that they are especially suitable for vaccine design.

Conclusion

The common characteristics of these lipopeptides are their non specific anti-infectious activity revealed by bacteriological and immunological studies : all behave as good candidates for the enhancement of the host defence against infectious diseases.

Lauroylpeptides and acylpeptides increase the resistance of immunocompromised mice infectious challenge and exert a synergic activity with antibiotics : their protective efficiency is obtained at doses ineffective when administered alone. This observation might be correlated to the stimulation of activities of phagocytic cells, especially of macrophages. Lipopeptides also stimulate tumor cytostatic and cytotoxic activities of macrophages as well as the NK functions ; their use in cancer therapy, either directly (for some acylpeptides) or in combination with chimiotherapy, surgery and radiotherapy, may be considered.

Lipopeptides of *E. coli* protein are of particular interest by their mitogenic activity on B-lymphocytes, even after a covalent linkage to an antigen such as viral epitopes. Their efficiency as specific viral vaccines in some experiments open the way to a new field of vaccine development.

References

1. Migliore-Samour D, Bouchaudon J, Floc'h F, Zerial A, Ninet L, Werner GH, Jollès P. Propriétés immunostimulantes et adjuvantes d'un lipopeptide de faible poids moléculaire. *CR Acad Sci Paris* 1979 ; 289 D : 473-6.
2. Tanaka H, Goto T, Kohsaka M, Aoki H, Imanaka H, Hashimoto M, Kitaura Y, Nakaguchi O, Hemmi K, Takeno H, Okada S, Mori J, Senoh H, Mine Y, Nishida M. Studies on FK-156 isolated from a *Streptomyces* : synthesis and immunostimulating activities of γ-D-glutamyl-(L)-meso-diaminopimelic acid derivatives. In : Yamamura Y, Kotani S, Azuma I, Koda A, Shiba T, eds. *Immunomodulation by microbial products and related synthetic compounds.* Proceedings of the International symposium, Osaka, July 27-29 1981, International Congress series, 563. Amsterdam-Oxford-Princeton : Excerpta Medica : 171-4.
3. Cybulla J, Brückner H, Jung G, Wipperfürth T, Bessler WG. The mitogenic principle of *Escherichia coli* lipoprotein : B-lymphocyte mitogenicity of N-palmitoyl-cysteine and N-palmitoyl-glutamic acid α-methyl esters. *Biochem Biophys Res Commun* 1980 ; 92 : 1389-96.
4. Migliore D, Jollès P. Contribution to the study of the structure of adjuvant active Waxes D from Mycobacteria : isolation of a peptidoglycan. *FEBS Lett* 1968 ; 2 : 7-9.

5. Werner GH, Maral R, Floc'h F, Migliore-Samour D, Jollès P. Adjuvant and immunostimulant activities of water soluble substances extracted from *Mycobacterium tuberculosis var hominis*. *Biomedicine* 1975 ; 22 : 440-52.
6. Ellouz F, Adam A, Ciorbaru R, Lederer E. Minimal structural requirements for adjuvant activity of bacterial peptidoglycan derivatives. *Biochem Biophys Res Commun* 1974 ; 59 : 1317-25.
7. Coon J, Hunter R. Selective induction of delayed hypersensitivity by a lipid-conjugated protein antigen which is localized in thymus-dependent lymphoid tissue. *J Immunol* 1972 ; 110 : 183-90.
8. Migliore-Samour D, Floc'h F, Maral R, Werner GH, Jollès P. Adjuvant activities of chemically modified water-soluble substances from *Mycobacterium tuberculosis*. *Immunology*, 1977 ; 33 : 477-84.
9. Migliore-Samour D, Bouchaudon J, Floc'h F, Zerial A, Ninet L, Werner GH, Jollès P. A short lipopeptide, representative of a new family of immunological adjuvants devoid of sugar. *Life Sci* 1980 ; 26 : 883-8.
10. Floc'h F, Poirier J. Immunopotentiating activities of a low molecular weight lipopeptide, RP 56142. Studies in infectious models. *Int J Immunopharmacol* 1988 ; 10 : 863-73.
11. Werner GH, Floc'h F, Bouchaudon J, Zerial A, Migliore-Samour D, Jolles P. Low molecular weight synthetic lipopeptides : a new class of immunopotentiating substances. In : Serrou B, Rosenfeld C, eds. *Current concepts in human immunology and in cancer immunomodulation*. Elsevier Biomedicine 1982 : 17 : 645-52.
12. Floc'h F, Bouchaudon J, Fizames C, Zerial A, Dutruc-Rosset G, Werner GH. Lauroyltetrapeptide (RP 40639) and related lipopeptides : a novel class of synthetic immunomodulating agents. *Drugs of the Future* 1984 ; 9 : 763-76.
13. Migliore-Samour D, Delaforge M, Jaouen M, Mansuy D, Jollès P. *In vivo* effects of immunomodulating lipopeptides on mouse liver microsomal cytochromes P-450 and on paracetamol-induced toxicity. *Experientia* 1989 ; 45 : 882-6.
14. Fizames C, Poirier J, Floc'h F. Immunomodulating and antitumor activities of a synthetic lauroyltripeptide (RP 56142). *J Biol Response Mod* 1989 ; 8 : 397-408.
15. Decock-Le Reverend, Loucheux C, Livera C, Pettit LD, Migliore-Samour D, Jollès P. The interaction of copper (II) with a lipotetrapeptide. *Inorg Chim Acta* 1987 ; 136 : 173-6.
16. Floc'h F, Poirier J, Fizames C, Woehrle R. Pimelautide (RP 40639) from experimental results to clinical trials : an illustration. In : Azuma I, Jollès G, eds. *Immunostimulants now and tomorrow*. Tokyo : Japonese Scientific Societies Press, and Berlin : Springer Verlag, 1987 : 183-204.
17. Gattegno L, Migliore-Samour D, Saffar L, Jollès P. Enhancement of phagocytic activity of human monocytic-macrophagic cells by immunostimulating peptides of human casein. *Immunol Lett* 1988 ; 18 : 27-32.
18. Migliore-Samour D, Bousseau A, Caillaud JM, Naussac A, Sedqi M, Ferradini C, Jollès P. Radioprotective effects of the immunostimulating lauroylpeptide LtriP (RP 56142) *Experientia* 1993 ; 49 : 160-6.
19. Poirier J, Bousseau A, Folliard F, Molinie B, Terlain B. RP 56142 as a inducer of cytokines. 7th International Congress of Immunology, Berlin, August 1989.
20. Hemmi K, Takeno H, Okada S, Nakaguchi O, Kitaura Y, Hashimoto M. Total synthesis of FK-156 isolated from a *Streptomyces* as an immunostimulating peptide : application of a novel copper chelate amino protection. *J Am Chem Soc* 1981 ; 103 : 7026-8.
21. Kitaura Y, Takeno H, Aratani M, Okada S, Yonishi S, Hemmi K, Nakaguchi O, Hashimoto M. Synthesis and RES — stimulating activity of bacterial cell-wall peptidoglycan peptides related to FK-156. *Experientia* 1982 ; 38 : 1101-3.
22. Mine Y, Yokota Y, Wakai Y, Fukada S, Nishida M, Goto S, Kuwahara S. Immunoactive peptides, FK-156 and FK-565 I. Enhancement of host resistance to microbial infection in mice. *J Antibiotics* 1983 ; 36 : 1045-50.
23. Sone S, Okubo A, Inamura N, Nii A, Ogura T. Synergism of synthetic acyltripeptide and its analogs with recombinant interferon-γ for activation of antitumor properties of human blood monocytes. *Cancer Immunol Immunother* 1988 ; 27 : 33-7.

24. Kolodziejczyk AM, Kolodziejczyk AS, Stoev S. New convenient synthesis of immunostimulating peptides containing meso-diaminopimelic acid. Syntheses of FK-565 and FK-156. *Int J Peptide Res* 1992 ; 39 : 382-7.
25. Gotoh T, Nakahara K, Nishiura T, Hashimoto M, Kino T, Kuroda Y, Okuhara M, Kohsaka M, Aoki H, Imanaka H. Studies on a new immunoactive peptide, FK-156 II. Fermentation, extraction and chemical and biological characterization. *J Antibiotics* 35 : 1982 ; 1286-92.
26. Goto T, Aoki H. The immunomodulatory activities of acylpeptides. In : Azuma I, Jollès G, eds. *Immunostimulants now and tomorrow*. Tokyo : Japonese Scientific Societies Press, and Berlin : Springer Verlag, 1987 : 99-108.
27. Mine Y, Watanabe Y, Tawara S, Yokota Y, Nishida M, Goto S, Kuwahara S. Immunoactive peptides, FK-156 and FK-565. III- Enhancement of host defense mechanisms against infection. *J Antibiotics* 1983 ; 36 : 1059-66.
28. Inamura N, Nakahara K, Kito T, Gotoh T, Kawamura I, Aoki H, Sone S. Activation of tumoricidal properties in macrophages and inhibition of experimentally-induced murine metastases by a new synthetic acyltripeptide, FK-565. *J Biol Response Mod* 1985 ; 4 : 408-17.
29. Sone S, Mutsuura S, Ogawara M, Utsugi T, Tsubura E. Activation by a new synthetic acyltripeptide and its analogs entrapped in liposomes of rat alveolar macrophages to the tumor cytotoxic state. *Cancer Immunol Immunother* 1984 ; 18 : 169-73.
30. Yi-Li W, Kaplan S, Whiteside T, Herberman RB. *In vitro* effects of an acyltripeptide, FK-565, on antitumor effector activities and on metabolic activities of human monocytes and granulocytes. *Immunopharmacol* 1989 ; 18 : 213-22.
31. Nakamura K, Nakahara K, Aoki H. Induction of colony-stimulating factor (CSF) by FK-156 and its synthetic derivative, FK-565. *Agric Biol Chem* 1984 : 48 : 2579-80.
32. Inamura N, Nakahara K, Aoki H. Augmentation of Interleukin 1 (IL-1) release by murine macrophages stimulated with FK-565. *Agric Biol Chem* 1984 ; 48 : 2393-4.
33. Yokota Y, Mine Y, Wakai Y, Watanabe Y, Nishida M, Goto S, Kuwahara S. Immunoactive peptides, FK-156 and FK-565 II. Restoration of host resistance to microbial infection in immunosuppressed mice. *J Antibiotics* 1983 ; 36 : 1051-8.
34. Kusumi T, Yamada A, Cao M, Tanaka A, Takenada H, Imanishi J. Enhancing effects of immunoactive peptide FR 48217 on immunological responses to vaccination by inactivated influenza virus. *Vaccine* 1989 ; 7 : 351-6.
35. Yokota Y, Watanabe Y, Mine Y. Inhibitory effects of FK-565 alone and in combination with zidovudine on retroviral infection by Friend leukemia virus in mice. *J Antibiotics* 1988 ; 41 : 1479-87.
36. Izumi S, Nakahara K, Gotoh T, Hashimoto S, Kino T, Okuhara M, Aoki H, Imanaka H. Antitumor effects of novel immunoactive peptides, FK-156 and its synthetic derivatives. *J Antibiotics* 1983 : 36 : 566-74.
37. Talmadge JE, Chirigos MA. Comparison of immunomodulatory and immunotherapeutic properties of biological response modifiers. *Springer Semi Immunopathol* 1985 ; 8 : 429-40.
38. Talmadge JE, Lenz B, Schneider M, Phillips H, Long C. Immunomodulatory and therapeutics properties of FK-565 in mice. *Cancer Immunol Immunother* 1989 ; 28 : 93-100.
39. Mine Y, Watanabe Y, Wakai Y, Kikuchi H, Nakahara K, Aoki H, Wakamiya N, Ueda S, Kato S. Adjuvant effect of FK-565 on vaccinia virus-induced tumor-specific immunity. In : Ishigami J, ed. *Recent advances in chemotherapy*. Proceedings of the 14th International Congress of Chemotherapy. Tokyo : University Tokyo Press, 1985 : 953-4.
40. Braun V. Covalent lipoprotein from the outer membrane of *Escherichia coli*. *Biochem Biophys Acta* 1975 ; 415 : 335-77.
41. Bessler WG, Ottenbreit BP. Studies on the mitogenic principle of the lipoprotein from the outer membrane of *Escherichia coli*. *Biochem Biophys Res Commun* 1977 ; 76 : 239-46.
42. Bessler WG, Resh K, Hancock E, Hantke K. Induction of lymphocyte proliferation and membrane changes by lipopeptide derivates of the lipoprotein from the outer membrane of *Escherichia coli*. *Z. Immunitäts-forsch* 1977 ; 153 : 11-22.

43. Baschang G. Muramylpeptides and lipopeptides : studies towards immunostimulants. *Tetrahedron* 1989 ; 45 : 6331-60.
44. Jung G, Carrera C, Brückner H, Bessler WG. The mitogenic principle of *Escherichia coli* lipoprotein : synthesis, spectroscopic characterisation, and mitogenicity of N-Palmitoyl-S-[(2R,S)-2,3-dipalmitoyl-oxypropyl]-(R)-cysteine methyl ester. *Liebigs Ann Chem* 1983 : 1608-22.
45. Wiesmüller KH, Bessler W, Jung G. Synthesis of the mitogenic S-[2,3-Bis(palmitoyloxy)propyl]-Npalmitoyl-pentapeptide from *Escherichia coli* lipoprotein. *Hoppe-Seyler's Z Physiol Chem* 1983 ; 364 : 593-606.
46. Prass W, Ringsdorf H, Bessler W, Wiesmüller KH, Jung G. Lipopeptides of the N-terminus of *Escherichia coli* lipoprotein : synthesis, mitogenicity and properties in monolayer experiments. *Biochem Biophys Acta* 1987 ; 900 : 116-28.
47. Bessler WG, Cox M, Wiesmüller KH, Jung G. The mitogenic principle of *Escherichia coli* lipoprotein : B-lymphocyte mitogenicity of the synthetic analogue Palmitoyl-tetrapeptide (Pam-Ser-Ser-Asn-Ala). *Biochem Biophys Res Commun* 1984 ; 121 : 55-61.
48. Johnson RB, Kohl S, Wiesmüller K, Jung G, Bessler WG. Synthetic analogs of the N-terminal lipid part of bacterial lipoprotein are B-lymphocyte mitogens *in vitro* and *in vivo*. *Immunobiol* 1983 ; 165 : 27-35.
49. Bessler WG, Johnson RB, Wiesmüller K, Jung G. B-lymphocyte mitogenicity *in vitro* of a synthetic lipopeptide fragment derived from bacterial lipoprotein. *Hoppe-Seyler's Z Physiol Chem* 1982 ; 363 : 767-70.
50. Lex A, Wiesmüller KH, Jung G, Bessler WG. A synthetic analogue of *Escherichia coli* lipoprotein, tripalmitoyl pentapeptide, constitutes a potent immune adjuvant. *J Immunol* 1988 ; 137 : 2676-81.
51. Hoffmann P, Heinle S, Schade UF, Loppnow H, Ulmer AJ, Flad HD, Jung G, Bessler WG. Stimulation of human and murine adherent cells by bacterial lipoprotein and synthetic lipopeptide analogues. *Immunobiol* 1988 ; 177 : 158-70.
52. Reitermann A, Metzger J, Wiesmüller KH, Jung G, Bessler WG. Lipopeptide derivatives of bacterial lipoprotein constitute potent immune adjuvants combined with or covalently coupled to antigen or hapten. *Biol Chem Hoppe-Seyler* 1989 ; 370 : 343-52.
53. Muller CP, Bühring HJ, Becker G, Jung, G, Tröger W, Saalmüller A, Wiesmüller KH, Bessler WG. Specific antibody response towards predicted epitopes of the epidermal growth factor receptor induced by a thermostable synthetic peptide adjuvant conjugate. *Clin Exp Immunol* 1989 ; 78 : 499-504.
54. Bessler WG, Suhr B, Bühring HJ, Muller CP, Wiesmüller KH, Becker G, Jung G. Specific antibodies elicited by antigen covalently linked to a synthetic adjuvant. *Immunobiol* 1985 ; 170 : 239-44.
55. Hoffmann P, Wiesmüller KH, Metzger J, Jung G, Bessler WG. Induction of tumor cytotoxicity in murine bone marrow-derived macrophages by two lipopeptide analogues. *Biol Chem Hoppe-Seyler* 1989 ; 370 : 575-82.
56. Hauschildt S, Hoffmann P, Beuscher HU, Dufhues G, Heinrich P, Wiesmüller KH, Jung G, Bessler WG. Activation of bone marrow-derived mouse macrophages by bacterial lipopeptide : cytokine production, phagocytosis and Ia expression. *Eur J Immunol* 1990 ; 20 : 63-8.
57. Hauschildt S, Bassenge E, Bessler W, Busse R, Mülsch A. L-arginine-dependent nitric oxide formation and nitrite release in bone marrow-derived macrophages stimulated with bacterial lipopeptide and lipopolysaccharide. *Immunology* 1990 : 70 : 332-7.
58. Seifert R, Schultz G, Richter-Freund M, Metzger J, Wiesmüller KH, Jung G, Bessler WG, Hauschildt S. Activation of superoxide formation and lysozyme release in human neutrophils by the synthetic lipopeptide Pam_3-Cys-Ser-$(Lys)_4$. *Biochem* 1990 ; 267 : 795-802.
59. Steffens U, Bessler W, Hauschildt S. B cell-activation by synthetic lipopeptide analogues of bacterial lipoprotein bypassing phosphatidylinositol metabolism and proteinkinase C translocation. *Mol Immunol* 1989 ; 26 : 897-904.

60. Hauschildt S, Wolf B, Lückhoff A, Bessler WG. Determination of second messengers and protein kinase C in bone marrow derived macrophages stimulated with a bacterial lipopeptide. *Mol Immunol* 1990 ; 27 : 473-9.
61. Offermanns S, Seifert R, Metzger JW, Jung G, Lieberknecht A, Schmidt U, Schultz G. Lipopeptides are effective stimulators of tyrosine phosphorylation in human myeloid cells. *Biochem J* 1992 ; 282 : 551-7.
62. Uhl B, Wolf B, Schwinde A, Metzger J, Jung G, Bessler WG, Hauschildt S. Intracellular localization of a lipopeptide macrophage activator : immunocytochemical investigations and EELS analysis on ultrathin cryosections of bone marrow-derived macrophages. *J Leukocyte Biol* 1991 ; 50 : 10-8.
63. Wolf B, Hauschildt S, Uhl B, Metzger J, Jung G, Bessler WG. Localization of the cell activator lipopeptide in bone marrow-derived macrophages by electron energy loss spectroscopy (EELS). *Immunol Lett* 1989 ; 20 : 121-6.
64. Schlecht S, Wiesmüller KH, Jung G, Bessler WG. Enhancement of protection against Salmonella infection in mice mediated by a synthetic lipopeptide analogue of bacterial lipoprotein in *S. typhimurium* vaccines. *Int J Med Microbiol* 1989 ; 271 : 493-500.
65. Wiesmüller KH, Jung G, Hess G. Novel low-molecular-weight synthetic vaccine against foot-and-mouth disease containing a potent B cell and macrophage activator. *Vaccine* 1989 ; 29-33.
66. Deres K, Schild H, Wiesmüller KH, Jung G, Rammensee HG. In vivo priming of virus-specific cytotoxic T lymphocytes with synthetic lipopeptide vaccine. *Nature* 1989 ; 342 : 561-4.
67. Bessler WG, Jung G. Synthetic lipopeptides as novel adjuvants. *Res Immunol* 1992 : 143 : 548-53.

9

The immunomodulating and therapeutic properties of AS101

B. SREDNI, M. ALBECK, Y. KALECHMAN

CAIR Institute, Department of Life Sciences,
Bar-Ilan University, Ramat Gan, 59200 Israel.

Product

Historical background

There has been growing interest in the potential of synthetic compounds to modify immune responses by imitation of cytokine action. The restorative properties of immunomodulators spring from their ability to induce the differentiation and proliferation of particular groups of cells. In cancer patients, immunotherapy is one of a variety of modalities proposed to either prevent or eliminate tumor metastases. The administration of various naturally occurring or synthetic biological response modifiers has been shown to enhance host immune reactivity and to elicit antitumor activity. However, the maximum tolerated dose of biological response modifiers, such as gamma-interferon (γ-IFN) and interleukin-2 (IL-2), is lower than the dose required to exhibit maximum biological activity.

Developing strategies to overcome the toxicity of biological response modifiers and, alternatively, developing and characterizing new agents that do not exhibit such side effects, could greatly improve the prospects for the use of immunotherapy in treating human patients.

We have developed a new synthetic compound, AS101, which is a low molecular weight organic tellurate compound soluble in organic solvents but only slightly soluble in water. Its development was based on the similarity in chemical configuration to the anti-tumor agent dichloroethylene diamineplatinum (cisplatin). The platinum atom has been replaced with tellurium, an element from the sixth group of the periodical table of elements (oxygen, sulfur, sellenium and tellurium), the first three of which have been reported to show immunomodulatory activity. Of the series of compounds which were synthesized and screened for their ability to stimulate proliferation and lymphokine production by lymphoid cells, only some of the tellurium compounds were active. The coumpound with the highest activity, ammonium trichloro (dioxoethylene-O,O')tellurate (coded AS 101), was chosen for continued studies *in vivo* and *in vitro*.

This review describes the marked immunomodulatory properties exhibited by AS101, its therapeutic potential in various immunological disorders in animal models, its minimal toxicity and the clinical trials on cancer and AIDS patients conducted in view of these properties.

Chemical properties of AS101

AS101 is prepared by refluxing TeCl4 with ethylene glycol in acetonitrile or by heating (80 °C) TeCl4 with NH_4Cl in ethylene glycol as solvent [1].

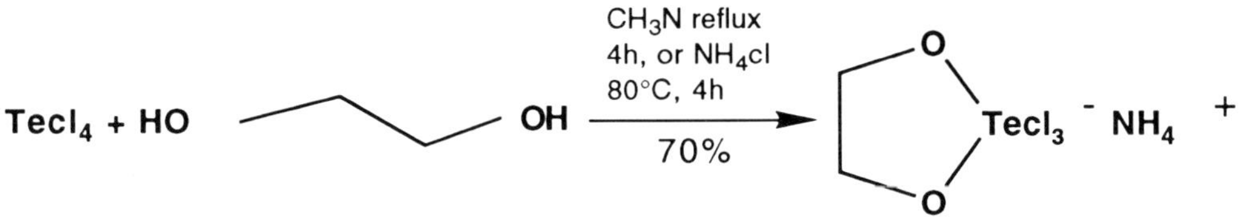

$TeCl_4$ + HO—CH$_2$CH$_2$—OH $\xrightarrow[70\%]{\substack{CH_3N\ reflux \\ 4h,\ or\ NH_4Cl \\ 80°C,\ 4h}}$ [dioxolane-$TeCl_3$]$^-$ NH_4^+

Replacing NH_4Cl by KCl (but not NaCl) results in the potassium salt of AS101. Refluxing $TeCl_4$ with ethylene glycol in benzene gives dichloro (dioxyethylene0'-0)tellurium (II) (AS103) which also exhibits immunomodulating properties. Other telluriums (III) (AS102) as well as some derivatives of higher homology of the ethylene glycol moiety in this series were found to have similar activity (Figure 1).

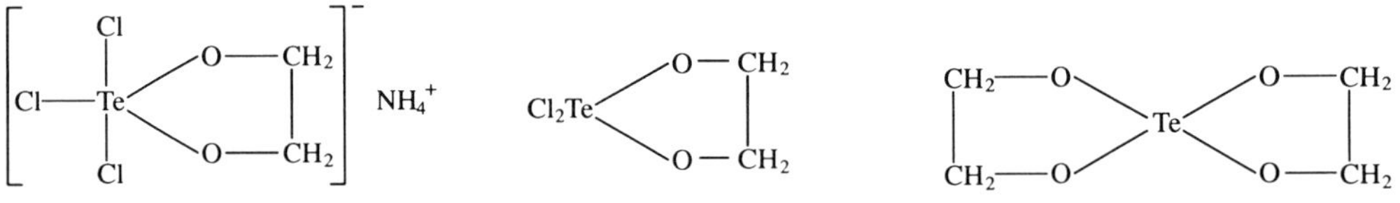

(I) AS101   (II) AS103   (III) AS102

Figure 1. Chemical structure of compounds.

Compounds such as diphenyltelluriumdichloride, triphenyltelluriumchloride and many other organotellurium compounds tested by us, did not express this property.

AS101 is a white crystalline solid soluble in DMSO and very slightly soluble in water. Its melting point is 234 °C (d), HNMR, d = 4.39 (5,4 H), 7.1 9 (t, 4H). AS102 and AS103 are white amorphous powders. AS102 is insoluble in most organic solvent. MP = 210 °C (d). HNMR, d = 4.45 (S, 4H). All three compounds have very good shelf life time (years in closed bottles).

Experimental and preclinical studies

Toxicology

Toxicological effects of AS101 were studied by administration of the compound intraperitoneally to rats for a period of 4 weeks [2]. Detailed clinical, clinicopathological and pathological studies were carried out in groups of rats treated with increasing concentrations of AS101. The highest concentration administered to the rats was about 120 times that of the proposed therapeutic dose for humans. The doses ranged from 3 to 24 mg/kg/week. Clinical signs relating to treatment with AS101 were darkening of the eyes, dark colored urine, hind limb paresis and paraphimosis. A garlic odor pervaded the room where the experiment was performed. Tellurium is methylated in the liver and removed from the body in the form of garlic smelling compounds like dimethyl telluride. This explains the aliceous smell in the animal room. The effect of AS101 on hematological parameters was demonstrated in the high dosage groups of both sexes, although the female dose groups appear to have been more adversely affected.

Effects noted included decreases in pack cell volume (PCV), hemoglobin concentration (Hb), erythrocyte counts and thrombocyte numbers. These declines were seen in female rats receiving 12 and 24 mg/k/week of AS101. A decrease in the above parameters was also evident in the male group, however, statistical significance was not achieved. An increased corpuscular volume (MC/I) was evident in the two higher-dose female groups. The immaturity of the erythrocytes was borne out by the increased reticulocyte count in both these groups.

An increased leukocyte count in the female dose group receiving 24 mg/kg/week of AS101 was accompanied by a concomitant increase in eosinophil numbers.

Clinical chemistry assays revealed that the effects of the compound noted on liver enzymes were almost exclusively related to the female group receiving 241 mg/kg/week of AS101. These included increases in activity of the enzymes alanine amino transferase and aspartate aminotransferases and gammaglutamyltransferase. Plasma alkaline phosphatase activity was increased in a number of female rats of the high dose group but was not of statistical significance. Decreased concentrations of plasma albumin were detected in the female high dose group. In the male dose groups receiving 24 mg/kg/week AS101 the only change relating to the liver was a significant increase in the activity of plasma gamma-glutamyl transferase. Changes in the electrophoretic pattern were evident in a treatment-related increase in the betta-globulin fraction in both sexes receiving 24 mg/kg/week.

Lesions observed sporadically in rats receiving 24 mg/kg/week of AS101 were replacement of the marrow cavity with hard tissue, reduction in size of the thymus, enlarged spleen, reduction in the quantity of the abdominal fat pads.

A high incidence of retinal degeneration and atrophy was seen in rats receiving 12 and 24 mg/kg/week of AS101. AS101 appeared to be initially toxic to the photoreceptor layer. A dose related degeneration of the outer retinal layers was observed in the groups of rats treated with 12 and 24 mg/kg/week.

In the liver, a dose-related increase in hepatocytic fatty vacuolation was apparent.

In conclusion, i.p. injection of rats with AS101 elicited a spectrum of toxicological effects, which in a number of instances have been documented in the literature and appear to be directly related to tellurium poisoning. Novel findings were ocular pathological changes and bone marrow changes accompanied by thrombocyte count reductions. In general the changes were limited to those rats receiving 12 and 24 mg/kg/week of AS101.

The therapeutic dose for man for AS101 has been proposed as 0.2 mg/kg/week. The toxicological changes elicited in rats were seen at doses of 60 and 120 times the therapeutic level. At the present time no severe adverse toxicological effects have been seen in man in the course of the clinical trials carried out.

Pharmacokinetic studies

The tissue levels of tellurium following administration of AS101 to mice was estimated on an atomic absorption spectrophotometer using a method developed for the identification of samples with low tellurium content [3]. This procedure involves the use of platinum as a chemical modifier to thermally stabilize tellurium in order to prevent the high volatility of the metal.

The parmacokinetic studies were conducted on male CBA mice (20-25 g) injected i.v. with 1.25 mg/kg of AS101 and placed in metabolism cages to collect urine. On day 4, mice were anesthetized and blood collected into heparinized tubes from the severed axillary vessels. Plasma was isolated; livers and kidneys were removed, rinsed, blotted dry and stored at $-20\,°C$ until processed for tellurium content.

Excretion of AS101 in mice amounted to 18 % of the administered i.v. dose in the first 24 hours. Levels of tellurium were undetectable in urine collected on subsequent days. Plasma, liver, and kidney of mice also had detectable levels of tellurium on day 4 post administration of AS101 (16.7 + 6.1 ; 249 + 24 ; 556 + 148 ng/g of tellurium, respectively). Urine and kidney had the highest tellurim concentration (555 + 147 ng/ml and 556 + 148 ng/g of tellurium, respectively).

The binding of AS101 to plasma *in vitro* was also studied. Human plasma was incubated at 37 °C with AS101 at a final concentration of 464 ng/ml (190 ng Te/ml). At selected time points, ultrafiltrates were obtained for tellurium determination. A separate aliquot was added to cold trichloro acetic acid (TCA) and subjectd to 12,000 g centrifugation. The resulting supernatants were analyzed for tellurium content. The data indicates that there is significant plasma protein binding of AS101 which is released on addition to TCA. Irreversible binding also occurs as evidenced by the monoexponential decay of tellurium in both plasma ultrafiltrates and plasma-TCA supernatants. The half life of this decay is 49.5 hours for the UF curve and 43.3 hours for the TCA curve.

Repeated administration of AS101 may result in changes in the pharmacokinetics of the drug. We therefore studied the pharmacology of Te in Beagle dogs receiving chronic administration of 0.5 mg/kg of AS101 as a short i.v. infusion 3 times a week for 3 or 6 months [4]. The levels were measured by flameless atomic absorption spectroscopy. Plasma pharmacokinetics of Te did not differ in dogs that had been dosed for either 3 or 6 months. Te levels in plasma decayed in a biphasic manner with half-lives of 27 ± 10 min and 138 ± 56 h for the initial and terminal phase respectively. Total clearance of the drug was 8 ± 2 ml/h/kg and the volume of distribution at steady state was 1.5 ± 0.6 % 1/kg. Urinary excretion in 72 h was 25 ± 6 %. Tissues from dogs sacrificed 72 h after the last dose indicated that the kidney had one of the highest concentrations (42 µlg/g at 3 months and 51 µg/g at 6 months). Lower concentrations were found in the heart (4.8 and 13.4), spleen (2.2 and 2.7), liver (1.0 and 1.4), and lung (0.37 and 0.51). Thus, only in the heart were Te levels grossly higher at 6 months compared to those at 3 months. In conclusion, it was found that after chronic administration of AS101 in dogs, Te is extensively bound to tissue and slowly excreted from the body.

Immunomodulating properties and mechanism of action

- **In vivo** *studies*

After showing the ability of AS101 to induce cell proliferation and cytokine secretion *in vitro* by both human and mouse cells, we tested the effects of *in vivo* administration of the compound [5, 6]. Groups of normal Balb/c mice were treated systemically with AS101 at 10 µg/animal, administered either as a single injection or as a continuous treatment of twice-weekly injections for 2 months. AS101 was able to induce IL-2 receptor expression on approximately 40 % of the spleen cells when administered as a continuous treatment, but not as a single dose. On the other hand, a single dose of 10 µg of AS101 injected into Balb/c mice caused a significant augmentation of IL-2 and colony stimulating factor (CSF) production in splenocytes explanted into culture and treated with mitogen. Maximal IL-2 production was obtained on day 1 and 3 post-injection, whereas for CSF activity, two separate peaks were observed on days 1 and 5. These two peaks represented the secretion of two different colony-stimulating factors, the first predominantly macrophage CSF (M-CSF) and the second maily granulocyte/macrophage CSF (GM-CSF) (Figure 2).

These studies were all conducted on normal mice. Numerous other *in vivo* studies were performed on mice subjected to various treatments or on mice with immunological disorders. These will be presented in the next section.

- **In vitro** *studies*

— **Animal cells** : AS101 was found to stimulate mouse spleen cells to proliferate and to produce lymphokines such as interleukin-2, (IL-2), and colony stimulating factor (CSF), which are regulators of lymphopoiesis and myelopoiesis [5, 6]. AS101 at 0.05-1 µg/ml induced optimal CSF production by mouse spleen cells, and optimal IL-2 production was found at 0.1-0.5 µg/ml AS101. The ability of AS101 to stimulate the secretion of CSF was not restricted to spleen cells. Much higher levels of CSF were secreted by bone marrow cells stimulated by AS101 [7]. The levels of CSF secreted by 0.5×10^6 BM cells were three times higher than the levels secreted by 5×10^6 spleen cells/ml. AS101 was also able to induce the secretion of interleukin-1 (IL-1). The secretion of IL-1 was analyzed in peritoneal exudate cells from Balb/c and C3H-HeJ mice injected with thioglycolate. AS101 at 0.5 µg/ml induced the secretion *in vitro* of very large amounts of IL-1 from both Balb/c and C3H/HeJ peritoneal exudate cells (PEC). At this concentration, IL-1 secretion was more than double that obtained after stimulation with LPS [7]. The LPS contamination of the substance was established by a Limulus assay and shown to contain less than 2 u/ml both in the AS101 preparation and in the peritoneal exudate-conditioned medium. The effect of AS101 induced supernatants could be ablated

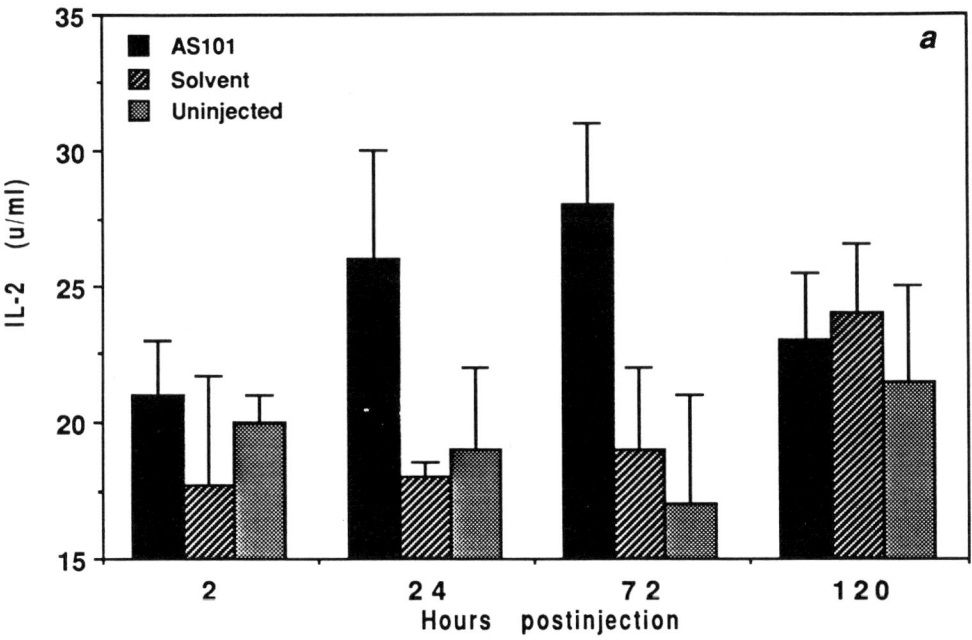
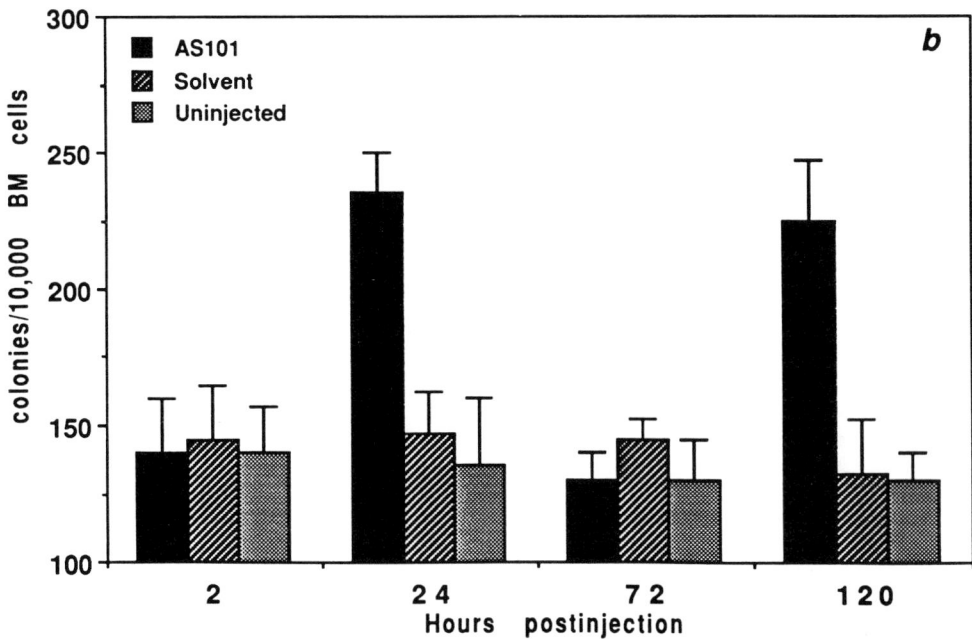

Figure 2. Effect of *in vivo* treatment with AS101 on subsequent *in vitro* lymphokine production by mouse spleen cells. Fifteen male Balb/c mice were injected once with 10 μg AS101/animal. Fifteen animals were sacrificed at each of the indicated times, and production of IL-2 (a) and CSF (b) by Con A-Stimulated pooled splenocytes was assayed in comparison to PBS injected mice.

by anti-IL1 antibodies. The effect of AS101 on macrophages was also demonstrated by the ability of the compound to stimulate mouse PEC cells, isolated by peritoneal puncture 72 h after i.p. thioglycolate injection, to secrete tumor necrosis factor (TNF) [8] (Table I).

Table I. Cytokine secretion by mouse cells stimulated by AS101.

AS101 µg/ml	IL-2 production u/ml	CSF production by spleen cells (colonies/10⁵ cells)	CSF production by BM cells (colonies/10⁵ cells)	IL-1 production by PEC cells (u/ml)	TNF production by PEC cells (u/ml)
1.0	4.0 ± 0.3	2.0 ± 0.1	36 ± 2	–	–
0.5	9.0 ± 2.0	2.0 ± 0.1	78 ± 6	22 ± 3	6 ± 0.5
0.1	12.0 ± 2.0	35.0 ± 3.7	102 ± 6	9 ± 2	3 ± 0.3
0.05	4.0 ± 0.3	38.0 ± 3.2	20 ± 2	–	–
0.01	0.5 ± 0.1	15.0 ± 2.0	0	–	–

Mice spleen cells or adherent PEC cells were incubated with various concentrations of AS101 for 24 hours. The supernatants were tested by biological assays for cytokines content.

— **Human cells**

(a) **Cytokine secretion**: AS101 can stimulate normal human mononuclear cells (MNC) to express IL-2 receptors, to produce IL-2 and to proliferate [5, 6]. Various concentrations of AS101 were tested in parallel for induction of all three functions. Concentrations of 0.1-0.5 µg/ml were found to be optimal. Proliferation was measured directly by incorporation of 3H-TdR into DNA. IL-2 production was assayed by proliferation of an IL-2 dependent cloned murine CTLL line. Induction of IL-2 receptors was measured by acquisition of responsiveness to exogenously supplied IL-2. Using another assay, approximately 25 % MNC from normal donors stained positively with monoclonal anti-IL-2 receptor antibodies after culture with 0.5 µg/ml of AS101 for 48 h, compared to only 2 % of cells incubated in medium alone (Table II).

Table II. Cytokine secretion and induction of IL-2 receptors by human cells stimulated by AS101.

AS101 µg/ml	IL-2 production u/ml	IL-1 production by PEC cells u/ml	TNF production by MNC u/ml	γ-IFN production by MNC u/ml	Induction of IL-2R (stimulation index)
1	1.8 ± 0.4	1 ± 0.5	–	–	7.0 ± 1.5
0.5	12.2 ± 5.3	13 ± 2	5.5 ± 1	37.5 ± 7.5	35.7 ± 8.6
0.1	14.3 ± 4.6	21 ± 3	2.0 ± 0.3	032.9 ±	12.9
0.05	1.1 ± 0.2	6 ± 2	–	–	2.9 ± 1.4
0.01	1.5 ± 0.4	1 ± 0.4	–	–	1.1 ± 0.3

Human MNC or adherent PEC cells were incubated with various concentrations of AS101 for 24 hours. The supernatants were tested by biological assays for cytokine content. Expression of functional IL-2 receptors was assayed by responsiveness to IL-2 of MNC incubated for 24 hours with the indicated concentrations of AS101.

AS101 has also the ability to stimulate human MNC to secrete γ-IFN and TNF when incubated with the cells for 96 h [8]. The secretion of these factors can be raised significantly when a PKC-inducer is inserted into the cultures with AS101 (see Mechanism of action). Since stimulation by AS101 was shown not to be restricted to lymphoid cells, we tested whether AS101 could also induce macrophages to secrete IL-1. For this purpose, we used peritoneal exudate cells obtained from end stage renal disease patients treated by peritoneal dialysis. Adherent cells were cultured with AS101 for 6 h and IL-1 was secreted by those cells in a dose dependent manner. It has been postulated in animal models that IL-2 and γ-IFN are secreted by a subpopulation of T helper cells named TH1 [9]. Although this subpopulation has not been identified in humans, the stimulation by AS101 of IL-2 and γ-IFN secretion by human MNC could be attributed to the activation of a selected helper subpopulation. When MNC were obtained from AIDS patients, AS101 was found to directly enhance the ratio of CD4 to CD8 positive cells *in vitro* as determined by immunocytofluorometry. After culture for 48 h with 1 µg/ml of AS101, the percentage of CD4 positive cells rose from the mean basal level of 24 to 42, the percent of CD8 positive cells remaining at the basal level of 39. MNC incubated in control medium remained at basal values, *i.e.* 87-88.

(b) **Inhibition of the reverse transcriptase activity and replication of human HIV type I by AS101** *in vitro*: Human immunodeficiency virus type I (HIV-I), the etiologic agent of acquired immune deficiency syndrome (AIDS), is a human lymphotropic retrovirus, cytopathic for helper/inducer T cells. HIV-I, similar to other retroviruses, requires virion-associated reverse transcriptase (RT) for replication of the virus and production of infectious viral particles. Thus, a therapy that interferes with RT activity might decrease the production of infectious virus and limit or prevent disease.

In an attempt to study whether AS101 has defined antiviral activity, the inhibitory effect of AS101 on the growth of HIV-I *in vitro* was investigated. Furthermore, in an attempt to identify biochemically the nature of the inhibitory activity, the extent of inhibition of RT was studied using purified recombinant HIV-I RT. The inhibitory effect of AS101 was studied on the different catalytic functions associated with HIV-I RT, namely RNA dependent DNA polymerase (RDDP), DNA dependent DNA polymerase (DDDP) and Ribonuclease H (RNase H) activities [10].

AS101 suppressed the production of HIV-I by PMNC under continuous-inhibition conditions. Treatment with increased concentrations of AS101, *i.e.* 0.1, 0.5, 1.0 and 5.0 µg/ml for 14 days, yielded 44, 58, 62 and 81 percent inhibition respectively (Figure 3). AS101 had no effect on PMNC viability, growth or morphology in this culture system. In AS101-treated cultures, maximal RT activity was achieved after 11 days post-infection while untreated infected cells continued to release viral particles to the culture medium, as was demonstrated by the increasing RT activity. To assume the reliability of the exogenous reaction for RT and to rule out non-specific inhibition of the reaction, different concentrations of AS101 were added to all free supernatants containing HIV-I prior to virus concentration. Following incubation for 1 hour at 4 °C and ultracentrifugation, RT activity was determined on viral pellets. The specificity and reliability of RT were confirmed and rated out the possibility of non-specific inhibition of RT reaction by the tested compounds. The antiviral effects of AS101 were confirmed in another viral assay which tests the expression of HIV-I antigens in treated culture fluids by ELISA. In fresh peripheral blood lymphocyte cultures infected with HIV-I and treated for 7 days, AS101 inhibited viral protein production by 85 % at 10 µg/ml.

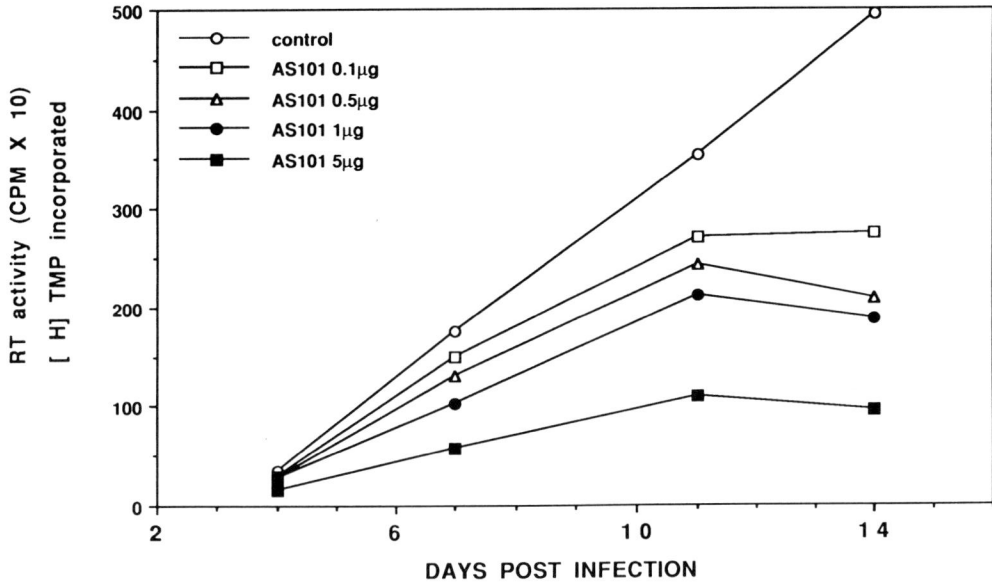

Figure 3. Inhibition of reverse transcriptase activity by AS101. Three days old PHA stimulated MNC were infected with HIV-1 and cultivated in medium containing various concentrations of AS101. The activity of RT in pelleted and disrupted virus from culture supernatants was measured after 4, 7, 11 and 14 days.

In assays determining the inhibitory effects of AS101 on RT-associated activities, it was found that RDDP activity was impaired by 90 % of its initial activity in the presence of 10 μg/ml of AS101. The calculated IC50 value for AS101 was 1 μg/ml. Inhibition of DDDP activity by AS101 was similar to that shown for RDDP activity. The calculated IC50 value was 1.8 μg/ml. AS101 inhibited RNase activity with IC50 value of 10 μg/ml.

The anti-HIV-I activity of AS101 reflected by inhibition of virus replication and by inhibition of the different catalytic functions associated with the viral RT, in the absence of drug-related toxicity to lymphocytes, strongly argues for its evaluation as a therapeutic agent for patients with AIDS-related complex or AIDS.

(c) **Immunoregulation *in vitro* of mononuclear cells from SLE patients** : Diverse alterations in the numbers and functions of immunoregulatory T cells have been documented in connective tissue diseases : they include imbalance in the percentage of T cell subpopulations, deficient T cell suppressor function, abnormal kinetics of the autologous mixed lymphocyte reactions and abnormalities in NK cell activity. Some of the changes could be attributed to decreased IL-2 activity which in systemic lupus erythromatosus (SLE) may be a cardinal immunoregulatory aberration. Current treatments for SLE use corticosteroids and/or immunosuppressors : they do not address the specific immunoregulatory disturbances that are involved but are directed at reducing the polyclonal activation of B cells.

When MNC from SLE patients were treated *in vitro* with AS101, it was found that AS101 increased the production of IL-2 by cells from both SLE patients and healthy controls, it raised the percentage of cells bearing IL-2 receptor from 2.1 ± 1.3 to 16.4 ± 4.5 in unstimulated T cells and from 26.1 ± 9.4 to 31.1 ± 8.6 in PHA-stimulated T cells from SLE patients. AS101 also improved the suppressor function of SLE patients' T cells by as much as two-fold while having little effect on the suppressor function of normal cells [11].

- *Mechanism of action*

The mechanism of action of AS101 in triggering lymphocyte stimulation resembles that of many other lymphocyte activators. Incubation of mouse splenocytes with AS101 triggers a rapid 2.5 fold increases in intracellular Ca^{2+}, as measured by the quin-2 acetoxymethyl ester assay [5]. In order to elucidate further the role of Ca^{2+} in the activation and IL-2 secretion of cells stimulated with AS101, we investigated the effect of EGTA (a chelator of extracellular Ca^{2+}), nifedipine (the Ca^{2+} channel blocker), and cyclosporin A (which selectively inhibits Ca^{2+} activated steps in the lymphocyte activation process). We found that these compounds inhibited both processes in a dose dependent manner [12].

It is now well known that antigen- and mitogen-mediated lymphocyte activation is correlated with the induction of Ca^{2+} influx and the activation of protein kinase C (PKC) [13]. At present, it is generally accepted that PKC is the cellular target for phorbol myristate acetate (PMA). These data led us to postulate that PMA [14] and AS101 might exert cumulative, perhaps synergistic effects on mouse spleen cells or human MNC, and that this could result in overt enhancement of lymphokine secretion and cell proliferation. It was found that significant enhacement of IL-2 secretion and cell proliferation of both human and mouse cells can be obtained by the synergistic effect of AS101 and the tumor promoter PMA. Co-operation between the two compounds also resulted in enhanced CSF production by mouse spleen cells. PMA alone induced proliferation of human MNC at high concentrations, while the same concentration of PMA did not affect IL-2 secretion. On the other hand, AS101 induced both IL-2 secretion and cell proliferation although its effect could be impressively elevated by cooperation with PMA. The effects of AS101 were compared with those of the calcium ionophore, A23187 (two structurally distinct compounds) on IL-2 and CSF secretion as well as on cell proliferation. The comparison was made when these compounds were inserted into the cultures either alone or in combination with PMA. An overt synergistic effect was evident when mouse spleen cells or human MNC were stimulated with either A23187 or AS101 in conjunction with PMA. The mechanism of action of AS101 is summarised in Figure 4. Recently, we have performed similar experiments with partially purified preparations of bryostatins, a group of natural compounds extracted from the phylum *Bryozoa*. These compounds are known to be nontumor promoting activators of PKC. We found evidence for a synergistic effect of the two compounds on the proliferation rate and the secretion of various cytokines such as IL-2, TNF, γ-IFN by either mouse cells or human MNC [8].

Since AS101 has been shown to possess multipotential stiumulatory activities, and to exhibit low toxicity, and bryostatin, in contrast to the phorbol ester PMA, has been shown to have no tumor promoting activity, we believe that a combined treatment with the two agents might increase the endogenous production of cytokines,

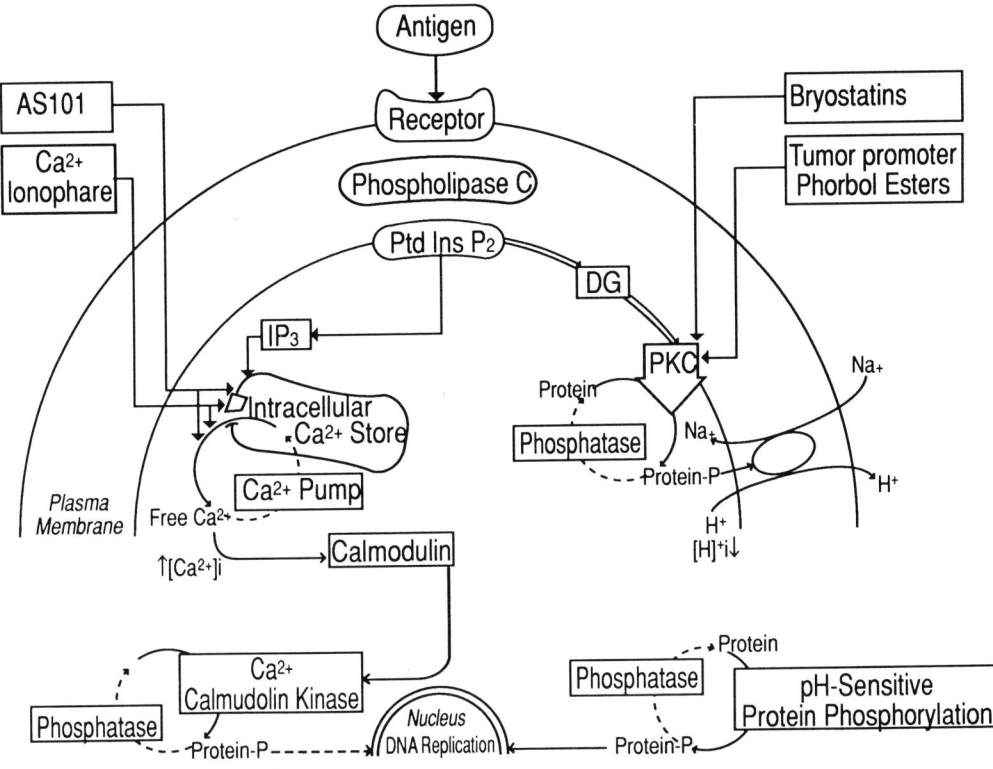

Figure 4. Mechanism of T cell stimulation by AS101.

thus improving the restoration of immune responses in conditions involving immune suppression.

Therapeutic effects on animal models with immunological disorders

• *Infections* : The immunoenhancing properties of AS101, especially the ability to stimulate the secretion of IL-2 and γ-IFN, prompted us to test the effects of the compound in *in vivo* models of viral infections. As IL-2 and IFN can activate natural killer (NK) cells to lyze viral infected cells, it could be hypothesized that this agent can exert an antiviral effect *via* induction of these cytokines.

Two models of mouse viral infection were chosen. In the first model, mice were infected with WestNile virus (WNV) which causes fatal damage to the central nervous system. The animals were treated with 10 μg/mouse of AS101 on day 1 and day 6 post-infection. The viability was recorded on day 8 post-infection, when no unprotected mice survived. AS101 could protect 60 % of the infected animals [6] (Table III).

In the second model, adoptive transfer of immune spleen cells was used to treat murine cytomegalovirus (MCMV) infected mice. In this model, mice are rendered more susceptible to MCMV infection by injection of cyclophosphamide, their mortality rate reaching 90-100 %. These mice can be protected by adoptive transfer of immune spleen cells from mice immunized with a sublethal dose of murine CMV. In this study we investigated the protective efficacy of adoptive transfer of immune spleen cells from mice treated *in vivo* with AS101 and a sublethal dose of MCMV. We found that this mode of treatment increases the rate of survival of infected mice to 80 % whereas only 25 % of mice treated with immune spleen cells from control mice survived (Table III).

Table III. Protection of viral-infected mice by AS101.

	West Nile virus			Murine cytomegalovirus	
Experiment No.	% survival		Experiment No.	% survival of infected mice, treated by passive transfer of :	
	PBS control	AS101 treated		PBS immunized spleen cells	AS101 treated immunized spleen cells
[1]	0	60	[1]	23	80
[2]	0	60	[2]	25	75

Mice were injected i.p. with 10³ LD50 of WNV. They were injected with AS101 on day 1 and 6 post-infection. Survival was recorded on day 8 postinfection when no unprotected mice were surviving. Two groups of mice were immunized with a sublethal dose of murine CMV and in addition one of the groups received i.p. injection of 20 119 AS101/injection on day 1,4,7,14. Thirteen days after the last AS101 injection, MCMV immunized mice were challenged with MCMV alone or MCMV + AS101. Spleen cells transfers were carried out 4 days after the second virus injection. They were transferred to mice treated with 250 mg/kg CTX and MCMV.

- *Tumor models*

Recent reports have demonstrated that manipulation of the immune system with various cytokines can mediate the regression of advanced metastatic cancer in mice and in humans. Despite encouraging results that seem to indicate the potential importance of this form of therapy, it has not yet been widely adapted. The main reason for this are the severe toxicities associated with high doses of cytokines used for treatment [15, 16]. The identification of AS101 as a new agent that does not exhibit serious side effects prompted us to investigate the effect of systemic administration of AS101 to tumor bearing mice.

Experiments were performed using three animal models.

(a) A model of Balb/c mice transplanted with a primary methylcholantrene-induced fibrosarcoma from balb/c strain. When the tumors were palpable, the animals were given 1 or 2 injections of 10 µg/animal of AS101. Tumor volumes were measured 13 days after transfer. We found that the volume of the tumor in untreated animals was 3-8 fold larger than in those treated with 10 µg of AS101 [6] (Table IV).

(b) A model of C57Bl mice transplanted with 3LL cells (Lewis lung carcinoma) into one hind footpad. When the tumors were palpable, the tumor-bearing footpads were amputated and twice weekly i.p. injections of AS101 or PBS were started. Survival of mice bearing metastases of Lewis lung carcinoma was followed for

Table IV. Therapeutic effects of AS101 in tumor models.

Methyl cholanthrene-induced fibrosarcoma			Lewis lung carcinoma		
Group	Number of treatments	Mean volume of tumor (cm² ± SD)	Weeks after amputation	PBS	% survival AS101 treated
1	0	3.9 ± 0.2	4	80	100
2	1	1.2 ± 0.4	5	80	100
3	2	0.5 ± 0.2	6	20	100
			8	20	80
			10	0	80
			12	0	60
			14	0	60

Mice were injected with methyl-cholanthrene-induced fibrosarcoma cells. When tumors were palpable, the animals were given 1 or 2 injections of AS101, 2 days apart. Tumors volumes were measured 13 days after transfer. Each group consisted of 30 mice. C57Bl mice (groups of 12) were injected with 3LL cells into one hind foodpad. On day 12 the tumor bearing foodpads were amputated and AS101 or PBS were injected twice weekly.

3 months and was significantly higher in the treated group than in the control group [5] (Table IV).

(c) A model of Balb/c mice transplanted i.p. with Madison lung carcinoma tumor cells. Based on our results on the chemoprotective properties of AS101 (see Chemotherapy), we wanted to examine whether AS101 could protect and enhance the impact of chemotherapy in this tumor model. Mice were treated with 250 mg/kg cyclophosphamide 12 days after tumor implantation. AS101 at 10 µg/mouse was given i.p. 3 times weekly, starting 1 day after tumor implantation. It was found that when mice were treated with cyclophosphamide at a dose of 250 mg/kg, their rate of survival was lower than that of control untreated mice. However, the combination of AS101 and CTX at that concentration increased the percentage of survival from 12.5 % to 87.5 % 43 days after tumor implantation [17] (Figure 5).

- *Autoimmunity*

Recently, an experimental model in which SLE was induced in mice by immunizing them with a pathogenic idiotype of human anti-DNA antibody 16/6 Id has been described. In preliminary studies it was noted that the production of IL-2 in the mice with induced SLE was diminished. Thus, the influence of IL2 production on the pathogenecity of SLE could be evaluated. This led us to consider treatment of mice with experimental SLE with the immunomodulator AS101 and to attempt to establish whether improved IL-2 production following treatment may have therapeutic effects on the course of the disease. It was found that 3 months after immunization with the anti-DNA idiotype (16/6 + Id) the ability of splenocytes to secrete IL-2 had decreased by 50 % and after 5 months by 75 %. Treatment of the SLE mice with AS101, every second day for 7 weeks, restored the ability of the splenocytes to secrete IL-2. Splenocytes derived from mice after 3 months of treated SLE had restored their ability to secrete IL-2 to normal levels, while splenocytes derived from 5 months of treated SLE, restored their ability to 83 % of normal control levels [18] (Table V).

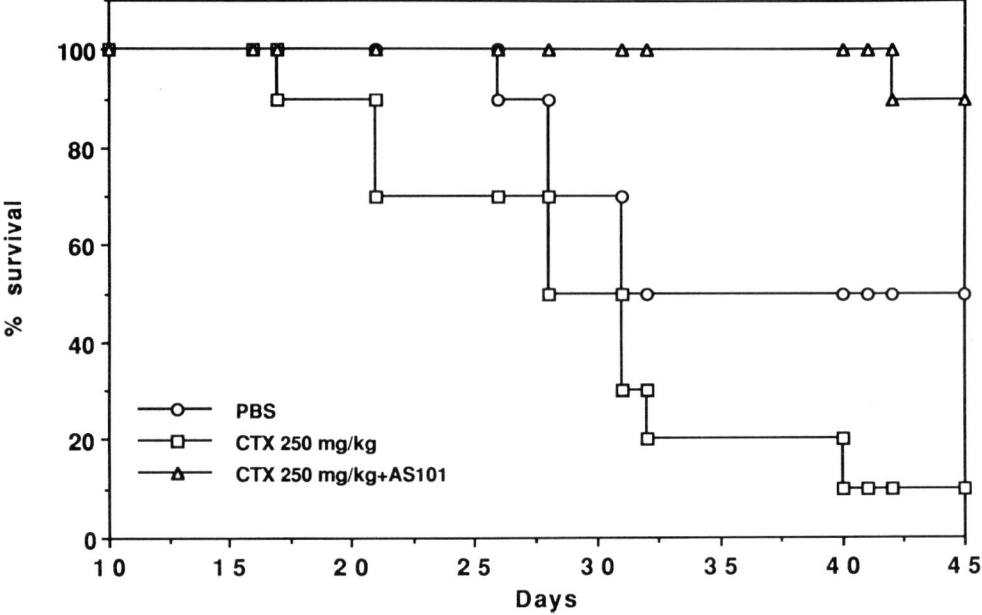

Figure 5. Effect of AS101 treatment with CTX on survival of tumor bearing mice. Mice were implanted I.P. with Madison lung carcinoma tumor cells and treated 12 days later with 250 mg/kg cyclophosphamide. AS101 at 1 011g/mouse was given i.p. 3 times weekly, starting one day after tumor implantation. The experiment included 20 mice/group.

Table V. Effect of AS101 treatment on IL-2 secretion by splenocytes from SLE mice.

Treatment in vivo	IL-2 production (u/ml)		
	Control mice	SLE mice after 3 months	SLE mice after 5 months
None	14.5 ± 2	7.0 ± 2	3.8 ± 1
AS101	ND	15.5 ± 3	12.0 ± 2

Mice in which SLE had been induced were killed 3 and 5 months after induction of the disease and subsequent to a 7 week treatment with AS101.

The expression of Tac antigen on splenocytes from 3 and 5 months after induction of SLE and treatment with AS101 was studied using anti-Tac antibody. It was found that treatment with AS101 augmented the number of Tac positive cells by more than 50 % both 3 and 5 months after disease induction and AS101 treatment.

Treatment of mice with AS101 injected into mice every second day for 7 weeks, did not affect the titres of autoantibodies in the sera of the mice, recorded 3 months after SLE induction. Elevated levels of antibodies to DNA, histones, cardiolipin Sm, RNP, SS-A (PO), SS-B (LA), 16/6 Id, anti 16/6 Id, were consistently found in the sera. Similarly, AS101 had no effect on the clinical parameters. Furthermore, no differences in the serological or clinical parameters were noted 5 months after disease induction. Although IL-2 production and Tac antigen expression in the treated mice were restored to normal levels by AS101, the serological parameters and the clinical course of the disease remained unaffected. We therefore believe that the low IL-2 production in SLE is the result and not the cause of SLE in mice and is most probably connected with and secondary to other immunological processes.

- *Radiotherapy. Protection from adverse effects of radiation*

The hemopoietic system is the primary critical tissue for radiation induced mortality in a dose range below the induction of the gastrointestinal syndrome. Damage of hematopoietic stem cells and precursor cells after exposure to whole body irradiation has been extensively examined in the last two decades. Damage caused by radiation is the outcome of exposure to radiation of patients suffering from various malignancies or alternatively exposure to harmful exogenous challenges. Radiation-induced destruction of the lymphoid and hematopoietic systems is the primary cause of septicemia and death. It is therefore of vital importance that AS101 was found to offer protection against the adverse effects of radiation by means of accelerating the restoration of functional hematopoietic cells.

We hypothesized that AS101 could exert radioprotective effects *via* induction of cytokines such as IL-1, which has been previously reported to have strong radioprotective properties [19], or other cytokines like GM-CSF or TNF which were also reported to synergize with IL-1 to exert their radioprotective effects. We found that injection of AS101 every other day for two weeks prior to a sublethal dose of 450 rads accelerated the rate of recovery of BM or spleen cellularity. The number of BM cells in the AS101 injected mice reached almost that of normal non-irradiated mice [7].

Table VI. Effect of AS101 on the recovery of hemopoietic cells from irradiated mice and their functioning.

	PBS treated	Irradiated AS101 treated		Non-irradiated control
		10 μg	30 μg	
Spleen cells × 10^7	1.8 ± 0.3	4.3 ± 0.5	3.8 ± 2	9 ± 1
BM cells × 10^6	14.0 ± 1	33.0 ± 3	25.0 ± 2	45 ± 3
CSF secretion by BM cells (colonies/10^5 cells)	60.0 ± 2	82.0 ± 3	59.0 ± 3	93 ± 4
No. BM-CFU-C	10.0 ± 2	51.0 ± 3	13.0 ± 3	120 ± 6
IL-2 secretion by spleen cells (u/ml)	6.0 ± 0.5	26.0 ± 3	24.0 ± 2	29 ± 3
Thymocytes proliferation (stimulation index)	12.3 ± 2	36.8 ± 3	34.6 ± 4	46 ± 5
Spleen cells proliferation (proliferation index)	15.7 ± 2	53.0 ± 6	48.0 ± 4	66 ± 7
BM CFU-S	11.0 ± 2	42.0 ± 3	14.0 ± 2	59 ± 3
Spleen CFU-S	3.0 ± 0.5	18.0 ± 3	32.0 ± 3	41 ± 4

Mice were injected every other day for 2 weeks with AS101 or PBS before receiving 450-rad irradiation. Nine days after irradiation various parameters were analyzed. IL-2 secretion and proliferation of spleen cells and thymocytes was analyzed two days after irradiation.

The same protocol of AS101 injections showed an increase in CSF production by BM or spleen cells. Following exposure to 450 rads, there was a dramatic decrease in the number of CFU-GM. Pretreatment of mice with AS101 increased twelve-fold the number of precursor cells (Table VI). These results provided sufficient grounds for reasoning that AS101, in enhancing the hematopoeitic functioning in sublethal irradiated mice, could also protect mice against lethal doses of irradiation. Indeed, we found that in mice treated with varying doses of AS101 prior to 840 rads of irradiation, there was a significant increase in survival rate (80 % compared to 30 % in control PBS injected mice) (Figure 6). Moreover, mice injected with AS101 and later on exposed to escalating doses of irradiation (780, 840, 950 rads) showed a shift in response from the higher to the lower doses of irradiation [7].

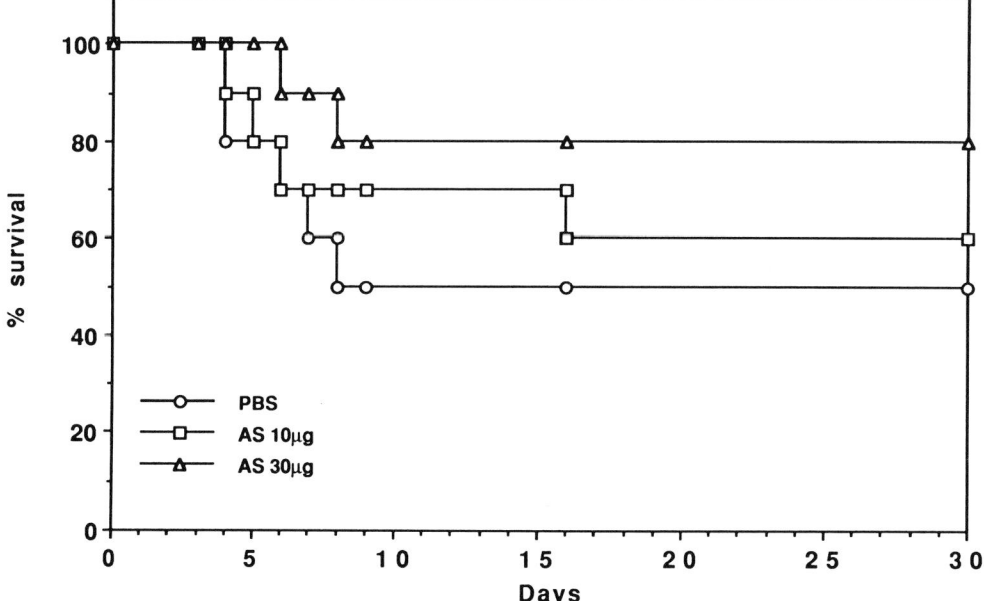

Figure 6. Radioprotective effect of AS101 on lethally irradiated mice. Balb/c mice were irradiated with 840 rad after being injected with different concentrations of AS101 or PBS for 2 weeks every other day. The experiment included 20 mice/group.

The recovery of spleen colony-forming units (CFU-S) in the bone marrow and spleen of AS101 treated mice was significantly faster than that of control PBS treated mice. The effect of AS101 on the recovery of endogenous CFU-S was also very significant. The number of these endogenous CFU-S has been found to have a close correlation to the survival rate of mice treated with radioprotective drugs. AS101 was found to increase the number of endogenous colonies either when it was injected prior to irradiation or immediately after irradiation. Each endogenous spleen colony from irradiated AS101 injected mice was found to include a higher number of CFU-S in AS101 treated mice.

AS101 was found to exert its radioprotective effects also on the T cell compartment. T cell and thymocytes proliferation in the presence of con A was significantly higher in AS101 treated irradiated mice than in PBS treated irradiated mice. IL-2 secretion by mouse spleen T cells was also significantly higher in AS101 treated mice.

AS101 was found to induce a higher number of CFU-S and CFU-GM into the S-phase of the cell cycle [20]. The late S phase of the cell cycle was reported in numerous studies to be the most radioresistant phase of the cell cycle. Therefore our finding that AS101 enhanced cell cycling of CFU-S and CFU-GM suggests that the rapid recovery of CFU-GM after irradiation could be a consequence of both enhanced survival of CFU-GM due to a large proportion of these cells in S phase of the cell cycle, and the differentiation of a greater number of CFU-S due to the survival of the latter following irradiation.

Our experimental results suggest that AS101 exerts its radioprotective effects by induction of large numbers of progenitor cells into the radioresistant S phase and by enhanced stimulation of CFU-S towards proliferation and self renewal. AS101 might exert these effects either directly or indirectly *via* cytokines like IL-1. It may be a useful agent for the restoration of hemopoiesis in patients after radiation therapy and may be beneficial in cases of overdose or accidental irradiation.

- *Chemotherapy. Protection from side effects of chemotherapy*

Chemical-induced cytoreduction is used therapeutically for the treatment of neoplasms and also to ablate bone marrow prior to BM transplantation. The efficacy of chemotherapy against advanced tumor depends on the dose intensity of the drugs utilized. Treatment with such agents, however, is limited by myelosuppression, immune suppression and other toxic effects on normal cells. Immunotherapy with cytokines like IL-1 and G-CSF may help to minimize the myelosuppressive effects of DNA-damaging agents. Since AS101 has been found to release these cytokines, we assumed that this agent might exert chemoprotective effects *via* induction of cytokines. We found that injection of AS101 every other day for two weeks prior to a sublethal dose of 250 mg/kg of cyclophosphamide (CTX) accelerated the rate of recovery of BM cellularity, BM colony forming units granulocyte-macrophage (CFU-GM) progenitor cells, and the secretion of CSF. AS101 was found to exert its chemoprotective effects also on the T cell compartment. T cell and thymocytes proliferation in the presence of conA was significantly higher in AS101 treated mice subjected to CTX at 250 mg/kg than in control PBS and CTX injected mice. IL-2 secretion by mouse spleen T cells was also significantly higher in AS101 treated mice (Table VII). These results provided sufficient grounds for reasoning that AS101 could also protect mice against lethal doses of CTX. Indeed we found that 90 % of mice treated with 25 µg AS101/mouse before receiving 300 mg/kg CTX survived 40 days following CTX treatment, while only 20 % survived in the PBS control group (Figure 7). Protection by AS101 was elicited in a dose dependent manner. At 400 mg/kg CTX, AS101 afforded similar results. These results prompted us to analyze the effect of AS101 in conjunction with lethal doses of CTX on tumor bearing mice (*see* Tumor section). These results suggest that chemo-immunotherapy protocols with AS101 have considerable potential for clinical application in minimizing adverse cytotoxicity resulting from alkylating agents.

The protection afforded by AS101 could also be demonstrated in *in vitro* BM cultures with various concentrations of ASTA-Z 7557, a potent derivative of CTX. This agent is commonly used to purge residual tumor cells possibly present in the mixture of BM cells used for autologous BM transplantation. In order to be effective, the chemical purge of the BM must fulfill two requirements : the treatment should eliminate the occult neoplastic cells, and it should not affect the hematopoietic cells that are necessary to ensure the recovery of the patient. ASTA-Z was found to spare CFU-S whereas CFU-GM are very sensitive to this agent. We found that prior incubation with AS101 protects CFU-GM from toxic effects of ASTA-Z [21].

Table VII. Effect of AS101 on the recovery of hemopoietic cells from cyclophosphamide treated mice and their functioning.

CTX treated Non-CTX treated	PBS treated	AS101 2.5 μg	Treated 10 μg	Control
BM cells × 10^6	33 ± 3	50.0 ± 4	46.0 ± 4	53 ± 6
CSF secretion by spleen cells (colonies/10^5 BM cells)	54.3 ± 9.1	156.5 ± 25.7	137.3 ± 27.6	180 ± 16
No. BM-CFU-C	14 ± 2.5	40.0 ± 3	42.0 ± 3	120 ± 11
IL-2 secretion by spleen cells (u/ml)	17.0 ± 3	31.0 ± 4	26.0 ± 3	39 ± 5

Mice were injected every other day for 2 weeks with AS101 or PBS before being injected i.p. with 250 mg/kg CTX. Nine days after CTX treatment various parameters were analyzed. IL-2 secretion and proliferation of spleen cells and thymocytes was analyzed two days after CTX treatment.

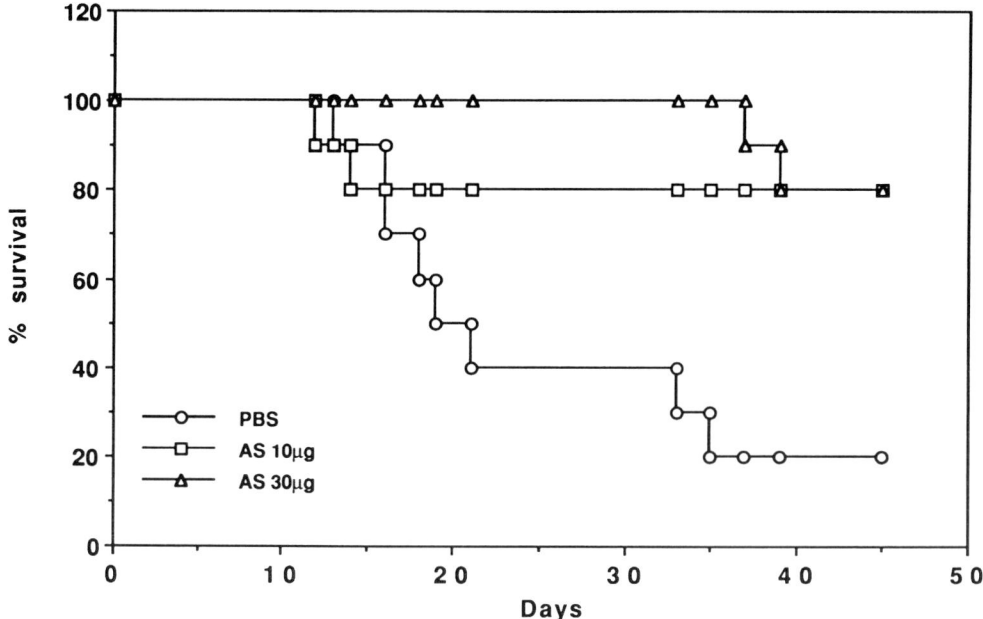

Figure 7. Protective effect of AS101 on lethally CTX treated mice. Balb/c mice were injected with 325 mg/kg cyclophosphamide after being injected with AS101 or PBS for 2 weeks every other day.

These data suggest that AS101 could be potentially useful in *ex vivo* purging of human BM when used concomitantly with ASTA-Z at concentrations known to spare CFU-S. This would increase the proportion of CFU-GM and thus decrease the risk of infections in BM transplanted patients.

We found that AS101 protection from toxic effects of ASTA-Z *in vitro* and CTX *in vivo* can be partially ascribed to increased aldehyde dehydrogenase (ALDH) activity induced by AS101. This enzyme catalyzes the reaction in which a metabolite with little cytotoxic activity is produced from 4-hydroperoxycyclophosphamide. The increase in ALDH activity was shown directly by measuring cellular toxicity of ASTA-Z and CTX in the presence of cyanamide — an inhibitor of ALDH. However, the chemoprotectiveness of AS101 was not limited to CTX, as it was also found to reconstitute — probably through other mechanisms — the number of spleen cells after 5-fluorouracil treatment [21].

Clinical studies

Phase I clinical trial in patients with advanced malignancies

The present phase I clinical trial was conducted in Israel on 60 patients with advanced cancer in order to define the maximal tolerated dose of AS101, to evaluate the toxicity of the compound, and to determine the optimal dose and schedule for immune modulation. AS101 was administered i.v. 2 or 3 times a week at doses 1-14 mg/m². Toxicity was minimal at doses 1-12 mg/m² (Table VIII) ; 14 mg/m² was found to be the maximal tolerated dose (MTD) when AS101 was injected thrice weekly. Immunological parameters were evaluated at all dose levels and the effect of low doses (1-3 mg/m² was compared to high doses (8-14 mg/m²). The production of IL-2, TNF and γ-IFN increased over baseline levels with significantly higher increases occurring at low doses. Increase in immunological parameters at 3 mg/m² is demonstrated in Figure 8. Analysis of WBC counts and T lymphocyte populations showed higher increases in the percent of CD^{3+} cells at low doses and similar effects at both low and high doses in the percent of CD^{4+} cells and WBC counts [22-24].

Natural killer and lymphocyte activating killer (LAK) cell activity was found to increase significantly in patients displaying IL-2 levels (Table IX). The long-term effect of AS101 was studied for patients undergoing 2 or 3 months of treatment. In the two-month-treatment period there was elevation during the first month in IL-2, γ-IFN, TNF and interleukin-2-receptor positive (IL-2R+) cells. During the second month, values of IL-2 and γ-IFN continued to increase or maintained the same level, whereas the values of TNF and the percent of IL-2R+ cells decreased slightly. In patients undergoing 3 months of treatment there was a continuous trend of increase in IL-2, percent of IL-2R+ cells and TNF during the whole study period. The comparative effects of 2 and 3 injections/week were studied during two months of treatment. It was found that the thrice weekly schedule was more effective with respect to cytokine secretion and percent of IL-2 receptor positive cells. According to this trial it appears that a regimen of 1-3 mg/m² of AS101 administered thrice weekly induces pronounced immune enhancement with tolerable toxicity. In view of theses findings a phase II study has recently been initiated.

Table VIII. Toxicity in patients treated with all doses of AS101.

Grade :	0 %	1 %	2 %	3 %	4 %	# Episodes
Garlic odor	—	—	—	100.0	—	458
Fever Pre :	83.8	15.8	0.4	—	—	988
2 hour :	78.7	19.2	2.1	—	—	988
4 hour :	69.5	25.9	4.6	—	—	988
8 hour :	67.2	30.0	2.8	—	—	988
Gastrointestinal						
— Oral (mucositis)	98.0	2.0	—	—	—	458
— Nausea/vomiting	77.7	12.4	9.0	0.4	0.4	458
— Diarrhea	97.8	1.7	0.4	—	—	458
— Constipation	79.9	17.7	2.2	0.2	—	458
Cutaneous	98.7	0.4	0.9	—	—	456
Alopecia	98.7	0.4	0.9	—	—	456
Allergic reactions	100.0	—	—	—	—	458
Pulmonary	74.3	9.8	7.2	7.2	1.5	459
Cardiac (rhythm)	98.5	1.5	—	—	—	460
Nervous system						
— Central	95.6	1.3	1.1	1.8	0.2	456
— Peripheral	90.8	0.4	6.4	0.7	1.8	455
Urinary tract						
— Cystitis	96.3	2.2	0.7	0.4	—	457
— Creatinine	95.9	2.7	0.3	1.1	—	370
— Protenuria	95.5	3.2	1.4	—	—	221
Bone marrow						
— WBC	99.2	0.8	—	—	—	387
— Platelets	99.5	0.3	0.3	0.5	—	382
Blood chemistries						
— Bilirubin	99.7	0.3	—	—	—	360
— SGOT	93.5	5.6	0.3	0.3	0.3	337
— SGPT	96.4	3.6	—	—	—	336
— LDH	83.6	8.5	2.6	2.6	—	305

Table IX. NK and LAK cell activity in patients exhibiting > 25 % and < 25 % increased in IL-2 secretion. All patients were included in the evaluation of cytotoxicity.

	NK activity		LAK activity	
Patient group displaying	Baseline	Response after treatment	Baseline	Response after treatment
At least 25 % increase in IL-2	10.31 N = 17	14.46 $p < 0.05$	9.40 N = 16	15.67 $p < 0.02$
Less than 25 % increase in IL-2	14.93 N = 27	14.67	15.92 N = 25	13.94

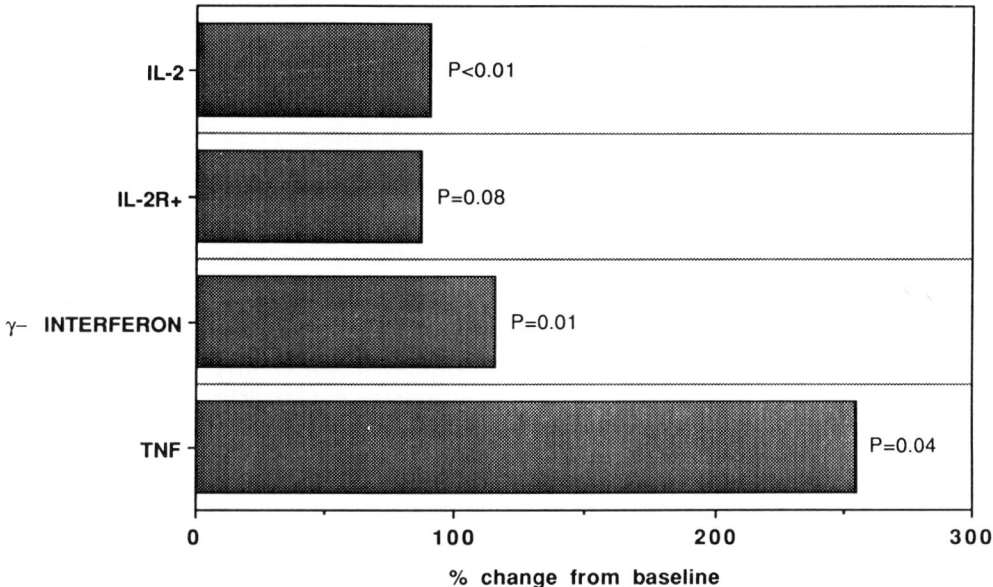

Figure 8. Cytokine production and IL-2 R expression of MNC of patients treated with 3 mg/m² of AS101.

Phase I clinical trials on AIDS patients

The treatment of HIV-related infections represents one of the greatest challenges of modern medicine. Three main strategies at halting the progression of the disease in infected subjects may be envisaged : antiviral treatment, immunorestoration, and combined therapy. AS101, as described in this review, is a compound with immunomodulating properties, HIV antiviral activity *in vitro*, and minimal toxicity. On the basis of these observations a phase I clinical trial on AIDS patients was conducted by Ruiz-Palacios *et al.* [25]. It included 48 patients answering the criteria of the CDC for AIDS. Patients were divided into 5 groups treated by escalating doses of AS101 (2, 3, 5, 8 and 13 mg/m²). All groups received treatment for 12 weeks and a follow-up was done for the next 24 months. Hematological and biochemical and immunological monitoring were performed twice prior to entry and the first 4 weeks every week and then every second week.

- *Toxicity monitoring*

None of the patients demonstrated any evidence of toxicity, with all parameters remaining stable throughout the study. Overall, there were no significant differences before and after treatment. The only universal effect was a garlic odor which is apparently a metabolite of AS101 secreted in the skin.

- *Immunological evaluation*

An enhancement of IL-2 production, response to IL-2 and induction of IL-2 receptors was observed in patients treated with AS101 doses of 2-8 mg/m². This increase stayed stable throughout the follow-up. Values observed for pervent of CD4 was increased significantly. The total CD4 in 3 mg/m² was also enhanced significantly. No important modifications of the CD8+ subset was observed. The increase in immunological parameters was usually observed after 4 weeks of treatment. 75 % AS101 treated patients that were p-24 positive reversed to negative.

Phase II clinical trials on AIDS patients

Forty-four patients (41 M, 3 F) were entered into the study in Saint-Antoine Hospital, Paris. CDC staging was stage IV for all of them. HIV antigenemia was positive in 50 % of the cases. Most patients were included because of toxicity and/or failure of AZT (80 %). Thirty-one patients were evaluable. Patients were treated with AS101 administered i.v. 3 times a week at 5 mg/m^2. Median duration of therapy was 4,5 months (1.5-14). Clinical improvement occurred in 54 % of the cases with weight gain and improvement of specific lesions was transiently observed during a median of 2 months. In four cases the disapperarance of cytopenia was observed. HIV antigenemia was positive in 17 patients, negative in 14. A negativation of antigenemia was never observed. T4 level increased (2-9 fold) in 30 % of the patients and T4/T8 ratio increased in 48 % of cases. Level of IL-2 increased in 48 tested patients. Toxicity was moderate : garlic smell of the breath (50 %), hair lightening (50 %), transient exathema (20 %) at the beginning of therapy [26].

*
* *

In conclusion, AS101 was safe and well tolerated. Positive results occurred in half of AIDS patients, yet these effects were not always sustained. In an effort to further help patients with advanced disease, a combined treatment of AS101 with AZT was given. Five male patients at stage IV entered the study. AS101 was given i.v. 3 times a week at 5 mg/m^2 and AZT was given *per os* 1 g/day. Four out of five had had previous toxicity of AZT (severe pancytopenia). One patient with pulmonary Kaposi sarcoma died from progression of KS ; the other four are alive. The median duration of the association was 3 months. Any clinical sign of intolerance was observed. One patient experienced neutropenia and AZT was stopped. Hematological tolerance in the other three was good. In three patients the clinical status improved [27]. In view of these studies a randomized phase II/III clinical trial in ARC and AIDS patients has already been initiated.

References

1. Albeck M, Tamari T, Sredni B. A synthesis and properties of Ammonium trichloro(dioxythylene-o, o')tellurate (AS1 01). A new immunomodulating compound. *Synthesis* 1989 ; 8 : 635.
2. Nyska A, Waner T, Pirak M, Albeck M, Sredni B. Toxicity study in rats of a tellurium based immunomodulating drug, AS101 : a potential drug for AIDS and cancer patients. *Arch Toxicol* 1989 ; 63 (5) : 386.
3. Siddik ZH, Newman RA. Use of platinum as a modifier in the sensitive detection of tellurium in biological samples. *Anal Biochem* 1987.
4. Engineer MS, Burditt T, Newman RA, Siddick ZH. Pharmacology of AS101 after multiple doses in dogs. *Proc Am Assoc Cancer Res* 1989 ; 30 : 584.
5. Sredni B, Caspi R, Klein A, Kalechman Y, Danzinger Y, Ben Ya'akov M, Tamari T, Shalit F, Albeck M. A new immunomodulating compound (AS101) with potential therapeutic application. *Nature* 1987 ; 330 : 6144.

6. Sredni B, Caspi RR, Lustig S, Klein A, Kalechman Y, Danziger Y, Ben Ya'akov M, Tamari T, Shalit F, Albeck M. The biological activity and immunotherapeutic properties of AS101, a synthetic organotellurium compound. *Nat Immun Cell Growth Regul* 1988 ; 7 : 163.
7. Kalechman Y, Albeck M, Oron M, Sobelman D, Gurwith M, Sehgal SN, Sredni B. The radioprotective effects of the immunomodulator AS101. *J Immunol* 1990 ; 145 : 1512.
8. Sredni B, Kalechman Y, Albeck M, Gross O, Aurbach D, Sharon P, Sehgal SN, Gurwith MJ, Michlin H. Cytokine secretion effected by synergism of the immunomodulator AS101 and the protein kinase-C inducer bryostatin. *Immunology* 1990 ; 70 (4) : 473.
9. Mosman TR, Coffman RL. Th1 and Th2 cells : different patterns of lymphokine secretion lead to different functional properties. *Annu Rev Immunol* 1989 : 7 : 145.
10. Vonsover A, Sredni B, Loya S, Horwith G, Kirsch TM, Albeck M, Gotlieb Stematsky T, Hizi A. Inhibition of the reverse transcriptase activity and replication of human immunodeficiency virus type 1 by AS101 *in vitro* (submitted).
11. Alcocer-Varela J, Alarcon-Segovia D, Sredni B, Albeck M. Effect of the new immunoregulator AS101 on *in vitro* functions of mononuclear cells from patients with systemic lupus erythromatosus. *Clin Exp Immunol* 1989 ; 77 : 319.
12. Sredni B, Kalechman Y, Shalit F, Albeck M. Synergism between AS101 and PMA in lymphokine production. *Immunology* 1990 ; 69 : 110.
13. Nishizuka Y. Studies and perspectives of protein kinase-C. *Science* 1986 ; 233 : 305.
14. Neidel JE, Kuhn LJ, Vandenbark GR. Phorbol diester receptor copurifies with protein kinase. *Proc Natl Acad Sci USA* 1983 ; 80 : 36.
15. Lee RE, Lotze MT, Skibber JM, Tucker E, Bonow RO, Ognibene FP, Carrasquillo JA, Rosenberg SA. Cardiovascular effects of immunotherapy with IL-2. *J Clin Oncol* 1989 ; 7 : 7.
16. Kozeny GA, Nicolas JD, Greekmore S, Hano JH, Fisher RL. Effects of IL-2 imunotherapy on renal function. *J Clin Oncol* 1988 ; 6 : 1170.
17. Kalechman Y, Albeck M, Oron M, Sobelman D, Gurwith M, Horwith G, Kirsch T, Maida B, Sehgal SN, Sredni B. The protective and restorative role of AS101 in combination with chemotherapy (in press).
18. Blank M, Sredni B, Albeck M, Mozes E, Shoenfeld Y. The effect of the immunomodulator agent AS101 on IL-2 production in SLE disease induced in mice by a pathogenic anti-DNA antibody. *Clin Exp Immunol* 1990 : 79 : 443.
19. Neta R, Douches S, Oppenheim JJ. Interleukin-1 is a radioprotector. *J Immun* 1986 ; 136 : 2483.
20. Kalechman Y, Gafter U, Sotnik Barkai 1, Albeck M, Gurwith M, Horwith G, Kirsch T, Maida B, Sehgal SN, Sredni B. Mechanism of radioprotection conferred by the immunomodulator AS101 (submitted).
21. Kalechman Y, Sotnik Barkai 1, Albeck M, Horwith G, Sehgal SN, Sredni B. The use and mechanism of action of AS101 in protecting bone marrow CFU-GM after purging with ASTA-Z (submitted).
22. Shani A, Gurwith M, Tichler T, Catane, R, Rozenszajn LA, Gezin A, Levl E, Schlesinger M, Kalechman Y, Michlin H, Shalit F, Farbstein H, Farbstein M, Albeck M, Sredni B. The immunologic effects of AS101 in the treatment of cancer patients. *Nat Immun Cell Growth Regul* 1990 ; 9 : 182.
23. Sredni B, Catane R, Shani A, Gezin A, Levi E, Schlezinger M, Kalechman Y, Michlin H, Shalit F, Rosenzajn LA, Farbstein H, Albeck M. Phase I study of AS101 (an organotellurium compound) in patients with advanced malignancies. In : Rubinstein E, Adam D, Lewis-Epstein E, eds. *Recent advances in chemotherapy*. Jerusalem, 1990 : 851.
24. Sredni B, Tichler T, Shani A, Catane R, Schlesinger M, Horwith G, Kirsch T, Maida B, Shalit F, Michlin H, Farbstein H, Farbstien M, Kalechman Y, Albeck M. Phase I clinical trial and immunomodulatory study of AS101 in patients with advanced malignancies (submitted).
25. Ruiz-Palacios GM, Ponce de Leon S, Alarcon-Segovia D, Alcocer-Varela J, Cruz A, Nares F, Ponce de Leon A, Rojas G, Sredni B. Tolerance and clinical response to AS101, a new immunomodulator in AIDS patients. IV international conference on AIDS, 1988.

26. Laporte JPh, Lebas J, Gonzales G, Meyohas M, Sredni B, Najman A, *et al.* AS101, a new immunomodulating compound in the treatment of AIDS. 5th International Conference on AIDS, 1989.
27. Laporte JPh, Frottier J, Dormont D, Imberi JC, Albeck M, Najman A. 5th International Conference on AIDS (Montreal), 1989.

10

Levamisole

M. ROCH-ARVEILLER

*Département de Pharmacologie, CNRS URA 595,
27, rue du Faubourg-Saint-Jacques, 75674 Paris Cedex 14, France.*

General characteristics

History

Levamisole, an isomer of tetramisole, was first described as an antihelminthic [1].

It was marketed under the name of Solaskil® in Western countries or as Decaris® in Eastern Europe and is active against nematodes and other round worms. It is still widely used as an antihelmintic in third-world countries and as an anti-parasitic agent in veterinary medicine, where it plays an important role in the treatment of livestock [2].

In 1971, Renoux and Renoux [3] showed that, in mice, tetramisole increases the protective effect of anti-brucellosis vaccine. This finding triggered a flow of papers dealing with experimental and clinical effects of levamisole. In the early days of immunotherapy, it was the first chemically defined substance to be used in the treatment of various chronic infections, cancers and rheumatoid affections, diseases for which an immunodeficiency is often invoked.

Structure

Levamisole, the levorotary isomer of tetramisole (2, 3, 5, 6-tetrahydro-6-phenylimidazo-(2-1b)-thiazole), has a molecular mass of 240.75 Da.

In its hydrochloride form, this white, crystalline powder is easily soluble in water and most organic solvents ; it is stable in acid medium, but undergoes hydrolysis in alkaline media and precipitates at pH 7.5. Under relatively mild conditions, including physiological conditions, it has recently been demonstrated [4] that levamisole may decompose to products which inhibit or enhance responses to Con A.

The inefficacy of the dextroisomer suggests the existence of enzymatic mechanisms needed to obtain an active molecule. Several metabolites result from thiazolidine hydrolysis and aromatic hydroxylation [5].

OMPI

The most interesting seemed to be 2-oxo-3-(2-mercaptoethyl)-5-phenylimidazolidine (OMPI), since it has been reported to (1) enhance the polymerisation of tubulin, and hence to increase cell microtubule integrity [5], (2) be more potent than levamisole in enhancing the clearance of i.v. injected colloidal carbon in mice [6], (3) protect cultured cells against necrosis induced by glutathione depletion [7], (4) prevent peroxidase-mediated inhibition of neutrophil motility and lymphocyte transformation [4]. These properties added to the generation of a sulphydryl compound, identified as OMPI, after incubation of levamisole with hepatic microsomes containing ADP-Fe and NADPH, *i.e.* under conditions of lipid peroxidation, provided a plausible explanation for the improved leukocyte reactivity seen under levamisole treatment. Levamisole hydrolysis seems to be specifically catalysed by α-ketoaldehydes and, in particular, glyoxal [7]. A prodrug hypothesis has thus been proposed for levamisole and Amery [8] and Amery and Gough [9] suggested that most pharmacological effects of levamisole are mediated by the *in vivo* formation of OMPI. However, OMPI rapid breakdown *via* methylation and oxidation has precluded its formal detection in *in vivo* metabolism experiments. Moreover for Graziani and De Martin [10], the metabolism of levamisole in rats proceeds *via* four major pathways of which the one leading to the formation of OMPI was the least important. Furthermore, certain dissimilarities between the effects of levamisole and OMPI, principally the lack of effect of OMPI on IL-1 production [11], do not conform with the prodrug hypothesis [12]. Detailed investigations on the *in vivo* formation of OMPI might be performed since Shu *et al.* [13] isolated a minor metabolite which has OMPI as a structural unit.

Toxicity

LD50 varies from 28 mg/kg (given intravenously to rats and mice) to 285 and 345 mg/kg for oral administration to mice and rats [14].

In the rat, a daily oral administration of 100 mg/kg of levamisole has no toxic effect, but a prolonged treatment of more than 20 mg/kg can induce convulsions in dogs and sheep [15].

Levamisole is neither mutagenic nor teratogenic.

Pharmacokinetics

Levamisole is rapidly absorbed in the gastrointestinal tract or at subcutaneous or intramuscular injection sites. Its plasma half-life is about 4 h in man, with the majority of metabolites being excreted in the urine and, to a lesser extent, in the feces [10, 16]. It is distributed throughout all body tissues and fluids, with a maximal level in the liver and the kidney, where it is metabolized. In man, a plasma peak of 0.5 mg/ml is reached 2-4 h after a single oral dose of 150 mg.

The amount of untransformed compound excreted in the urine is less than 5 %. Traces of levamisole are found in tears, bronchial mucus and mother's milk in the first hours following treatment [10, 17].

Administration. Side effects

In man, a standard daily dose of 150 mg is usually administered orally. Levamisole is often prescribed for 2 or 3 consecutive days per week, or every week. Except in cases of significant side effects, this therapy is prescribed for at least one year. Some studies include observations over a 7-year period [18]. It seems preferable to adjust the dose administered to patient's weight, while keeping in mind the increase of gastrointestinal side effects for doses higher than 2.5 mg/kg/d which has been refered as an optimal active dose [8] recommended by the manufacturer (Janssen R & D Company) for different clinical trials [19, 20]. It has been suggested that levamisole given two weeks was less toxic and more effective than levamisole given weekly. Levamisole exemplifies the concept that exquisitely precise timing and optimum dosages are necessary to obtain positive effects [21, 22].

The host's immunological response at the time of treatment must also be taken into consideration. The beneficial effect of levamisole is especially important in subjects markedly immunodepressed as a result of surgical shock or radiotherapy. To achieve maximal efficacy, levamisole therapy must be started very soon after surgery, at the time of the strong immunodepression caused by surgical shock [23]. However, a recent study on 297 cancer patients did not show better results in subjects treated earlier [18]. Moertel et al. [24] recommend administering levamisole to patients only after the acute period of post-operative care.

Incidence and types of side effects

Side effects are considered to be negligible for some authors [25, 26], whereas others report that their importance necessitated to termination of treatment in 21 % of the cases [27]. All of these effects are reversed in the 8 days following the end of the treatment.

Hematological side effects require the strict control of the white blood count throughout the treatment period.

Granulocytopenia progressing to agranulocytosis is observed in 4.9 % of the patients afflicted with rheumatoid arthritis, 2 % of those with cancer and 0.2 % of the others. It is independent of the mode of levamisole administration and of association with medications other than cortisone [28-31]. This effect is linked to the anti-free radical activity of the sulfur atom and is more common in HLA-B 27 women suffering from rheumatoid arthritis [32].

Pseudoflu symptoms, including fever, rash and stomatitis, are described in 20 % of the arthritis patients and 8.8 % of the others. Coadministration with prednisolone (5-10 mg) can reduce this effect [33].

Gastrointestinal disturbances, including vomiting and diarrhea, are noted frequently (15.8 % of the arthritis patients, 18.9 % of the others) with a bitter, metallic taste in the mouth [34].

Other side effects have also been reported [35] : sensory stimulation (excitation, insomnia, headhaches, vertigo), neurosensory disorders (13.6 % of the arthritis patients, 9.3 % of the others), dermatitis [33] possibly in association with vascular lesions and cardiorespiratory difficulties [36].

Levamisole induces an Antabuse alcohol reaction sometimes even requiring the prohibition of the use of alcohol-containing cosmetic lotions [37].

Experimental immunopharmacology

Most of the experimental studies on levamisole were carried out between 1970 and 1980 in the mouse and the rat and indicate that it can enhance humoral and cell-mediated immunity [38-40]. In addition, levamisole stimulates the functions of monocyte/macrophages [41] or other cells such as murine hepatic non parenchymal cells or bone marrow cells from the same mice [42].

However, this substance can be either immunosuppressive or immunostimulatory, depending upon the dose given and the time of administration after exposure to the antigen [43]. Results may vary according to the pathophysiological status of the cells at the onset of the experiment. It is generally accepted that responses are stronger and more constant in immunodepressed animals than in young and healthy ones [44].

Effect on lymphocytes

In vivo or *in vitro* treatment increases the percentage of peripheral blood lymphocytes and the number of their receptors for sheep red blood cells [43]. This can be demonstrated on cells incubated *in vitro* with levamisole or cells from patients treated with the drug [45].

The expression of these receptors seems to indicate an effect on lymphocyte maturation [37]. Levamisole treatment or *in vitro* incubation increases lymphocyte blastogenesis, especially in cell cultures using subliminal amounts of antigens or mitogens [46].

In addition, levamisole enhances the cytotoxic activity of T lymphocytes [47], the production of lymphokines [48] and suppressor T cell activity [49, 50]. All influence on B lymphocytes is undoubtly indirect, resulting from the stimulation of macrophages and T lymphocytes. However, elevated B-cell activity is inhibited by levamisole, as indicated by reduced IgG and IgM and circulating immune complex levels after long-term treatment [12].

The extent of modifications of lymphocyte functions varies with the strain, sex and age of the animals tested. Sansoni et al. [51] and Biniaminov and Ramot [52] have contested the stimulatory effect of levamisole on T lymphocytes and their functions.

Effect on phagocytes

Levamisole modulates the motility of macrophages [53] and polymorphonuclear leukocytes (PMN) [54]. For some authors [55, 56], spontaneous migration and that directed by the chemotactic peptide N-formyl-methionyl-leucyl-phenylalanine (fMLP), or zymosan- activated serum are increased. However, Pike and Snyderman [57] showed that levamisole does neither affect the spontaneous migration of monocytes nor exert any effect on PMN. Giroud et al. [58] observed an inhibition of normal rat PMN chemotaxis and a stimulation of the chemotaxis of PMN harvested after induction of an inflammatory reaction and depressed by it.

Levamisole also increases phagocytosis by cultured macrophages and produces a slight increase in the bactericidal potency of macrophages stimulated by lymphocytes [59].

Mechanisms of action

The structure of levamisole portends certain properties linked to the presence of the imidazole ring, with its cholinergic activity and others associated with the presence of sulfur.

Role of the imidazole ring

Incubation of lymphocytes or macrophages with levamisole (or imidazole) increases the intracellular level of cyclic guanosine monophosphate (cGMP) [60].

This action, in turn, would be responsible for (1) the enhanced proliferation of lymphocytes [61] and macrophages [59] (2) the heightened cytotoxicity [42, 47] (3) the increased migration of phagocytes [60] (4) the production of cytokines [48, 62, 63]. It has been suggested that one possible immunological mechanism behind the activity of levamisole might be its ability to induce or enhance the generation of immunomodulatory proteins. Kimball et al. [11] recently demonstrated that levamisole may exert immunobiologic activity as a result of its ability to enhance the release of immunologic mediators, such as IL-1, from activated macrophages. This property may contribute to restoration of depressed immune responses and to levamisole ability to serve as adjunctive immunotherapy of cancer [41, 64].

By augmenting the cGMP level, cholinergic substances favor the lymphocyte proliferation triggered by an antigenic stimulus. Considering that this effect does not result from a direct inhibition of cGMP phosphodiesterase [61], it may be speculated that levamisole interacts with acetylcholine membrane receptors. An interaction of levamisole with muscarinic receptors could give rise to the increased intracellular levels of cGMP. Yet we know that levamisole interacts with nicotinic receptors. Otherwise, the drug owes its antihelminthic activity to a specific agonistic binding with nicotinic receptors on the muscle of the nematode *Caenorhabditis elegans* and possibly of other roundworms [65]. By analogy, it may be speculated that levamisole exerts an important effect on mammalian cholinergic receptors. However, unless mRNA transcripts of such receptors can be demonstrated in leukocytes, the hypothesis that levamisole exerts some of its immunological effects by interaction with cholinergic receptors remains largely speculative [12].

Nevertheless, the imidazole core seems to be responsible for levamisole effects on the central nervous system and the neuromuscular system of vertebrates, and may cause convulsions.

Role of the sulfated ring

This cyclic moiety is responsible for the production of a serum factor capable of potentializing leukocyte responses. In transfer experiments, this factor increases the immune response to sheep red blood cells in mice. In addition, it induces the regression of tumors in spontaneous AKR leukemia, even in mice that do not respond directly to treatment [66]. Furthermore, this factor is not specific from one species to another.

In the *nude* mouse, levamisole, like the similar molecule diethylthiocarbamate (DTC), induces *in vitro* thymocyte differenciation and enhances *in vivo* immune responses. Sulfated molecules trigger the release of a serum factor which stimulates the production of thymic hormones and T-cell differenciation.

A recent study by Chicault *et al.* [67] shows the importance of the thiol group in protein interactions. According to these authors, the SH groups of proteins (among which serum albumin is one of the most important) would be attracted by S_1 and N_4 atoms of levamisole, thereby orienting the molecules and giving rise to other disulfide bridges. Levamisole would be a catalyst responsible for changes in the membrane structure and the position of SH groups and S-S bonds in the proteins. Models proposed by Noelle and Lawrence [68] and Petty [69] suggest that the position of the thiol group on the cell surface determines the T-cell response. It can thus be hypothesized that levamisole activating properties are associated with the presence of the thiol group. Levamisole and its main metabolite OMPI, can be considered as modulators of the SH groups or S-S bonds of their target cells.

These elements are in agreement with the observations of Schmidt and Douglas [56] who suggested that levamisole can restore depressed monocyte functions by changing their cell membrane structures and modulating the externalization of certain receptors, for example those of IgG or C3.

Inhibition of the action or production of endogenous immunosuppressive factors

Levamisole is known to possess anti-anergic properties in individuals with a defective immune status. A first group of hypotheses describes levamisole as an inducer of an endogenous immuno-enhancing humoral substance and three distinct serum factors have been described [70].

An other set of hypotheses proposes that levamisole blocks naturally occurring immunosuppressive factors. Activated murine T-cells are able to produce antigen-non-specific immunosuppressive cytokines. Among them, the soluble immune response suppressor (SIRS) acquires suppressive activity after conversion to an oxidized form, termed $SIRS_{ox}$ which is known to disrupt microtubular assembly [70]. Levamisole blocks the oxidative conversion of SIRS and dose-dependently reverses inhibitor effects demonstrated *in vitro* and *in vivo*.

This activity would lead to conservation of microtubule assembly, resulting in a « desuppression » of immune reactivity and enhancement of the functions of T-cells and monocytes.

However, the role of SIRS/SIRSox in imbalances of immune homeostasis remains to be confirmed [12].

Levamisole was also found to block the action of another immunosuppressive factor, namely SAF (suppressor activating factor) [70].

Metabolic effects

Levamisole could be an enzymatic inhibitor of the activity of the hexose monophosphate shunt in phagocytes [53]. However, no effect was noted on the activities of glucose-6-phosphate dehydrogenase, glutathione reductase and peroxidases. Furthermore, levamisole could be a captor of oxygen free radicals formed during phagocyte activation and, in this way, it could increase the response of these cells to chemoattractants and inactivate the peroxidation system. This would explain, at least in part, the enhanced chemotactic response of phagocytes [71].

Levamisole is a specific inhibitor of the fumarate reductase of nematodes, thus explaining its ability to paralyze them, and a powerful inhibitor of certain mammalian alkaline phosphatases [25, 72]. It is also capable of modifying inducible aryl-hydroxylases and inhibiting the aerobic glycolysis of tumors.

Thus, levamisole has many effects on cell metabolism. Moertel *et al.* [24] even postulate that its antitumoral activity could be uniquely linked to biochemical modifications completely independent of immunological effects.

Genetic and epigenetic factors

All the experimental and clinical results show that the effects produced by levamisole are closely dependent upon the dose administered. Experiments in mice indicate that the responses are under polygenic control, independent of the major histocompatibility complex and modified by a component linked to the Y chromosome, and dependent upon epigenetic factors appearing with age [14].

Therapeutic indications

Given its early recognition as an immunomodulator, levamisole has been used in the treatment of many diseases, particularly those revealing an immune deficit or recurrent infections.

Parasitoses and associated disorders

The first indication of levamisole as an antihelminthic is still valid.

Its immunostimulatory activity can increase defenses against associated infections [73] and favor healing of parasite-induced wounds [74].

It is also used to treat nematodiasis and shistosomiasis [75].

Rheumatoid diseases

Levamisole was used, above all, in the treatment of rheumatoid arthritis. Its activity can be compared to that of D-penicillamine but is lower than that of gold salts [33]. The absence of nephrotoxicity makes it preferable to other medications.

The regimen generally prescribed is 150 mg (in a single oral dose) per week for 6 months. Stronger doses engender side effects without improving efficacy. Patients with marked immune deficiencies seem to react better to low doses of levamisole than those who have normal responses. For this reason, the existence of a natural killer (NK) cell toxicity defect could be considered as a criterion for the selection of patients susceptible of responding to levamisole [76].

Kidney diseases

Levamisole has been used to treat chronic kidney diseases [77, 78], particularly in children in whom a functional T-lymphocyte defect was strongly suspected. This medication has no effect on the clinical manifestations or the evolution of IgA glomerulonephritis [79]. It can, however, improve the status of some children who relapse often during steroid-obtained remissions [80] and a recent study shows that levamisole is effective in maintaining a steroid-free remission in patients with high-dose steroid dependency. No action is evidenced if no prior immunodepression is established and levamisole cannot stimulate immunity to a level above normal [63].

Liver diseases

Levamisole has been used to treat chronic [81] and acute hepatitis [82] and chronic HBsAg-positive diseases [83].

This molecule does not seem to be effective against this type of disease. However it has recently been described that levamisole reduces the incidence of metastases to the liver [42].

Infectious diseases

Levamisole has been administered as an immunostimulant in chronic bronchial infections (especially in the USSR) or to avoid secondary infections after surgery. The treatment had no influence, in the latter case, on the number of postsurgical deaths, but a significant decrease in the number of febrile episodes in the group given levamisole was observed [84].

Levamisole has also been used to treat viral diseases, varicella [85], *Salmonella* [86] and *Brucella* infections [87], tuberculosis [88] and leprosy [89].

Used alone or in combination with antibiotics, its efficacy remains to be demonstrated in the treatment of infectious diseases.

Nervous disorders

In the USSR, levamisole has also been recommended for the treatment of juvenile schizophrenia [90, 91].

Cancers

The majority of trials were conducted on different types of cancers, including digestive tube (colorectal, stomach, intestinal), breast, lung, malignant melanomas and leukemias. The regimen is recommended alone or in association with radiotherapy [20] or chemotherapy [24]. For some authors, levamisole delays the appearance of metastases [92] whereas for others it has no effect [93]. The major conclusion derived from experimental observations were that levamisole was more active on slowly growing tumors, and that beneficial effects could be expected in particular when it was used as an adjuvant to cytoreductive treatment [22]. Recently the addition of levamisole to 5-fluorouracil (5-FU) to improve the clinical outcome of colorectal cancer patients has been extensively explored [94]. The significant advantage was maintained for 5-FU plus levamisole treatment for both recurrence-free interval and survival [94].

Levamisole efficacy seems clearer when marked immunodepression is evidenced before the treatment. Our increasing knowledge of immunology and the availability of recombinant interleukins, monoclonal antibodies and cloned lymphoid cells should enable us to monitor the immune status of patients more reliably and allow more defined experimental and clinical investigations on levamisole and other immunotropic agents.

Several reviews [12, 22, 23, 72, 95] summarized the clinical studies undertaken with levamisole in the treatment of cancer.

Conclusion

Synthesized and marketed (Solaskil®, Specia) for its antiparasitical properties, levamisole is still expansively administered to human and animals, particularly in the treatment of livestock.

The recent evidence that levamisole is an effective immunoadjuvant in specific diseases stages of colon cancer and melanoma will certainly promote new clinical trial. For Greenspan and Erlich [95], the combination of levamisole with leucovorin, BCG, interferons and other immune modifiers remains an open door for investigations.

References

1. Thienpont D, Vanparijs OFJ, Raeymaekers HM, Vandenberk J, Demoen PJA, Allewun FTN, Marsboom RPH, Niemeggers CJE, Schellekens KHL, Janssen PAJ. Tetramisole (R 8299) a new, potent broad spectrum antihelmintic. *Nature* 1966 : 209 : 1084-6.
2. Janssen PAJ. The levamisole story. *Progress research*. In : Jucker E, ed. Basel and Stuttgart : Verlag, 1976 : 347-83.
3. Renoux G, Renoux M. Effet immunostimulant d'un imidothiazole dans l'immunisation des souris contre l'infection par *Brucella abortus*. *CR Acad Sci Paris, série D* 1971 ; 272 : 349-50.
4. Hanson AK, Nagel DL, Heidrick ML. Immunomodulatory action of levamisole. I. Structural analysis and immunomodulating activity of levamisole degradation products. *Int J Immunopharmacol* 1991 ; 13 : 655-68.
5. De Brabander M, Aerts F, Gueuns G, Van Ginckel R, Van de Veire R, Van Belle H. OMPI : a sulfhydryl metabolite of levamisole that interacts with microtubules. *Chem Biol Interact* 1978 ; 28 : 45-9.
6. Van Ginckel R, de Brabander M. The influence of a levamisole metabolite (DL-2-oxo-3(2-mercaptoethyl)-5-phenylimidazolidine) on carbon clearance in mice *Reticuloendoth Soc* 1979 ; 25 : 125-31.
7. Van Belle H, Janssen PAJ. α-ketoaldehydes specific catalysis for thiol formation from levamisole. *Biochem Pharmacol* 1979 ; 28, 1313-8.
8. Amery WK. Double blind levamisole trial in resectable lung cancer. *Ann NY Acad Sci* 1976 ; 277 : 260-8.
9. Amery WK, Gough DA. Levamisole and immunotherapy : some theoretic and practical considerations and their relevance to human disease. *Oncology* 1981 ; 38 : 168-81.
10. Graziani G, De Martin GL. Pharmacokinetic studies on levamisole : on the pharmacokinetics and relative bioavailability of levamisole in man. *Drugs Exp Clin Res* 1977 ; 2 : 235-9.
11. Kimball ES, Clark MC, Schneider CR, Persico FJ. Enhancement of *in vitro* lipopolysaccharide-stimulated Interleukin-1 production by levamisole. *Clin Immunol Immunopathol* 1991 ; 58 : 385-98.
12. Van Wauwe J, Janssen PAJ. On the biochemical mode of action of levamisole : an update. *Int J Immunopharmacol* 1991 ; 13 : 3-9.
13. Shu YZ, Kingston DGI, Van Tassell RL, Wilkins TD. Metabolism of levamisole, an anticolon cancer drug by human intestinal bacteria. *Xenobiotica* 1991 ; 21 : 737-50.
14. Renoux G. Immunomodulateurs. Giroud JP, Mathé G, Meyniel G, eds *Pharmacologie clinique* Exp Sci Fse (2ᵉ édition), 1988 : 1873-93.
15. Forbes LS. Toxicological and pharmacological relations between levamisole, pyrantel and diethylcarbamazine and their significance in helminthic chemotherapy. *Southeast Asian J Trop Med Public Health* 1972 ; 3 : 235-41.
16. Heykans J, Wynants J, Scheijgrond H. The absorption, excretion and metabolism of levamisole in man. Janssen Pharmaceutica. *J Clin Reprod*, Nov. 1975.
17. Adams JG. Pharmacokinetics of levamisole. *J Rheumatol* 1978 ; 5 (suppl. 4) : 437-42.
18. Arnaud JP, Bruyse M, Nordlinger B, Martin F, Pector JG, Zeitoun P, Adloff A, Duez N. Adjuvant therapy of poor diagnosis colon cancer with levamisole : results of an EORTC double blind randomized clinical trial. *Br J Surg* 1979 ; 66 : 507-9.
19. Lichtenfeld JL, Wiernik PH. Levamisole in a phase I trial. *Cancer Treat Rep* 1976 ; 60 : 963-4.
20. Perez CA, Bauer M, Emami BN, Byhadt R, Brady LW, Scotte-Doggett RL, Gardner P, Zinninger M. Thoracic irradiation with or without levamisole (NSC- 177023) in unresectable non-small cell carcinoma of the lung : a phase III randomized trial of the RTOG. *Int J Radiat Oncol Biol Phys* 1988 ; 15 : 1337-46.
21. Amery WK, Butterworth BS. The dosage regimen of levamisole in cancer : is it related to efficacy and safety ? *Int J Immunopharmacol* 1983 ; 5 : 1-9.
22. De Brabander M, De Cree J, Vandebroek J, Verhaegen H, Janssen AJ. Levamisole in the treatment of cancer : Anything new ? (Review). *Anticancer Res* 1992 ; 12 : 177-88.

23. Windle R, Wood RFM, Bell PRF. The effect of levamisole on postoperative immunosuppression. *Br J Surg* 1979 ; 66 : 507-9.
24. Moertel CG, Fleming TR, McDonald JS, Haller DG, Laurie JA, Goodman PJ, Ungerlieder JS, Emerson WA, Tormey DC, Glick JH, Veeder MH, Mailliard JA. Levamisole and fluorouracil for adjuvant therapy on resected colon carcinoma. *N Engl J Med* 1990 ; 322 : 352-8.
25. Laurie JA, Moertel CG., Fleming TR, Wieand HS, Leigh JE, Rubin J, McCormack GW, Gerstner JB, Krook JE, Maillard J, Twito DI, Morton RF, Tschetter LK, Barlow JF. Surgical adjuvant therapy of large bowel carcinoma : an evaluation of levamisole and the combination of levamisole and fluorouracil. *J Clin Oncol* 1989 ; 7 : 1447-56.
26. Renoux G, Renoux M. Influence de l'administration de lévamisole sur la réactivité des lymphocytes T de cancéreux avancés. *Nouv Presse Med* 1976 ; 5 : 67-70.
27. Parkinson DR, Cano PO, Jerry LM, Capek A, Shibata HR, Mansell PW, Lewis MG, Marquis G. Complications of cancer immunotherapy with levamisole. *Lancet* 1977 ; 1 : 1129-32.
28. Mielants H, Veys E. A study of the hematological side-effects of levamisole in rheumatoid arthritis with recommendations. *J Rheumatol* 1978 ; 5 (Suppl. 4) : 77-83.
29. Symoens J, Veys E, Mielants M, Pinals P. Adverse reactions to levamisole. *Cancer Treat Rep* 1978 ; 62 : 1721-30.
30. Teerenhovi L, Heinoven E, Grohn P, Klefstrom P, Mehtonen M, Tilikanen A. High frequency of agranulocytosis in breast cancer patients treated with levamisole. *Lancet* 1978 ; 2 : 151-2.
31. Williams IA. Levamisole and agranulocytosis *Lancet* 1976 ; 1 : 1080-1.
32. Diez RA. HLA-B27 and agranulocytosis by levamisole. *Immunol Today* 1990 ; 11 : 270.
33. Veys EM, Mielants H, Verbruggen G. Gold salts, levamisole and D-penicillamine as a first choice slow-acting antirheumatic drugs in rheumatoid arthritis ; a long-term follow up study. *Clin Exp Rheumatol* 1987 ; 5 : 111-6.
34. Chicault M, Luu Duc C, Boucherle A. Drug protein interactions. On the protein-protein interaction induced by levamisole *in vitro*. A mechanism hypothesis. *Arzneim Forsch/Drug Res* 1988 ; 38 : 1387-9.
35. Onuaguluchi G, Igbo IN. Comparative local anœsthetic and antiarrhythmic actions of levamisole hydrochloride and lignocaine hydrochloride. *Arch Int Pharmacodyn* 1987 ; 289 : 278-89.
36. Anthony HM, Mearns AJ, Mason MK, Scott DG. Levamisole and surgery in bronchial carcinoma patients : increase in deaths from cardiorespiratory failure. *Thorax* 1979 ; 34 : 4-12.
37. Renoux G, Modulation of immunity by levamisole. *J Pharmacol Exp Ther* 1978 ; 2 : 397-423.
38. Chirigos MA. *Control of Neoplasia by modulation of the immune system*. New York : Raven Press, 1977.
39. Fischer GW, Oi VT, Ampaya EP, Kelley JL, Bass JW. Enhanced host defense mechanism with phenylimidothiazole. *Pediatr Res* 1974 ; 8 : 4-7.
40. Renoux G, Renoux M. Immunology effect of phenylimidothiazole (tetramisole) on the graft-versus host reactions. *CR Acad Sci Paris, série D* 1972 ; 274 : 3320-3.
41. Renoux G, Renoux M. Immunostimulation par le lévamisole, cibles et mécanismes. *Nouv Presse Med* 1978 ; 7 : 197-201.
42. Johnkoski JA, Hsueh CT, Doerr RJ, Cohen SA. Augmentation of the immune response of the murine liver by levamisole *Am J Surg* 1992 ; 163 : 202-7.
43. Renoux G, Renoux M. Modulation of immune reactivity by phenylimidothiazole salts in mice immunized. *Immunology* 1974 ; 113 : 779-90.
44. Bruley-Rosset M, Florentin I, Kiger N, Davigny M, Mathe G. Effects of *Bacillus* Calmette-Guerin and levamisole on immune responses in young adult and age-immunodepressed mice. *Cancer Treat Rep* 1978 ; 62 : 1641-50.
45. Brunner CJ, Muscoplat CC. Immunomodulatory effects of levamisole. *Am Vet Med Assoc* 1980 ; 176 : 1159-62.

46. Levy J. Correlations of clinical and laboratory effects of treatment by levamisole in autoimmune disease. *Cancer Treat Rep* 1978 ; 62 : 1715-9.
47. Faanes RB, Dillon P, Choi YS. Levamisole augments the cytotoxic T-cell response depending on the dose of drugs and antigen administered. *Clin Exp Immunol* 1977 ; 27 : 502-6.
48. Whitcomb ME, Merluzzi VJ, Cooperband SR. The effect of levamisole on human lymphocyte mediator production *in vitro*. *Cell Immunol* 1976 ; 21 : 272-7.
49. Balaram P, Padmanabhan TK, Vasudevan DM. Role of levamisole immunotherapy as an adjuvant to radiotherapy in oral cancer. II Lymphocyte subpopulations. *Neoplasma* 1988 ; 35 : 235-42.
50. Sampson D, Peters TG, Lewis JD. Dose dependence of immunopotentiation and tumor regression induced by levamisole. *Cancer Res* 1977 ; 37 : 3526-9.
51. Sansoni P, Rosetti A, Tridente G, Buttirini U. The effect of levamisole on peripheral T lymphocytes of patients with malignant lymphoma. *J Immunopharmacol* 1982 ; 83 : 223-32.
52. Biniaminov M, Ramot A. *In vitro* restoration by levamisole of thymus-derived lymphocyte function in Hodgkin's disease. *Lancet* 1975 ; 1 : 464.
53. Wright DG, Kirkpatrick CH, Gallin JI. Effects of levamisole on normal and abnormal leukocyte locomotion. *J Clin Invest* 1977 ; 59 : 941-50.
54. Rabson AR, Anderson R, Glover A. Defective neutrophile motility and recurrent infections. *In vitro* and *in vivo* effects of levamisole. *Clin Exp Immunol* 1978 ; 33 : 142-9.
55. Anderson R. Levamisole stimulation of neutrophil chemotaxis and chemokinesis by protection of both the leucoattractant and the cellular chemotactic response from inactivation by the peroxidase/hydrogen peroxide/halide system. *All Appl Immunol* 1981 ; 65 : 257-65.
56. Schmidt ME, Douglas SD. Effects of levamisole on human monocyte function and immunoprotein receptors. *Clin Immunol Immunopathol* 1976 ; 6 : 299-305.
57. Pike MC, Snyderman R. Augmentation of human monocyte chemotactic response by levamisole. *Nature* 1976 ; 261 : 136-7.
58. Giroud JP, Roch-Arveiller M, Muntaner O, Bradshaw D. Action comparée du lévamisole, du muramyldipeptide et de la tuftsine sur le chimiotactisme des polynucléaires de Rat. *Nouv Rev Fr Hematol* 1980 ; 22 : 69-76.
59. Hadden JW, Englard A, Sadlick JR, Hadden EM. The comparative effects of isoprinosine, levamisole, muramyldipeptide and SM1213 on lymphocyte and macrophage proliferation and activation *in vitro*. *Int J Immunopharmacol* 1979 ; 1 : 17-27.
60. Anderson R, Glover AM, Koornhof HJ, Rabson AR. *In vitro* stimulation of neutrophil motility by levamisole maintenance of cGMP levels in chemotactically stimulated levamisole-treated neutrophils. *J Immunol* 1976 ; 117 : 428-32.
61. Hadden JW, Hadden EM, Coffey RG, Corrales-Lopez E, Sunshine G. Levamisole and imidazole : *in vitro* effects on lymphocyte proliferation and cyclic nucleotide levels. *Cell Immunol* 1975 ; 20 : 98-103.
62. Redondo JM, Lopez-Guerrero JA, Fresno M. Potentiation of interleukin 2 activity by levamisole and imidazole. *Immunol Lett* 1987 ; 14 : 111-6.
63. Turriziani M, Giuliani A, Bulgarini B, De Vecchis L. Role of levamisole as immunomodulant in mouse lymphoma model. *Immunopharmacol Immunotoxicol* 1991 ; 13 : 425-45.
64. Renoux G, Renoux M. Roles of the imidazole or thiol moiety on the immunostimulant action of levamisole. In : Chirigos MA, ed. *Control of neoplasia by modulation of the immune system*. Raven Press, 1977 : 67-80.
65. Lewis JA, Fleming JT, Mc Lafferty S, Fleming J, McGee T. Choligernic receptor mutants of the nematode *Caenorhabditis elegans*. *Mol Pharmacol* 1987 ; 31 : 185-93.
66. Renoux G, Renoux M, Guillaumin JM, Kassel RL, Fiore N. L'action antitumorale du lévamisole (LMS) dans la leucémie spontanée AKR et sa stimulation des réponses aux érythrocytes sont médiatisées par des facteurs sériques. *Ann Immunol* 1975 ; 126 : 99-104.

67. Chicault M, Luu Duc C, Boucherle A. Drug protein interactions. Comparative studies of levamisole and structural analogs or agents with immunomodulatory effect on the mechanism of protein aggregation. *Arzneim Forsch/Drug Res* 1990 ; 40 : 55-7.
68. Noelle RJ, Lawrence DA. Modulation of T cell function. II Chemical basis for the involvement of cell surface thiol-reactive sites in control of T-cell proliferation. *Cell Immunol* 1981 ; 60 : 453-69.
69. Petty HR. A sulfhydryl redox model of antibody-dependent phagocytosis. *Mol Immunol* 1985 ; 22 : 1001-3.
70. Amery WK, Bruynseels JPJ. Levamisole, the story and the lessons. *Int J Immunopharmacol* 1992 ; 14 : 481-6.
71. Anderson R, Glover A, Rabson AR. The effect of chemotactic factors and agents which inhibit neutrophil movement on anaerobic glycolysis and hexose monophosphate shunt activity. *Immunology* 1978 ; 35 : 141-9.
72. Stevenson HC, Green I, Hamilton JM, Calabro BA, Parkinson DR. Levamisole : known effects on the immune system, clinical results, and future applications to the treatment of cancer. *Clin Oncol* 1991 ; 9 : 2052-66.
73. Coles GC, Giordano DJ, Tritschler JP. Efficacy of levamisole against immature and mature nematodes in goasts with induced infections. *Am J Vet Res* 1989 ; 50 : 1074-5.
74. Makled MK, Rifaasr M, Azab M, Makhlouf S, El Missiry AG, Khalil N. Determination of healing response by immunostimulant therapy (levamisole) in cutaneous leishmaniasis. *Chemioterapia* 1987 ; 6 (supp) : 214-6.
75. Makled MK, Gindy MS, Abdel Wahab MF, El Missery AG, Bebars MA, Soffar SA. Parasitological and clinical effect of levamisole in intestinal bilharziasis. *J Egypt Soc Parasitol* 1985 ; 15 : 299-303
76. Barada RA, O'Brien W, Horwitz DA. Defective monocyte cytotoxicity in rheumatoid arthritis : a correlation with disease activity and reversal by levamisole. *Arthritis Rheum* 1982 ; 25 : 10-6.
77. Mehta KP, Ali U, Kutty PM, Kolhatar U. Immunoregulatory treatment for minimal change nephrotic syndrome. *Arch Dis Child* 1986 ; 61 : 153-8.
78. Niaudet P, Drachman R, Gagnadoux MF, Broyer M. Treatment of idiopathic nephrotic syndrome with levamisole. *Acta Paediatr Scand* 1984 ; 73 : 637-41.
79. Belovezhdov N, Robeva R. Controlled therapeutic trial in IgA glomerulonephritis. *Vutr Boles* 1982 ; 21 : 49-53.
80. Drachman R, Schlesinger M, Alon U, Mor J, Etzioni A, Shzpira H, Ottali M, Drukker A. Immunoregulation with levamisole in frequently relapsing steroid responsive nephrotic syndrome. *Acta Paediatr Scand* 1988 ; 77 : 721-6.
81. Arnold W, Meyer Zum Buschenfelde KH. Aktuelle stand der therapie chroniischer leberentzundungen. *Leber Magen Darm* 1981 ; 11 : 73-80.
82. Dienstag JL, Isselbacher KJ. Therapy for acute and chronic hepatitis. *Arch Intern Med* 1981 ; 141 : 1419-23.
83. Chadwick RG, Jain S, Cohen BJ, Scott GM, Thomas HC, Sherlock S. Levamisole therapy for HbsAg-positive chronic liver disease. *Scand J Gastroenterol* 1980 ; 15 : 973-8.
84. Ausobsky JR, Evans M, Pollock AV. Levamisole and postoperative complications : a controlled clinical trial. *Br J Surg* 1982 ; 69 : 447-8.
85. Tamphaichitra D. Efficacy of acyclovir combined with immunopotentiating agents in the treatment of varicella zoster. *J Antimicrob Chemother* 1987 ; 19 : 255-62.
86. Fedianin IP, Golub TV, Solozhenkin VG, Rostovsteva GA. Decaris as a stimulator of immunogenesis in *Salmonella* infection in infants. *Pediatria* 1988 ; 4 : 93-4.
87. Mukozova LA. Effect of levamisole on the cellular and humoral immunity indices in patients with chronic brucellosis. *Zh Mikrobiol Epidemiol Immunobiol* 1988 ; 10 : 45-9.
88. Feuereisl R, Papezova E. Treatment of patients with pulmonary tuberculosis with antitubercular preparations and levamisole. *Probl Tuberk* 1988 ; 3 : 31-3.
89. Kahr HK, Bhatia VN, Kumar CH, Sirumban P, Roy RG. Evaluation of levamisole, an immunopotentiator, in the treatment of lepromatous leprosy. *Indian J Lep* 1986 ; 58 : 592-600.

90. Sekirina TP, Mikheva TV, Koliaskina GI, Tsutsul'kovkaia MI, Orlova VA. Use of levamisole in the combined therapy of patients with slowly juvenile schizophrenia. *Zh Nevropatol Psikhiatr im ss Korsakova* 1988 ; 88 : 90-4.
91. Semenov SF. Clinico-immunological aspects of using levamisole in psychiatric practice. *Zh Nevropathol Psychiatr im ss Korsakova* 1988 ; 88 : 100-7.
92. Louffi A, Shakr A, Jerry M, Hanley J, Shibata H. Double blind randomized prospective trial of levamisole/placebo in stage I cutaneous malignant melanoma. *Clin Invest Med* 1987 ; 10 : 325-8.
93. Badmanabhan TK, Balaram P, Vasudevan DM. Role of levamisole immunotherapy as an adjuvant to radiotherapy in oral cancer. I. A three year clinical follow up. *Neoplasma* 1987 ; 34 : 627-32.
94. Grem JL. Levamisole as a therapeutic agent for colorectal carcinoma. *Cancer Cells*, A Review 1990 ; 2 : 131-7.
95. Greespan EM, Erlich R. Levamisole and the new area of chemoimmunotherapy. *Cancer Invest* 1991 ; 9 : 111-24.

11

Cyclosporine

F. DE LA TOUR DU PIN, H. HUMBERT, F. DEVAUX, H. PHAM-GIA

Laboratoires Sandoz, 14, boulevard Richelieu, 92500 Rueil-Malmaison, France.

The novel immunomodulatory properties of Cyclosporine (cyclosporine A, Sandimmun), a fungal derivative isolated from *Tolypocladium inflatum*, were discovered by Borel *et al.* (Sandoz Laboratoires de Recherche, Basel) [1, 2] and reported in 1976. The product was marketed in transplantation between 1981 and 1984, then later in autoimmune diseases, in many countries under the name of Sandimmune, or Sandimmun.

General characteristics

Cyclosporine A is a cyclic polypeptide composed of 11 amino acids with a molecular weight of 1,202.6 g (C_{26}, H_{111}, N_{11}, O_{12}) (Figure 1). It is purified to a fine white cristalline powder that is highly lipophilic; it is poorly water-soluble (0.04 mg/g) and, in contrast, highly soluble in organic solvents, such as methanol (> 500 mg/g). Cyclosporine A is generally stable in all its different formulations.

Toxicology

Acute toxicity studies carried out in rat, mouse and rabbit have demonstrated the low level of toxicity of intravenous and oral administrations of cyclosporine. The results are summarized in Table I.

Intravenous administration to dogs has resulted in anaphylactic reactions caused by Cremophor EL, a constituent of the injectable solution.

The results of toxicity studies after repeated oral and intravenous administrations of cyclosporine (13 weeks and 2 years, p.o., in rat 13 weeks, p.o., in monkey; 52 weeks, p.o., in dog; 4 weeks, i.v., in rat and monkey) have usually shown weight loss, often associated with reduced food intake, vomiting and diarrhea, primarily in dog and sometimes in monkey after intravenous administration The kidney and, to a lesser extent, the liver can be considered the target organs in rat, dog and monkey, with the rat being the most sensitive species.

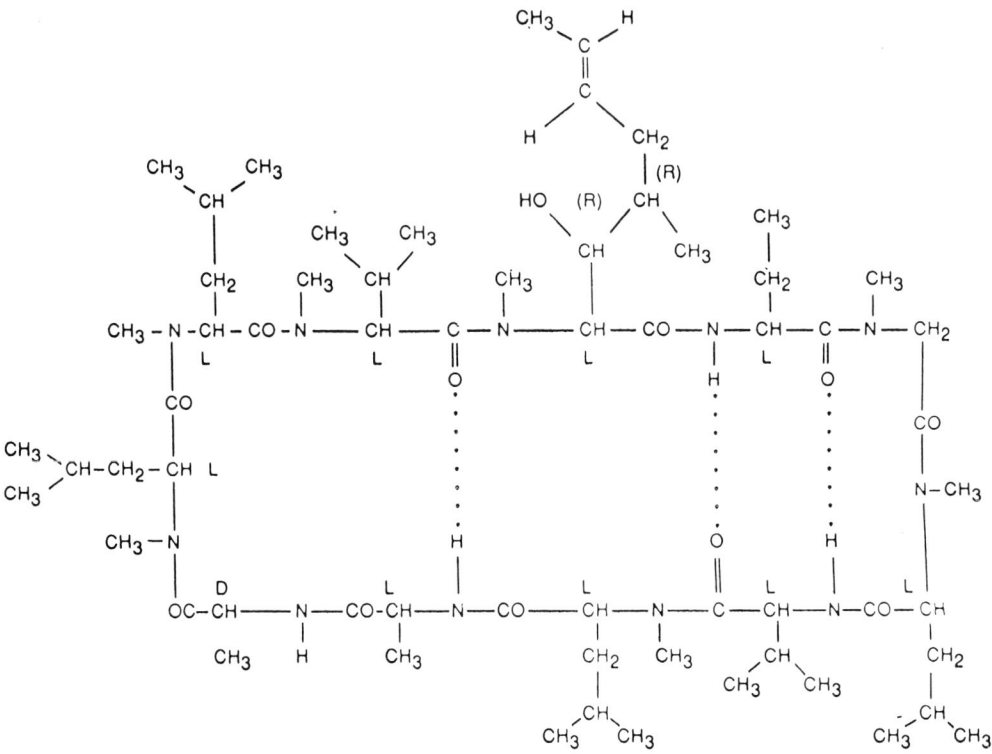

Figure 1. Developed chemical formula of Cyclosporine.

Table I. Acute experimental toxicity of Cyclosporine.

Species	DL 50 (mg/kg)	
	i.v.	p.o
Mouse	107	2300
Rat	25	1500
Rabbit	10	>1000

Histological examination of the kidney shows modifications of the proximal tubule system. The histological modifications of the liver observed in monkey indicate cholestasis.

The renal and hepatic dysfunctions demonstrated biochemically and histologically have been proven to be reversible when the treatment was stopped in the majority of animals.

Hematological analyses reveal a dose-dependent decrease in the number of leukocytes, sometimes with the lymphocyte level being diminished due to atrophy of the lymphatic system, a consequence of the immunosuppressive activity of the product.

Reproductive studies show that Cyclosporine does not affect the fertility of either males or females and is not toxic to fetuses or embryos at doses well-tolerated by the mothers. In addition, at doses toxic to the mothers, cyclosporine has no teratogenic activity.

In vitro *and* in vivo gene-toxicity studies demonstrate, by their negative results, an absence of mutagenetic potential.

No carcinogenic potential has been found in the rat. In contrast, in the mouse, an increased frequency of malignant lymphomas is observed at high doses.

Pharmacokinetics

In animals

The pharmacokinetics of Cyclosporine have been studied in many animal species : the absorption rate varies, depending upon the species (35 % in rat — 50 % in dog), and the maximal concentration is attained 2-4 h after administration. Cyclosporine diffuses widely throughout tissues and organs. The tissue/blood concentration ratio can reach a value of 10. The highest levels are found in liver and kidney : muscle and brain have values lower than that of blood.

The product is strongly bound to erythrocytes (50 %) in blood, while it is bound primarily to lipoproteins in plasma (> 90 %) [3]. Metabolism of the drug conserves the structure of the cyclic oligopeptide. The principal metabolic pathways are hydroxylation and N-demethylation reactions. Numerous metabolites have been detected, however, only a few (M1, M17 and M21) have levels comparable to that of the parent molecule [4].

Elimination is mainly biliary, with more than 60 % found in bile in the rat after intravenous administration. Elimination is biphasic, with an initial half-life of about 4 h and a second one of 21 and 45 h in rat and dog, respectively.

In humans

Many studies have been carried out on the pharmacokinetics and the metabolism of Cyclosporine in healthy volunteers and patients. The major findings are given below.

- *Distribution in blood*

Cyclosporine distribution in the blood is dependent upon numerous parameters [4]. It is strongly bound to red blood cells and this binding is temperature dependent. Thus, on the average, for a blood concentration equal to 100 %, the concentration in plasma separated at 37 °C is about 50 % that of plasma separated at 22 °C is about 200 %. Cyclosporine binding to erythrocytes is saturable for concentrations greater than 1,000 ng/ml. More than 90 % of the Cyclosporine present in plasma is bound to proteins, particularly lipoproteins (mainly high-density lipoproteins (HDL)). A modification of the lipoprotein composition would obviously affect the distribution of the molecule in the blood (this protein binding is not concentration dependent).

Changes in the hematocrit lead to variations in the erythrocyte/plasma distribution. In all cases, the ratio of the concentration in plasma separated at 37° C over the blood concentration is hardly influenced by changes in the hematocrit, but this ratio is dependent upon small variations in the temperature at the time of separation.

In order to standardize the follow-up procedures for patients by reference to a well-defined range of concentrations, it is recommended that the product be dosed in the blood.

- *Metabolism*

Approximately 27 metabolites have been characterized, either by their retention time in high-performance liquid chromatography (HPLC) or by their molecular weight. The structures of only 12 of them have been determined. The principle metabolic pathways undergo monohydroxylation and *N*-demethylation [5].

More than 90 % of the metabolites are found in circulating erythrocytes and lymphocytes. The activity and toxicity of these metabolites have been evaluated in many studies with contradictory results. However, from these various findings, it seems that the different metabolites are only slightly active or inactive. In regard to toxicity, and notably that of the little or unknown metabolites, no definitive conclusion can be drawn. Nevertheless, the toxicity of the major metabolites studied in animals can be eliminated. Since the metabolites seem to contribute little or not to the activity or toxicity, the dosage of the unchanged product in the blood appears to be the most appropriate analysis.

- *Absorption and bioavailability*

The absorption of Cyclosporine is influenced by many factors, such as gastric motility, the presence of biliary salts, administration concomitant with other medications.

The influence of nutrition has been the subject of several studies whose results have not always been in agreement. When differences could be demonstrated, they were always moderate. As for many other active molecules, a nycterohemeral effect, with a slowed absorption when administered in the evening, is noted.

Cyclosporine is absorbed rapidly, with a maximal plasma concentration being attained 2-4 h after administration.

The product is intensely metabolized : the bioavailability reflects the level of absorption and first-pass liver extraction. Mean absolute bioavailabilities as disparate as 18 % and 60 % have been reported. It is evident that the pathological state of the patients given Cyclosporine can influence the bioavailability of the drug. On the average. The absolute bioavailability is about 30 %. Monitoring or the blood levels enables individual adjustment of the dose administered.

The bioavailability of orally administered cyclosporine is linear in the dose range of 350-1,400 mg.

A new formula of Cyclosporine A (Neoral®) is already on the market in some European countries, and should be introduced in 1995, in France. Bioavailability of the active product is increased, hepatic function and intestinal absorbtion is greatly improved.

- *Tissue distribution*

The distribution or metabolites and unaltered product has been studied *postmortem* in different tissues. The highest concentrations of Cyclosporine and/or its metabolites are found, in decreasing order of importance, in liver, adipose tissue, spleen, kidney, muscles and blood.

In all cases, the high concentration observed in fat is contradictory to the fact that obese patients should receive doses based on their ideal weight in order to obtain levels equivalent to those of other patients [6].

In pregnant women, the circulating Sandimmune levels are the same as those found in maternal cord blood. High concentrations are noted in the placenta [7]. Mother's milk has levels a little lower than those in maternal blood. In all cases, breast-feeding should be avoided by patients taking Sandimmune.

- *Elimination*

For the most part, elimination occurs *via* the biliary pathway. Renal excretion of Cyclosporine and its metabolites represents only 6 % of the dose administered. Thus, an alteration of renal function does not, or at least not significantly, modifies elimination of the active ingredient.

Elimination is carried out in two phases, with a final half-life of about 10-15 h. This elimination and its resultant half-life are influenced by several factors including interaction with other medications, liver function status and patient's age. Thus, children under 10 years of age undergo more rapid clearance than adults and require higher mg/kg doses.

In light of the importance of the biliary excretion of this compound, any hepatic disorder will affect its pharmacokinetics.

Hence, very large increases of the metabolic fractions are seen in patients with cholestasis. This observation mandates a closer monitoring of patients having received a liver transplant or suffering from some form of liver dysfunction.

- *Interactions*

Numerous pharmacokinetic interactions have been reported for Cyclosporine, resulting in an increase or decrease of Cyclosporine whole blood levels [8-10]. The exact mechanism of these interactions has not yet been elucidated in the majority of cases. The different hypotheses proposed to explain them include modifications of absorption and/or competition with cytochrome P-450 and/or alterations of biliary excretion.

When Cyclosporine is given in conjunction with another medication to tranplant patients, it is recommended that the Cyclosporine and creatinine levels be monitored during the days following administration in transplanted patients. In autoimmune diseases, this is not compulsory : follow-up by creatinine levels and BP being usually sufficient.

Immunomodulatory properties and mechanism of action

In vivo and ex vivo studies

In 1976, Jean-Francois Borel and his coworkers [1, 2] published the first results demonstrating Cyclosporine modulation of humoral immunity in the mouse. After immunization with sheep red blood cells, the formation of hemagglutinating antibodies is inhibited in a reproducible and dose-dependent manner by the administration of Cyclosporine. This agent, in comparison with other immunosuppressors. has a better therapeutic index and lower hematopoietic toxicity. The extent of humoral response inhibition affecting the different classes of antibodies is even greater in the case of a primary immunization. It also depends upon the nature of the antigen ; Cyclosporine is especially active against thymus-dependent antigens.

The lack of Cyclosporine efficacy in the experimental model of the athymic *nude* mouse further demonstrates that the modulation of this humoral immunity is indeed dependent upon a previous action on cellular immunity [3]. This mechanism is confirmed *in vivo* in rodents by the inhibition of delayed hypersensitivity reactions and the suppression of local graft-*versus*-host and host-*versus*-graft reactions. In the animal models of allogeneic organ grafts, to which we shall return later, *ex vivo* investigations have shown that pretreatment of animals with Cyclosporine blocks the development of effector cytotoxic T cells.

In vitro studies

Investigations with animal and human cells have evaluated the different stages of the immune response. The dose-dependent, early and reversible inhibition of T-lymphocyte proliferation in response to mitogenic or alloantigenic stimulation confirms the major impact of Cyclosporine on cellular immunity without lymphotoxicity. Cyclosporine blocks, in particular, the proliferation of resting T cells and is less effective against activated lymphocytes. In animals and man, Cyclosporine prevents the appearance of cytotoxic T cells without affecting the effector mechanisms of mature cells and provokes the induction of suppressor T cells. These immunosuppressive effects seem to be primarily linked at the level of the helper T cell to a functional interruption of the system of interleukin 2 and its receptor, which controls the growth and differentiation of T-lymphocytes. Cyclosporine is associated with the inhibition of the synthesis of several other cytokines involved in the cascade of immune reactions (Figure 2).

In addition to interleukin 2, the central element of this regulation, interleukins 3, 4 and 5, interferon-gamma, granulocyte-macrophage colony-stimulating factor (GMCSF) tumor necrosis factors (TNF) alpha and beta [11, 12] are also implicated. These cytokines participate in a network of communications between them and cooperation with other cell groups : monocytes, macrophages and B lymphocytes.

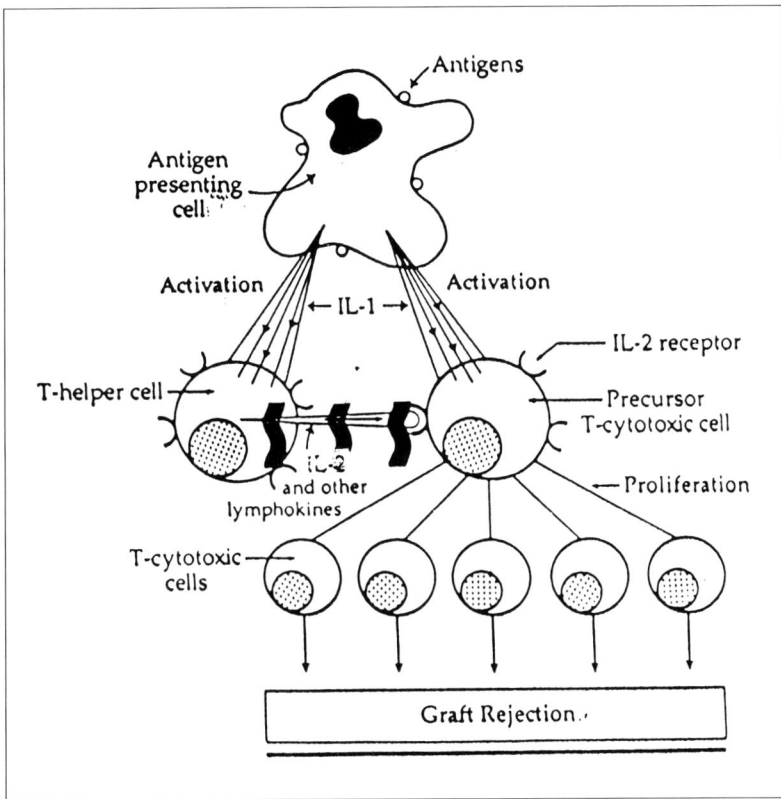

Figure 2. Cyclosporine mechanism of action. Cyclosporine prevents differentiation and proliferation of T-cytotoxic lymphocytes by selectively intervening at two critical stages of development. It impedes the production and release of Il-2 and many other lymphokines responsible of proliferation of effector T-cytotoxic lymphocytes and other cells with immune functions, and may also inhibit interleukin-2 receptor (IL-2R) expression on both T-helper and T-cytotoxic lymphocytes, effectively limiting their activation and proliferation.

Molecular mechanisms of action

After antigen binding to the T cell receptor, Cyclosporine acts on the early events in T cell activation. It blocks the mobilization of intracellular ionized calcium reserves, which constitute one of the effector mechanisms of this activation. Calmodulin, a nuclear and cytoplasmic protein dependent upon intracellular calcium, is a moderate-affinity, non-specific Cyclosporine vector. On the other hand, cyclophilin, another transport protein, is specific, ubiquitous and exhibits high affinity. It is found in the cytoplasm and nucleus as well as in numerous target tissues, for example, hematopoietic organs. brain, liver and kidney, and has enzymatic (peptidyl-prolyl-*cis-trans*-isomerase) activity [13]. Cyclosporine inhibits *in vitro* the activity of this enzyme, which is responsible for the *cis*-to-*trans* isomerization of proline-bearing proteins. It could thus interfere with their spatial configurations at the level or intranuclear passage.

In fact, in the nucleus, interleukin 2 gene deletion experiments and those in transgenic mice demonstrated that the specific inhibition of Cyclosporine acts upon proteins comprising the exon activation factors, situated at the 5'-end of the sequence coding for the gene. This molecular mechanism of action also seems to be valid for interleukin 4 and interferon-gamma.

Therapeutic effects in animal models of immune disorders

Infections

The results obtained in animal models vary according to the experimental protocol used. Thus, for mice inoculated with herpes simplex virus, interference with the specific immune protection does not occur after oral administration of Cyclosporine, but does after intraperitoneal injection. For cytomegalovirus or hepatitis or influenza virus, the results vary according to the animal model and the dosage administered.

In all cases, the percentage of infections, their severity and mortality are lower than those seen with other immunosuppressors. Similar results are noted in bacterial and fungal infections. The demonstration in several animal models of an antiparasitic activity against cerebral forms of malaria, schistosomiasis and leishmaniasis should be emphasized.

Tumors

Cyclosporine has a cytostatic effect, inhibiting the proliferation of certain tumor cell lines of lymphocytic origin (mostly T cells), but also of non-lymphocytic or hematopoietic origin. However, the doses required to inhibit tumor proliferation are 10-times higher than those needed to block lymphocyte growth *in vivo*.

Cyclosporine's ability to reverse anti-cancer chemotherapy resistance phenomena, under the control of *MDR* genes for certain tumors, should also be noted.

Transplantation

The first experimental findings on the effect of Cyclosporine on transplanted organs were reported in 1976 by J.F. Borel *et al.* [1, 2], who demonstrated the prolonged survival of an allogeneic skin graft in mice. The most classic models are kidney and heart allografts in rat and dog or bone marrow grafts in rodents. Tangible differences exist between the results obtained, depending upon the organ grafted and the animal species used.

Generally speaking, Cyclosporine provides clear therapeutic progress, as compared to other immunosuppressors (steroids, azathioprine, methotrexate, total lymphoid irradiation). It has been shown to be even more effective when administered soon after the presentation of alloantigens and when it is a first graft. It enabled some new allografts, impossible before, to be performed successfully in animals : lung, small intestine and pancreas. Thanks to this drug, similar procedures have been established for multiple-organ transplant, for example heart-lung or kidney-pancreas.

For xenografts, on the other hand, progress has been made, but early and late rejections remain numerous.

Autoimmunity

Investigations have been carried out using several animal models of induced or genetic, organ-specific or non-specific, autoimmune diseases. Cyclosporine can be used to prevent the appearance of the disease (prediabetes in the NOD mouse or BB rat) or as a curative therapy for an existing disease (autoimmune uveitis in the guinea pig). It provides three types of therapeutic benefits :

(1) short-term prevention of sometimes fatal evolution (experimental allergic encephalomyelitis) ;
(2) immediate improvement of the functioning of organs whose deficiency is associated with a major handicap (arthritis, uveitis) ;
(3) long-term prevention of the appearance of degenerative complications (diabetes, nephritis).

Inflammatory pathologies

In acute inflammation induced in the rat, Cyclosporine is not effective : there is no anti-inflammatory or anti-pyretic effect. In contrast, chronic inflammation, simulated as induced arthritis in the rat, is sensitive to preventive and curative Cyclosporine treatments, with a therapeutic index similar to that of nonsteroidal anti-inflammatory drugs (NSA1Ds).

Associated treatments

Combining methotrexate with Cyclosporine to treat bone marrow grafts in the dog improves graft-*versus*-host tolerance for major histocompatibility differences. In contrast, associating Cyclosporine with total irradiation before kidney transplant in the dog paradoxically seems to lead to poorer tolerance than that obtained with the two treatments administered separately.

Other pharmacological properties

Hematopoietic system

Cyclosporine does not modify, in any way, the number of leukocytes or thrombocytes. It does not interfere with the chemotactic properties or the oxidative metabolism of granulocytes. It inhibits the *in vitro* expression of genes coding for interleukin 3 and GMCSF, but does not have any deleterious effect on hematopoiesis, confirming that its role is limited to T-lymphocytes.

Central nervous system

In the mouse, very high doses of Cyclosporine (500 mg/kg in one dose) acutely decrease the animal's activity and appetite and are associated with ptosis and piloerection. These effects are reversible and are not observed at lower doses.

First clinical application

Organs transplantations

The first clinical trials began in 1978 with kidney (Calne, Cambridge) and bone marrow grafts (Powles, London), then heart transplants (Shumway, Stanford ; Cabrol, Paris) and liver grafts (Starzl, Pittsburgh ; Bismuth, Paris) in 1981.

Applications were accepted as of 1981 in Switzerland, in 1983 and 1984 by health authorities of the principal Western countries (Germany, USA, UK, Scandinavian nations, Belgium, France).

For **renal transplantation**, Cyclosporine (Sandimmune) presents a real benefit (without being revolutionary) in terms of graft survival : $+10+20$ % actuarial survival at one year, depending upon the center. The decisive advantage is represented by steroid-sparing, with fewer bacterial infections and resumed or maintained growth in children. Survival at 5 years or more speaks eloquently (70-75 %). In addition, the product enables transplantation in « high risk » patients.

The dual therapy of Cyclosporine and low doses of prednisone or Cyclosporine and azathioprine is most commonly used. It is often preceded by a short-term (usually about 2 weeks) three-ways, or even four-ways, immunosuppression by polyclonal or monoclonal antibodies or corticosteroids. Some groups only start Cyclosporine treatment after the end of this « risk » period. Cyclosporine is prescribed in monotherapy for long-term maintenance in some centers, except for patients at high risk of rejection : the Canadian multicenter trial and Munich Kidney Transplant Center have adopted this approach and have been able to successfully withdraw corticosteroids 3-6 months after transplantation in a certain number of patients.

For **cardiac transplantation**, Cyclosporine represented in 1981-1982 a quasi-revolutionary therapy. The mid-term (1-2 years) success rate, rarely achieved with previously used immunosuppression protocols, surpasses 85 % at times. At 5 years (long-term), this success rate is still between 60 % and 70 %.

In most centers, immunosupressor protocols consist of an initial phase of three- or four-way association (lasting about 3 weeks), with Sandimmune usually being introduced around the third day post-transplantation. The combination of moderate doses of prednisone, or azathioprine (if the tendancy towards rejection is higher) remains the standard regimen.

For **liver transplantation**, Cyclosporine also plays a significant role in the therapeutic arsenal, when introduced in 1981-1982 ; it increases greatly the immediate and long-term success rates. The product is introduced (orally) several days post-transplantation, generally after an initial phase of intravenous perfusion. The percentages of a long-term graft survival are, at 5 years post-transplantation, generally comprised between 65 % and 70 %.

In children, for **kidney liver and heart transplantation,** Cyclosporine is an essential factor for the quality of life, eliminating the need for high doses of steroids.

This list is not exhaustive : Cyclosporine is also used in lung and heart-lung transplantation and other « solid » (pancreas) or « multi-organ » grafts.

Bone marrow grafts

The primary contribution of Cyclosporine, alone or more frequently associated with methotrexate, is the reduction in the frequency and especially the severity or graft-*versus*-host disease (GVHD), whose severe acute forms are decreased by half (30 % *versus* 60 %), as compared to control groups without Cyclosporine. Unlike organ transplants, the length of treatment is limited for bone marrow (an average of 6 months).

Pharmacological and therapeutic monitoring of patients

The necessity of precise monitoring of blood Cyclosporine levels in these above-cited indications, is clearly established. Measurements are made using radioimmunoassays, usually with whole blood. Generally the blood levels determined using a monoclonal antibody directed against the active substance (without its metabolites) should fall in the range 100-300 ng/ml. This control enables the adjustment of the treatment to each patient, since large interindividual variations due to age, time since transplantation, therapeutic regimen (associations) used and organ transplanted have been observed. The daily oral maintenance treatment is usually between 2 and 8 mg/kg.

Cyclosporine therapeutic margin is rather narrow, but a better knowledge of its « minimum efficacy » has reduced, compared to its initial trials, the frequency and severity of side effects [14, 15]. *Drug Monitoring*, Sandoz, Basel, 1989, evaluated Cyclosporine's major side effects in the context of organ transplantation : kidney dysfunction (51.7 %), high blood pressure (38.4 %), hypertrichosis (32.9 %), benign neurological perturbations, *e.g.*, tremors or paresthesias (25.9 %), liver dysfunction (18.4 %) and gingival hyperplasia (14.8 %).

The term kidney dysfunction most often refers to moderate and reversible modifications of glomerular filtration and proximal tubule reabsorption. Histological lesions (arteriolar and tubular, interstitial fibrosis) are more rarely observed in biopsies. High blood pressure, although frequent, is rarely severe and responds to antihypertensive drugs : the responsibility of therapy with corticosteroids is often cited. Close monitoring of blood levels guarantees both the efficacity and the innocuousness of the treatment in transplant patients.

New therapeutic applications

The therapeutic potential of Cyclosporine in certain diseases of autoimmune origin and in which T-lymphocytes and the lymphokines play a pathogenic role has been the object of many studies over the past few years, which are summarized in G. Feutren synthesis [16] in psoriasis, nephrotic syndrome, rheumatoid arthritis and autoimmune uveitis. Official approval of these indications is now obtained in most countries. Other clinical trials, not as promising or as advanced, have been under-taken : insulin-dependent diabetes, non-transplantable severe aplastic anemia, Crohn's disease and primary biliary cirrhosis. Finally, investigations have begun for multiple sclerosis and some forms of myasthenia : so far the results have been disappointing, despite positive conclusions drawn in some centers.

Psoriasis

Cyclosporine, in addition to its effect on activated T-lymphocytes, can also interfere in the proliferation of keratinocytes. An international phase III clinical report, based on 842 patient files, concluded that the product was effective, as a second-line treatment, in the severe forms of the disease and in cases failing to respond to classical treatments, at an initial dose of 2.5 mg/kg/d that can be increased to a maximum of 5 mg/kg/d.

Creatininemia and blood pressure must be monitored, but dosage of Cyclosporine blood levels is not routinely necessary.

The percentage of lasting remissions (6 months and longer) reaches 81 %, but termination of treatment leads to the reappearance of the symptoms. Renal insufficiency, uncontrolled hypertension and a history of malignant tumors are contraindications for the initiation of this therapy.

Nephrotic syndrome

Cyclosporine is considered to be an effective second-line treatment, especially in patients refractory to or intolerant of corticosteroid therapy. The efficacy is clearer in corticodependent patients and enables partial or total steroid-sparing. The percentage of remissions varies according to the form of the nephrotic syndrome, with an average of 60 % complete remissions. This percentage is about 45 % for steroid-resistant minimal-change nephropathy, 49 % for steroid-resistant focal glomerulosclerosis ; 80 % in steroid-dependent minimal-change nephropathy. The administration protocol is similar to that recommended for psoriasis, with higher initial doses.

Rheumatoid arthritis

The results in multicenter clinical studies, in various countries, give a good general appraisal of Cyclosporine efficacity. On 5 mg/kg/d of Cyclosporine, the overall responder rate was 54 %.

The essential criteria were : articular score, intensity of spontaneous pain, functional capacities. The progressive adaptation to the dose and the monitoring of creatininemia and blood pressure are necessary precautions. The benefit in terms of « quality of life » in this invalidating disease is emphasized by the authors of the different clinical studies.

Uveitis

Intermediate or posterior non infectious uveitis have a chronic evolution, with inflammatory acute periods resulting in a visual severe deficiency. Corticoid resistance leads to trial of immunosuppressive therapy. Positive results on experimental models, then in clinical trial, underlines efficacity of Sandimmune® on intermediate and posterior uveitis, in their corticodependant or corticoresistant varieties. Initial dosage at 5 mg/kg/d should be maintained till control of inflammatory process and improval of visual acuity, then adjusted to therapeutical answer.

References

1. Borel JF, Feurer C, Gubler HU, Stahelin H. Biological effects on Cyclosporine A : a new antilymphocytic agent. *Agents Actions* 1976 ; 6 : 468-75.
2. Borel JF, Wiesinger D. Effects of cyclosporin A on murine lymphoid cells. In : Lucas DO, ed. *Regulatory mechanisms in lymphocyte activation* New York : Academic Press, 1977 : 716-8.
3. Kahan BD. Cyclosporin — Therapeutic drug monitoring. Hawk's Cay, January 14-17, 1990, Florida. *Transplant Proc* 1990 ; 22 : 1097-359.
4. Maurer G. Metabolism of cyclosporine. *Transplant Proc* 1985 ; 17 (4/Suppl. 1) : 19-26.
5. Humbert H. Metabolites of cyclosporine : blood and tissue levels. Biological activity ? *Nucl Med Biol* 1990 ; 17 : 723-7.
6. Flechner SM, Kolbeinsson ME, Tam, Lum B. The impact of body weight on cyclosporine pharmacokinetics in renal transplant recipients. *Transplantation* 1989 ; 47 : 806-10.
7. Flechner SM, Katz AR, Rogers AJ, Van Buren C, Kahan BD. The presence of cyclosporine in body tissues and fluids during pregnancy. *Am J Kidney Dis* 1985 ; 5 : 60-3.
8. de La Tour du Pin F. Interactions de la cyclosporine avec la thérapeutique anti-infectieuse. *Lettre Infectiol* 1989 ; 4 : 318-22.
9. Yee GC, McGuire TR. Pharmacokinetic drug interactions with cyclosporin (Part I) *Clin Pharmacokinet* 1990 ; 19 : 319-332.
10. Yee GC, McGuire TR. Pharmacokinetic drug interactions with cyclosporin (Part II). *Clin Pharmacokinet* 1990 ; 19 : 400-15.
11. Andrus L, Lafferty KJ. Inhibition of T-cell activity by cyclosporin A. *Scand J Immunol* 1982 ; 15 : 449-58.
12. Morris PJ. Cyclosporin A. Overview. *Transplantation* 1981 ; 32 : 349-54.
13. Fischer G, Wittman-Lieboldt B, Lang K, Kiefhaber T, Schmidt FX. Cyclophilin and peptidyl-prolyl-*cis-trans*-isomerase are probably identical proteins. *Nature* 1989 ; 337 : 473-6.
14. Krups P, *et al*. Side effects and safety of Sandimmun in long-term treatment of transplant patients. In : *Cyclosporine in auto-immune diseases*. Springer Publ., 1985 : 43-9.
15. Cockburn I, *et al*. An interim analysis of the on going long term safety study of cyclosporin in renal transplantation. *Transplant Proc* 1988 ; 20 ; (S3) : 519-29.
16. Feutren G. The use of Cyclosporine in auto-immune diseases. In : Bach JF, ed. *T-cell-directed immunointervention. Frontiers in pharmacology and therapeutics.* Oxford : Blackwell Publ 1993 ; 101-8.

12

FK506 : a powerful new drug for T cell-directed immunointervention

A.W. THOMSON, J. WOO, A. ZEEVI, N. MURASE,
J.J. FUNG, S. TODO, T.E. STARZL

Pittsburgh Transplantation Institute and Departments of Surgery and Pathology, University of Pittsburgh School of Medicine, Pittsburgh, Pennsylvania, USA.

Product

Historic background of FK506

Manipulation of the immune system and, in particular, drug-based immunosuppression, has been the key ingredient in successful organ transplantation. The first steps along this pathway were with steroids and relatively non-specific cytotoxic agents, as summarized elsewhere [1-3]. This primitive era of immunosuppression came to an end with the discovery of the T cell specific immunosuppressant Cyclosporin A (CsA) in the early 1970s [4]. This breakthrough has spawned a basic and clinical literature so vast that it almost defies the efforts that have been made at collation and synthesis [5-7]. Clinically, improvements in both allograft survival rates and patients' quality of life have been achieved [8] using CsA alone [9] or in combination with steroids [10] and/or other immunosuppressive modalities.

The long-term administration of immunosuppressive drugs that is necessary to counteract rejection following transplantation (including use of azathioprine, corticosteroids and CsA) is usually associated with toxic side effects. Although CsA is regarded as the most successful primary immunosuppressive drug to prevent rejection, its nephrotoxicity remains a significant and difficult problem in patient management [11-13]. In certain cases, treatment of patients with CsA has to be terminated due to its unacceptable nephrotoxicity. In addition, administration of CsA may be associated with other side effects, including hypertension, hirsutism, hepatotoxicity and diabetogenicity [11, 14, 15] and CNS disturbances [16]. Most of these toxic effects were already described in the first report by Calne *et al.* [9] and Starzl *et al.* [10] and completely annotated by Kahan [8] a decade later.

As a result, the search for novel, less toxic agents that have a higher therapeutic index or lower risk : benefit ratio and act at specific target sites within immunocompetent cells is of prime importance in the search for useful prototypes for human immunosuppression.

During routine screening of the fermentation broths of *Streptomyces* for specific inhibitory effects on mouse mixed lymphocyte reactions, Goto and Kino [17-19] of the Fujisawa Pharmaceutical Co., Ltd., Osaka, Japan, 1982-1983, identified strain no. 9993 that was designated *Streptomyces tsukubaensis*, and appeared to possess potent immunosuppressive properties. The product isolated from the fungal strain was designated FK-900506 (or later FK506). Although according to structure and function, FK506 was classified as a macrolide antibiotic, it had no growth inhibitory effect on bacteria or yeast and showed only limited antifungal activity against *Aspergillus fumigatus* and *Fusarium oxysporum* [18].

Preliminary investigations showed that FK506 was very effective in suppressing immune responses both *in vivo* and *in vitro* and that the effective concentration was usually 10 to 100 times lower than CsA [17-19]. These initial studies were presented publicly for the first time by Ochiai at the 11th International Congress of the Transplantation Society held in Helsinki in August, 1986, and published the following March [20] By this time, further confirmatory *in vitro* studies from other laboratories began to appear [21]. Since then, there has been rapid progress in elucidating the immunosuppressive properties of FK506 in various animal models and also its mode of action (reviewed by Thomson [22]). Within 2 further years, additional intensive studies in several laboratories throughout the world led to the experimental clinical application of FK506 in human organ transplantation at the University of Pittsburgh [23]. Further detailed documentation of the molecular action immunosuppressive properties, pharmacology, toxicology and early clinical experiences with FK506 can be found in the proceeding of the First International Congress on FK506 and in a recent comprehensive review of the drugs properties [24].

Physico-chemical properties of FK506

FK506 is a white crystalline powder at room temperature ; it is highly soluble in non-polar solvents, such as methanol, ethanol and chloroform but it is insoluble in polar solvents. The molecular formula of FK506, deduced by elemental analysis and mass spectrometry, is $C_{44}H_{69}NO_{12}$-H_2O (molecular weight 822) [25]. Infrared spectral analysis showed the presence of hydroxy groups (3530 cm^{-1}), carbonyl groups (1750, 1730, 1710 cm^{-1}) and an amide group (1650 cm^{-1}). Further detailed structural analysis by nuclear magnetic resonance revealed two ketones, one lactone, one hemiketal, three O-methyls and five C-methyls with the remainder being 12 methylenes and 13 methines. The structures of FK506, CsA and rapamycin (a close structural analogue of FK506) are shown in Figure 1. Both FK506 and rapamycin share a similar structure, *i.e.* a lactone ring with sugar substituents, totally different from that of CsA, a cyclic peptide comprising 11 amino acids.

FK506 is relatively stable under normal conditions and has a melting point of 127-129 °C. Full activity of FK506 can still be detected after storage for 6 months at 40 °C, 3 months at 82 % relative humidity, 3 months under 500 Lux fluorescent light exposure and 24 months at room temperature [25]. Reports of its synthesis began to appear in 1989 [26, 27].

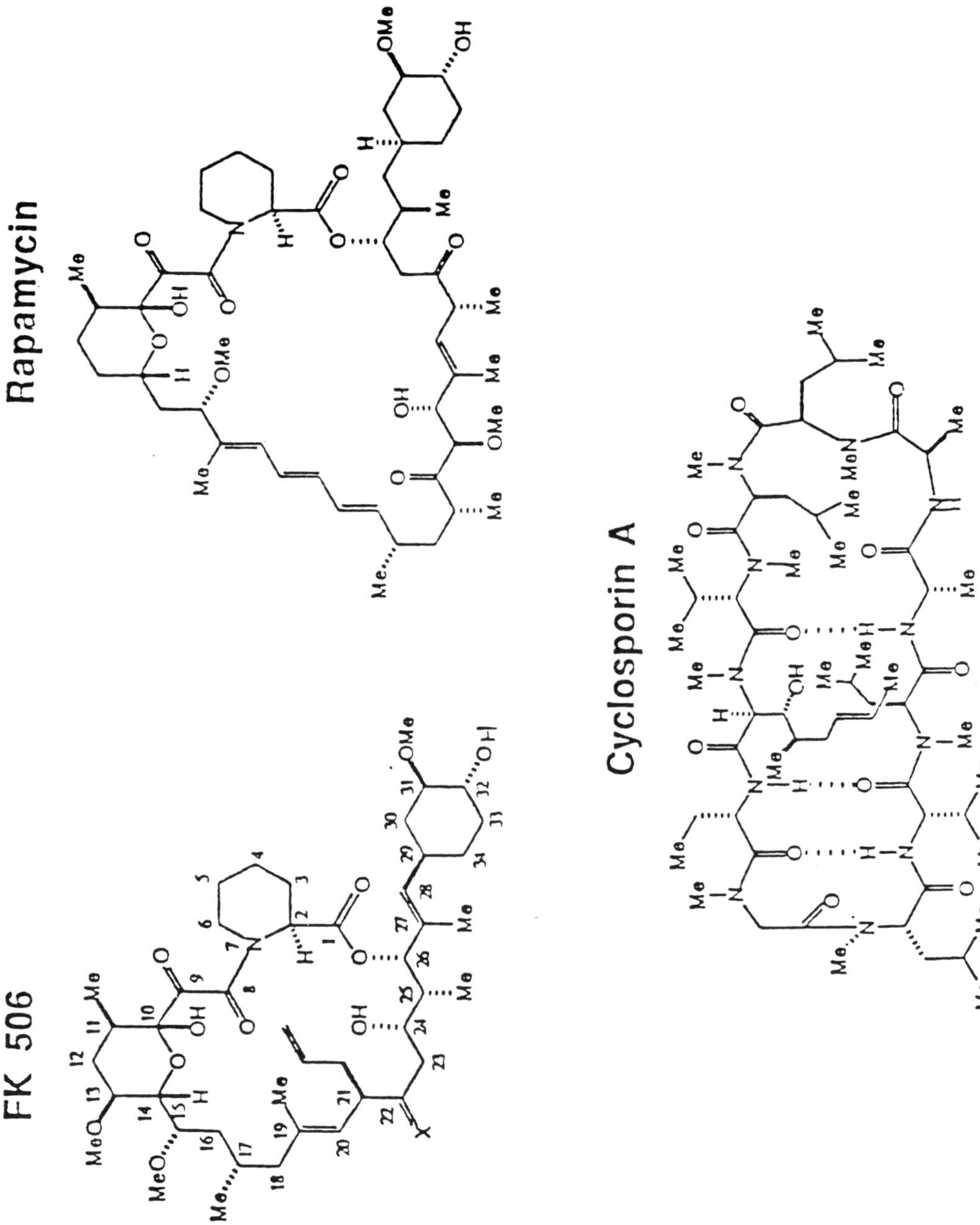

Figure 1. Structures of Cyclosporin A, FK506 and the close structural analogue of FK506, Rapamycin.

Experimental and preclinical studies

Toxicology

Such a powerful anti-lymphocytic agent as FK506 is likely to have structural effects on lymphoid tissue. Striking but reversible thymic medullary atrophy accompanying the immunosuppressive action of FK506 in rodents [28, 29] has been observed. This phenomenon is associated with a cytopathic effect on thymic epithelial cells, which express self major-histocompatibility complex (MHC) antigens and secrete thymic hormones, and with reduced numbers of mature thymocytes [30, 31]. FK506 may therefore have the capacity to interfere with self MHC recognition by thymocytes and T cell differentiation and maturation. A recent study suggests however that, during FK506 treatment, rat thymocytes may retain their potential for peripheral mobilization [32].

FK506 shows differential toxicity in animals [22]. It is well tolerated at therapeutic dosage by rodents, although minor renal impairment and hypoglycemia have been reported in rats [28, 29]. However, in dogs, FK506 can be severely toxic, causing anorexia and vascular lesions that may affect various organs, especially the heart and gastrointestinal tract [33-35]. A syndrome of lethal emaciation was described in canine recipients of kidneys and livers [36, 37]. Hepatocellular swelling, renal proximal tubular cell vacuolation, and pancreatic acinar cell degeneration have also been attributed to FK506 [38]. Calne *et al.* [39] reported lethal emaciation and hyperglycemia in FK506-treated baboons who had received renal allografts but major side effects were not observed in baboons given high doses of FK506 in other centers [40, 41].

The most alarming histopathologic finding was widespread arteritis in studies from Cambridge, England [35, 42]. Todo *et al.* [38] confirmed the presence of these lesions after transplantation but demonstrated their presence also in dogs treated with CsA or nothing. The possibility that arteritis was a nonspecific finding in the traumatized dog [43] was consistent with Ochiai's observation after canine renal transplantation that the lesions were inversely related to the FK506 dose and therefore the control of rejection [44]. Nevertheless, the specter of arteritis was a dominant concern in the early clinical trials.

Pharmacokinetics

Precise pharmacokinetic studies rely on the accuracy and sensitivity of the assay employed. Most studies on the quantitation of FK506 have used an enzyme-linked immunosorbant assay (ELISA), in which either a monoclonal or polyclonal antibody is used, with sensitivity down to 20 pg/ml [45]. A modified ELISA, using a mouse monoclonal anti-FK506 antibody for quantitation of FK506 in human plasma has been described [46].

Monitoring of plasma FK506 concentrations by a FK506 ELISA kit [45] showed that, at immunosuppressive doses (1.0 mg/kg, *per os*) in the dog, the serum trough level was between 0.08 and 0.4 ng/ml, while at non-immunosuppressive dosage, a lower trough plasma concentration was observed, indicating that the effective, prophylactic serum trough level was between 0.1 and 0.4 ng/ml [47]. Co-administration of FK506 with CsA can reduce the threshold effective FK506 trough level and this may offer an explanation for the synergy exhibited between these two drugs [47], which was reported earlier in *in vitro* models [21, 48] and in intact animals by Murase *et al.* [49] and by Todo *et al.* [31, 33]. In canine kidney recipients undergoing rejection, reduction in serum creatinine level and the attenuation or disappearance of the cellular infiltrate during rejection was observed in FK506-treated animals and was shown to correlate with an increase in FK506 trough level [47].

FK506 is not rapidly absorbed after oral administration but once it is absorbed, it is distributed in various organs, including lung, spleen, heart and kidney [50]. The majority of FK506 is metabolized by liver and is then excreted in bile, urine and faeces within 48 hours of administration [50, 51]. Activity of cytochrome P-450, the enzyme that metabolizes CsA, has been demonstrated both *in vivo* [50] and *in vitro* [52] to be downregulated by the presence of FK506, implying a possible mechanism whereby FK506 affects the pharmacokinetics of CsA which also depends on this same degradation system [53]. In addition, FK506 also possesses hepatotrophic effects *(see below)*, similar to those of CsA [54, 55]. For a review of the pharmacokinetics of FK506, the reader is referred to a recent survey [56].

- **Other pharmacological properties**

The hepatotrophic qualities of FK506 include the augmentation of the regeneration that occurs after partial hepatectomy [54] and protection of the liver from the hepatocyte injury caused by Eck-fistula (portacaval shunt) [57]. These observations mean that both CsA and FK506 are growth regulators, a finding of considerable interest as evidence mounts of the pleiotropic actions of these drugs. These actions are apart from the immunosuppressive properties of FK506. Increases in [^{3}H]-thymidine incorporation and percentage of mitosis beyond those occurring naturally, in 70 % hepatectomized rats, were observed in FK506 treated rats. Serum from unoperated FK506-treated rats (4 days with therapeutic doses) was found to cause an increase in mitosis in hepatocyte culture, although FK506 added directly to the hepatocyte culture system had no influence on the hepatocyte mitosis response [58, 59]. The same was true with the serum of T cell deficient nude rats, and these rats also displayed augmented regeneration under FK506 treatment. Using the Eck-fistula model in dogs that allows hepatocyte renewal and hypertrophy to be studied separately, hepatocyte proliferation is augmented by FK506 and normal cellular characteristics (cell size and morphology) are obtained [55, 60]. These results are compatible with the hypothesis that some circulating growth factor(s) is/are induced by FK506 and this may account for the significant improvement in hepatic function following treatment with FK506 after liver transplant [61]. It also introduces the possibility that FK506 could be used to promote liver healing after injury from ischemia [62] or from a variety of disease processes [55].

Immunomodulating properties and mechanisms of action

The reader is referred to several recent reviews for extensive coverage of the literature [22, 24, 63].

- **In vivo *and* ex vivo *studies***

Most early studies employed to evaluate the immunosuppressive properties of FK506 *in vivo* used models of organ graft rejection ranging from skin allografts to multi-visceral transplants in various experimental species, including rodents, dogs and primates, with CsA being used as the standard for direct comparison [22, 64].

These studies, however, shed little light on the mode of action of FK506 *in vivo*. Results from our laboratory have shown that a short course of treatment with FK506 can inhibit the delayed type hypersensitivity (DTH) response to sheep red blood cells (SRBC) in mice (Figure 2), alleviate the production of serum anti-SRBC antibody and anti-MHC class I alloantibody in rats [65], and attenuate the *ex vivo* responsiveness of rat splenic lymphocytes to polyclonal T cell mitogens. Early studies by Kino and colleagues showed that treatment of mice with FK506 resulted in suppression of the production of antibody plaque-forming cells against SRBC, the generation of DTH responses against methylated bovine serum albumin and the development of graft-vs-host reactions [19].

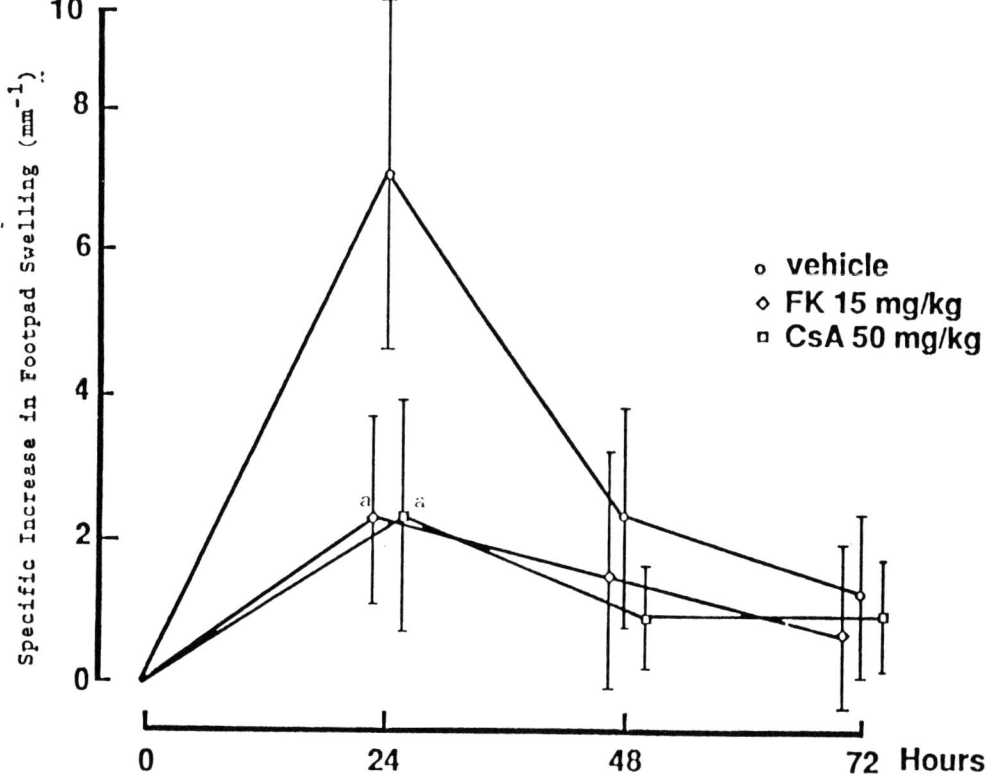

Figure 2. Influence of FK-506, 15 mg/kg/day, and CsA, 50 mg/kg/day on murine delay type hypersensitivity (DTH) to SRBC. Animals (MFI mice) were immunized with 16 SRBC, i.v., on day 0 and challenged on day 4 s.c. in the footpad with 18 SRBC. Increase in footpad swelling was assessed 24, 48 and 72 hours later by measuring the increase in dorsoventral thickness of the test and the control footpad. Results are expressed as specific increase in footpad thickness (10^{-1} mm, means ± 1 S.D.). a, $p < 0.01$ compared with vehicle-treated control.

As with CsA, the mechanism of action of FK506 is not fully characterized. The possible role of suppressor cells and their activity in FK506-treated animals have been particularly intriguing. Flow cytometric analyses of lymphocytes have revealed that treatment of rats with a short course of FK506 beginning on the day of immunization results in a transient increase in splenic $OX-8^+$ ($CD8^+$) cells with a concomitant decrease in $W3/25^+ : OX-8^+$ ($CD4^+ : CD8^+$) ratios [66], a phenomenon similar to *in vitro* observations on PHA-stimulated, cultured human blood lymphocytes (unpublished observation). Interestingly, a role for suppressor cells in FK506-treated animals is further implicated by the transfer of unresponsiveness using spleen cells from FK506-treated, long-term allograft survivors to naive recipients [20], and by the dependence on the spleen for the immunosuppressive properties of FK506 in mice [53]. Separate studies, however, have demonstrated that FK506 prevents the development of suppressor cells *in vitro* [67] and thus the role of suppressor cells in inducing immunosuppression in FK506-treated animals is still unresolved.

An analysis of the reasons for acceptance of heart and liver grafts has minimized the role of any single change, including that of suppressor cells, clonal deletion or classical enhancement [68]. Ochiai *et al.* [69] suggested that a serum soluble factor may contribute to FK506's immunosuppressive action in allograft recipients. Such a suppressor factor(anti-idiotypic antibody) has been observed in serum of CsA-treated animals following alloimmunization [70]. Thus, transfer of serum from allografted, drug-treated rats was found to prolong allograft survival in naive recipients [69]. However, Murase *et al.* [71] have failed to reproduce this observation. The difficulty in explaining exactly how grafts are accepted is reminiscent of the preceding literature with CsA [7]. One neglected possibility is that the graft itself undergoes change, in which case the process of graft acceptance is apt to be more complex and dynamic than currently envisioned [72, 73].

Although the role of suppressor cells in FK506 treated animals is unresolved, there is little doubt that immunosuppression *in vivo* is a direct result of inhibition of $CD4^+$ helper T cell activities. Flow cytometric studies have revealed that the increase in number of circulating, activated $CD4^+$ lymphocytes during a SRBC-induced immune response is significantly reduced [74]. In addition, severe depression of *ex vivo* Con A-induced spleen cell proliferation and alloantigen-induced lymph node cell proliferation was found in FK506-but not CsA-treated animals.

An important difference between FK506 and CsA *in vivo* concerns the ease of reversibility of the suppression of the humoral immune response. Early studies by Borel and his colleagues showed that cessation of treatment led to rapid reversibility of the immunosuppressive effect of CsA [5]; suppression of antibody production in FK506-treated animals, on the contrary, is not reversed following withdrawal of the drug 2 weeks earlier [74]. Most likely, these drug differences are quantitative only, and merely in illusion produced by the short (2 weeks) observation. However, the possibility of clonal depletion (in particular, B-cell clonal depletion) in these immunosuppressed animals should be mentioned. This may be a secondary effect of insufficient lymphokine production by helper T cells to maintain the growth and differentiation of activated B cells. This concept is supported by a recent *in vitro* finding that inhibition of anti-IgM-activated B-cell proliferation with FK506 resulted in cell death [75].

Apart from affecting cells within the secondary lymphoid organs, it was mentioned earlier that thymic medullary atrophy is a characteristic feature during FK506-treatment in rats [28, 29]. Further detailed study has shown that medullary epithelial cells are damaged and phagocytosed by thymic macrophages, within which remnants of epithelial cells are readily detected [33, 76]. Besides, FK506 treated rats demonstrate a reduction in the incidence of mature, medullary thymocytes and cells expressing MHC class I antigen [35, 76]. Since the thymus is the environment for development of T cells, any effect of FK506 on thymocyte maturation and differentiation may affect the distribution and responsiveness of lymphocyte populations in other lymphoid organs. The question of graft acceptance has been further complicated by recent experiments showing repopulation of lymphoid tissue within intestinal grafts of FK506-treated rats predominantly by recipient cells [73].

- **In vitro** *studies*

Animal cells

Preliminary studies showed that FK506 was a strong inhibitor of responses to polyclonal T cell mitogens, such as PHA or Con A. In murine studies, the IC_{50}s to inhibit Con A-induced spleen lymphocyte transformation were 0.7 nM and 30 nM for FK506 and CsA respectively [21]. Both drugs act at the time of commitment of lymphocytes from Go to Gl of the cell division cycle [77]. Since the mixed-lymphocyte reaction (MLR) is regarded as the *in vitro* model that most closely resembles *in vivo* allograft rejection, it has been used extensively to evaluate the immunosuppressive potency of FK506. It was reported that FK506 strongly inhibited alloantigen-induced lymphocyte transformation, with IC_{50}s of 0.07 nM and 20 nM for FK506 and CsA respectively, in murine cell cultures [21]. Using murine antigen-specific T cell clones, it was also demonstrated that FK506 was very effective in suppressing lymphocyte proliferative responses following antigen stimulation. Fifty percent inhibition of antigen-induced transformation of cloned T-lymphocytes (BC.21) by FK506 and CsA was achieved at 0.2 nM and 20 nM, respectively [21]. However, FK506 (up to 100 nM) was found to be ineffective in suppressing bacterial lipopolysaccharide (LPS)-induced mouse spleen cell transformation [78]. In contrast, recent findings have shown that anti-IgM induced B-cell proliferation [75, 78] and *Staphylococcus aureus* Cowan I (SAC) induced B cell differentiation [79] are strongly inhibited by FK506. This suggests that, as with CsA, there are FK506 sensitive and insensitive B-cell populations.

Studies by Eiras *et al.* [80] demonstrated an apparent variation in sensitivity to FK506 of lymphocytes from different animal species, ranging from highly sensitive rat lymphocytes to least sensitive baboon lymphocytes, with the sensitivity of human lymphocytes near the range of rat lymphocytes. The reasons for this interspecies variability are, at present, unclear.

Human cells

FK506 was found to be very effective in suppressing both alloantigen- and T cell mitogen- induced lymphocyte proliferation, with IC_{50}s of 0.21 nm and 20 nm for FK506 and CsA respectively, in suppressing human MLR, and IC_{50}s of 8.6 nm and 750 nm respectively, in inhibiting PHA-induced lymphocyte proliferation [67]. Compared with PHA-induced responses, those induced by alloantigen are more FK506 sensitive [67, 81-83], while CD28-induced responses are FK506 insensitive [84]. This reflects inherent differences between CD3 and CD28 activation pathways and their differential sensitivity to FK506. Delay in the addition of FK506 to mitogen-stimulated cultures results in reduction of antilymphocytic activity [85], suggesting the influence of FK506 on early events in T cell activation, including cytokine gene transcription, cytokine secretion, cytokine-receptor expression, protein kinase C (PKC) activities and Ca^{2+} mobilization that occur within the first 2 hours.

Synergistic effects between low doses of FK506 and CsA have been observed in the suppression of human MLR [48, 81, 86]. This phenomenon however, was lost

Table I. Summary of effects of FK506 on T cells.

	Effect	References
In vitro CMI		
MLR (human, mouse)	↓	[19, 21, 67]
Con A, PHA-induced lymphocyte proliferation	↓	[21, 67, 175]
Tc induction	↓	[21, 67]
Tc function	↓	As above
Ts induction	↓	[67]
In vivo CMI		
DTH (MBSA)	↓	[18]
Graft *versus* host disease	↓	As above
Host *versus* graft popliteal lymph node assay	↓	[53]
T-dependent humoral response:		
alloantibody	↓	[65]
anti-SRBC Ab	↓	[87]
Ex vivo Con A-induced spleen cell proliferation	↓	As above
Lymphokine production		
IL-1	?	
IL-2	↓	[19, 21]
IL-3	↓	[19]
IL-4	?	
IL-5	?	
IL-6	−	[91]
IFN-γ	↓	[19]
GM-CSF	↓	[19]
Lymphokine growth factor receptor expression		
IL-2R	↓	[19, 67, 175]
Tf-R	↓	[67]
MHC antigen expression		
HLA-DR on activated T cells	↓	[175]
HLA-DR on monocytes	−	As above
Gene expression		
IL-1α, β	−	[92]
IL-2	↓	As above
IL-3	↓	As above
IL-4	↓	As above
GM-CSF	↓	As above
TNF-α	↓	As above
IFN-γ	↓	As above
c-myc	↓	As above
c-fos	−	As above
Tf-R	−	As above
IL-2R α-chain	−	As above
TNFβ	−	As above
MHC class I HLA B-7	−	As above
FKBP	?	
TcRβ-chain	↑	[85]

Abbreviations: ↓, decrease; ↑, increase; −, no change ?, unclear
CMI: cell-mediated immune response
DTH: delayed-type hypersensitivity
TfR: transferrin receptor
FKBP: FK506 binding protein

at higher drug concentrations [78] and a narrow therapeutic window was suggested for FK506 and CsA combination [86].

Cytotoxic T lymphocyte (CTL) activity and suppressor T cell generation during human MLR were found to be inhibited by FK506. On the other hand, the cytolytic activity of CTL against target cells during the effector phase was FK506 resistant [21, 67], indicating that FK506 only affected the early induction phase of CTL development but had no effect on antigen recognition by CTL or the cytolytic mechanism. Moreover, Zeevi *et al.* [82] have shown that FK506 has no effect on human CTL differentiation and maturation from pre-effector to effector CTL. Recently, we have observed that concentrations of FK506 which strongly inhibit T cell proliferation do not inhibit soluble antigen (PPD) processing or presentation by human blood monocytes [87]. There is some evidence, however, that FK506 may inhibit alloantigen processing/presentation in human MLR [88]. FK506 metabolites isolated *in vitro*, using human liver microsomes, showed 10 % or less of the immunosuppressive activity of FK506 [89]. Bioassay of FK506, based on inhibition of alloreactive cloned T cell proliferation, may be useful in interpreting immunoassay levels with unknown specificity for biologically inactive forms of FK506 [82, 90].

- *Molecular activity mechanism*

Based on the inhibitory effect of FK506 on various mitogen- and alloantigen-induced T cell responses in culture (discussed above), it is believed that FK506 exerts its influence on CD4+ helper T cells with consequent effects on other cell types (Table I). Results from various studies using cytokine-dependent cell lines have shown that FK506 is effective in suppressing the production of IL-2 [19, 91], IL-3 and γ-IFN [19, 91] *in vitro*. The concentrations of FK506 required to inhibit cytokine production were close to those found to inhibit lymphocyte proliferative responses, *i.e.* IC_{50}s at 0.06 nM, 0.3 nM and 0.25 nM for IL-2, IL-3 and γ-IFN, respectively. This indicated that the inhibition of cytokine production may contribute at least in part to FK506's action on T cell activity. On the other hand, FK506 (up to 10 nM) was found to be ineffective in suppressing PHA-induced B-cell-stimulating factor, *i.e.* IL-6 (BSF-2) production by human peripheral blood mononuclear cells and the response to IL-6 driven proliferation of clone B-cells [80]. This further suggests a specific, immunosuppressive effect of FK506 on T-cell activation.

Apart from its effect on T lymphocyte proliferation, several studies have demonstrated that FK506 strongly inhibits the expression of IL-2 receptors (IL-2R). In the human MLR, expression of IL-2R (Table II) and transferrin receptor (TfR) was suppressed by FK506 in a dose dependent manner [67, 81]. That FK506 failed to inhibit IL-2R mRNA expression [92] suggests that inhibition of the corresponding cell surface receptor may be post-transcriptional.

Several reports have shown that FK506 strongly inhibits expression of mRNA for early T cell activation genes, including IL-2, IL-3, IL-4, IFN-γ, TNF-α, GM-CSF, c-myc [92, 93] and krox 24 [77]. A common activation signal, either its generation or transmission, is inhibited by FK506 as the gene expression is unaffected by the nature of the inducers used.

Kinetic studies revealed that FK506, like CsA, acted within 2 hours of cell stimulation and complete inhibition of IL-2 mRNA synthesis, occurred in cells exposed to FK506 for as little as 5 minutes [92]. Incubation of resting T cells with FK506 or CsA for 15 minutes before activation resulted in complete inhibition of IL-2 mRNA expression, suggesting the presence and the full functional activity of the cytosolic FK-binding protein (FKBP) *(see below)* in unstimulated cells.

Table II. Influence of various FK506 concentrations on IL-2R expression by alloactivated human lymphocytes.

FK506 (ng/ml)	Percent positive cells			Mean fluorescence channel		
0	38.3	±	5.5	182.7	±	2.5
0.1	18.1	±	6.6[a]	173.1	±	9.7
0.5	6.4	±	0.6[b]	152.3	±	11.1
0.75	2,1	±	2.9[b]	134.3	±	0.5[a]

Results are means ± 1 SD obtained from three separate experiments.
a, $p < 0.05$; b, $p < 0.02$ compared with untreated cells.

The inhibition of gene expression by FK506 is specific to early genes, with no inhibition of constitutively expressed TCR-β, class I MHC HLA-B7 gene or GPDH gene or late-phase genes like IL-2Ra, TfR and TNF-β [85, 92]. Inhibition and superinduction, respectively, of krox 20 and krox 24 mRNA by FK506 in murine lymphocytes [77] is of interest, since these genes encode proteins which are likely to regulate gene expression. No inhibition on IL-1α or IL-1β mRNA expression in LPS stimulated human monocytes was observed [92].

Results from experiments designed to look at the effect of FK506 prior to gene transcriptional events showed that FK506 did not affect Ca^{2+} mobilization [94], phosphatidylinositol turnover [95] or PKC activities [96] following binding of the antigen receptor, and the target of FK506 is probably a later event elicited by this pathway, and/or a separate activation pathway distinct from phosphoinositol breakdown.

Following its entry into the cytosolic compartment, FK506 binds with high affinity to a cytosolic, FK506 binding protein (FKBP) or « Fujiphilin » that is specific for FK506 [26, 27, 97]. By using HPLC gel filtration, a heat-stable cytosolic component that had a smaller molecular weight (M.W. 10 to 12 kDa) than the CsA-binding protein, cyclophilin (M.W. 17,737 Da), was found to bind to FK506 [97]. This binding protein is distinct from cyclophilin, since no specific binding of FK506 to purified calf thymus cyclophilin can be detected [97], and anti-cyclophilin IgG bound to bovine and human cyclophilins but did not crossreact with bovine or human FKBPs [27]. Cloning of FKBP [98, 99] has revealed that, despite their common enzymatic properties, FKBP and cyclophilin have dissimilar sequences. Further detailed analysis showed that unlabeled FK506 displaced the radioligand (32-[1-^{14}C]-benzoyl-FK506) from the FKBP binding complex in a concentration-dependent manner [26]. CsA, however, was not displaced from the CsA/cyclophilin complex, even by a 500-fold molar excess of FK506, indicating that FKBP and cyclophilin are two cytosolic components that bind specifically to FK506 and CsA respectively. The displacement of FKBP from a FK506 binding affinity matrix by the immunosuppressive macrolide antibiotic rapamycin, which is structurally related to FK506, provides further evidence for the specificity of this protein for binding to compounds that have structures related to FK506 only [26].

The first 16 residues of human FKBP were found to be identical to the corresponding bovine sequence but unrelated to any known sequence [26]. These FK506 binding proteins appear to represent a previously unidentified class of conserved proteins or « immunophilins » that may play an important role in lymphocyte activation [26, 100]. Their natural ligands have not been identified. cDNA of FKBP from human lymphocytes has been synthesized and binds with mRNA species of ~ 1.8 kb isolated from brain, lung, liver, and placental cells and leukocytes [98, 100], demonstrating the presence of this protein in various tissues. The level of FKBP mRNA in leukemic (Jurkat) T cells is, however, unaffected by cell activation through phorbol esters and ionomycin [100]. Proteins with high sequence homology with FKBP and which demonstrate PPIase activity have been identified in other animal species (including lower eukaryotes), showing that this class of proteins is widely distributed among unrelated organisms and implying their function may not be restricted to the mediation of immune system [3, 55, 99].

Recent findings have shown that cyclophilin has peptidyl-prolyl *cis-trans* isomerase (PPIase or rotamase) activity [101, 102]. PPIase catalyses the slow *cis-trans* isomerization of proline peptide bonds in oligopeptides and accelerates slow, rate-limiting steps in the folding of several proteins. This *cis-trans* isomerization, which is strongly inhibited by CsA [102], may represent a previously unidentified, fundamental molecular mechanism in various intracellular signal transduction processes [103] during T cell activation.

Although FKBP is antigenically distinct from cyclophilin, it possesses PPIase [104] activity, though several-fold lower than cyclophilin [26, 97]. FKBP catalyses the *cis-trans* isomerization of the Ala-Pro bond in the peptide N-succinyl-Ala-Ala-Pro-Phe-p-nitroanlide [77, 105]. Differences in FKBP isomerization activity, however, were observed when peptides with different amino acid substitutions were used [105]. Inhibition of FKBP's PPIase activity is specific to the binding to FK506 or rapamycin, while inhibition of cyclophilin's PPIase activity is specific to CsA [27, 106]. Since FKBP, like cyclophilin, also possesses PPIase activity and PPIase activity was found to be involved in visual signal transduction in *Drosophila* [97] implies that the PPIase activity of both proteins plays a critical part in T cell activation.

Both high affinity FKBP ligands, FK506 and rapamycin, inhibit T cell proliferation at subnanomolar concentrations. The cytoplasmic concentration of FKBP (Jurkat cells), however, may approach 5 nM. Therefore, inhibition of the rotamase activity of FKBP is probably an insufficient requirement for mediating the actions of these drugs in T cells, as only a small fraction of the enzyme would be inhibited at effective drug concentrations [107]. With the advance of molecular immunology, the nucleic acid sequence of the IL-2 enhancer (regulatory) region has been identified and five different *cis*-acting transcriptional segments of this region that bind different nuclear factors have been investigated [108-110]. Among them, the *trans*-acting nuclear factor NFAT- 1, which is only present in activated T cells [111], is believed to be important in signal transduction before cellular replicative events occur. Recent study has shown that the binding of nuclear factors to the transcriptional elements is suppressed by CsA and FK506 (Figure 3), thereby inhibiting IL-2 gene activation and leading to inhibition of lymphokine production [112, 113].

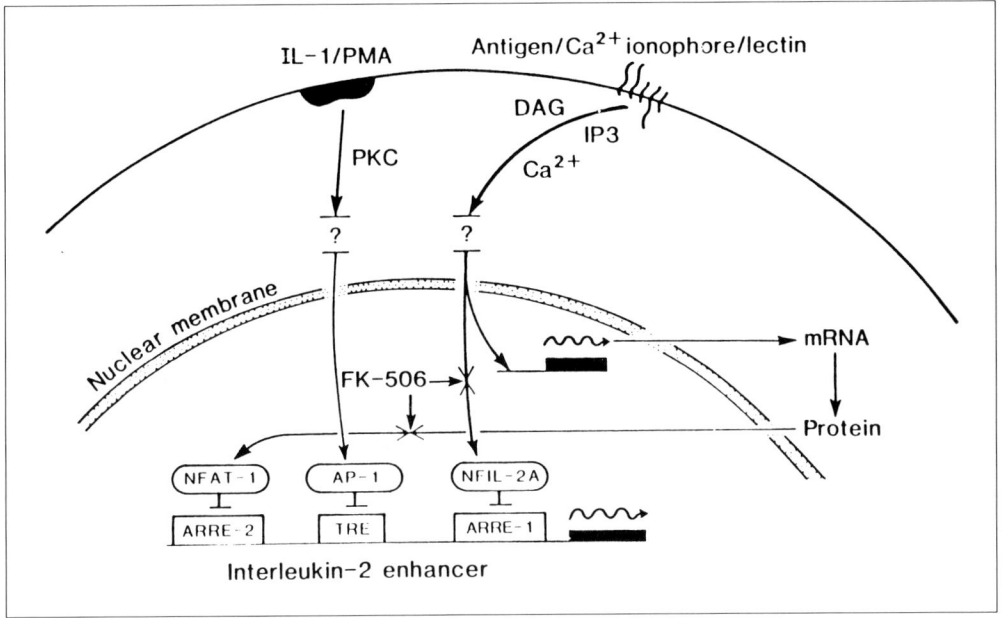

Figure 3. Proposed targets of FK506 within activated, CD4+ cells. For further details and references, see text.

Further recent insight into the molecular mechanisms of their immunosuppressive effects result from the formation of active complexes between the drug and its respective isomerase. These drug-immunophilin complexes interfere with signal transduction within the cell. Schreiber and his colleagues have shown that complexes of FK 506 and FKBP or of CsA and cyclophilin bind specifically to three polypeptides, — calmodulin, and the two subunits of calcineurin (a Ca^{2+}-activated, serine-threonine protein phosphatase) [114]. FK506 or CsA promotes the interaction of the normally non-interacting immunophilin and calcineurin. The drug -immunophilin complexes block the Ca^{2+}-activated phosphatase activity of calcineurin, which appears to be the target of these complexes [114]. Neither FK 506, CsA, FKBP, nor cyclophilin alone inhibits the phosphatase activity of authentic calcineurin.

An additional important observation has been that the drug-immunophilin complexes block Ca^{2+}-dependent assembly of NF-AT by inhibiting translocation of the pre-existing component of NF-AT from the cytoplasm to the nucleus [115]. The nuclear component of NF-AT is transcriptionally inactive in all cells other than activated T lymphocytes and is induced by signals from the TCR. Its appearance is not blocked by FK506 or CsA. It is thought that FK506 or CsA blocks dephosphorylation by calcineurin of the cytoplasmic component of NF-AT which is required for its translocation to the nucleus. In the absence of both nuclear and cytoplasmic components, binding of NF-AT to DNA and transcriptional activation of the IL-2 gene and other genes are suppressed. Whilst transcription directed by NF-AT is blocked in T cells treated with FK 506 or CsA, little or not effect is observed on other transcription factors, such as NF-KB or AP-1 [115].

Further details of the molecular action of FK506 may be found in recent reviews by Schreiber and Crabtree [116], Sigal and Dumont [117] and Liv [118].

Therapeutic effects in animals models of immunological disorders

- *Transplant*

Rodent skin grafts

Inamura et al. reported that short courses of FK506 administration (0.32 mg/kg, i.m. or 1.0 mg/kg, p.o.) could significantly prolong skin allograft survival across the MHC barrier between F344 (RT1^{1V1}) and WKA (RT1^k) rats. This could also be achieved with CsA at the much higher dose of 32 mg/kg [119]. Significant prolongation of skin allograft survival by FK506 administration was also found in other histoincompatible strain combinations, like ACI (RT1^a) to WKA and with minor histocompatibility differences *i.e.* Lewis (RT1^l) to F344. Healthy, functioning grafts could be maintained with a FK506 dose 1/10 of the initial therapeutic dose and with treatment only twice a week.

Rodent heart grafts

In heterotopic cardiac transplantation, long-term graft survival can be achieved by treatment with FK506 at 0.32 mg/kg, i.m. or 1.0 mg/kg, p.o. in F344 to WKA strain combination [33, 120], or 1.28 mg/kg i.m. in ACI (RT1^a) to Lewis (TR1^l) [49]. However, using a different strain combination, DA (RT1^a) to PVG(RT1^U), long-term graft survival was not observed and median survival time (MST) fell between 22 to 30 days postoperatively [121].

By using the ACI to Lewis strain combination, it was further demonstrated that a temporary, donor-specific unresponsiveness was developed in these long-term graft survival recipients, since a second graft from a third party donor was rejected faster than a second graft homologous to the first graft [49, 68]. Prolongation of the second graft was observed without any further administration of FK506 [44]. The effective administration of FK506 in preventing cardiac allograft rejection seems to be schedule-dependent, with reduction of median survival time (MST) following reduction of treatment frequency per week [49, 53, 68]. In addition, maximum prolongation of cardiac allograft survival was reported when treatment was given from days 4 to 6 postoperatively in the ACI to Lewis strain combination [49], at which time signs of cardiac graft rejection begin to occur.

Rodent liver grafts

Long-term liver allograft survival can be achieved in some strain combinations without the application of immunosuppressive agents. However, the administration of immunosuppressants to prolong liver graft survival between certain strain combinations, like PVG to Lewis and ACI to Lewis is necessary. Like prolongation of cardiac allograft survival, FK506 at 0.3 mg/kg or higher (1.28 mg/kg) significantly prolonged liver allograft survival [71, 72] and no signs of acute rejection, such as portal tract inflammation or endothelialitis, was observed when FK506 was given at 1.0 mg/kg [122]. Results of experimental transplantation in rats [49, 68, 71] are summarized in Table III.

Other rodent grafts

Apart from being effective in controlling rejection of commonly transplanted organs as discussed above, FK506 was also effective in promoting survival of those organ transplants that were regarded as a stringent test of any immunosuppressive agent. Thus, FK506 was effective in suppressing rejection of limb [123, 124], islet [125], heterotopic [126] and orthotopic small intestine, and multivisceral and intestinal [72, 73] allografts, thus demonstrating its broadly effective immunosuppressive action in comparison with currently employed immunosuppressants. FK506 also is superior to CsA for the prevention [27] and reversal of GVHD after bone marrow transplantation [28].

Table III. Results of allotransplantation obtained in rats (ACI to Lewis).

Prolongation of heart/liver allograft survival after a short course of FK506				
	MST			
	Days 0-2	Days 4-6	Days 0-13	No FK506
Heart[a]	36.0	91.0	87.0	6.0
Liver[a]	> 100	> 100	> 100	10.0

Combination of FK506 and CsA in heterotropic heart transplantation	
Treatment[b]	MST (Days)
Untreatment	6.0
FK 0.02	8.0
FK 0.04	10.5
CsA 2.5	10.0
FK 0.02 + CsA 2.5	26.0
FK 0.04 + CsA 2.5	35.0

Specificity of unresponsiveness developed in FK506-treated cardiac transplanted animals				
First Graft			Second Graft[d]	
Donor	FK[c]	MST (days)	Donor	MST (days)
ACI/BN	−	< 13	−	−
ACI	+	91.0	−	−
−	+	−	ACI	10.0
−	+	−	BN	34.0
ACI	+	63.5	ACI	45.0
ACI	+	54.0	BN	14.0

a : dose of FK506 is 1.28 mg/kg/day ; b : mg/kg/day ; c : 1.28 mg/kg intramuscularly on days 4, 5 and 6 after first ACI heart allografting ; d : 2 secondary grafting at 2 weeks after first grafting. Data from [49, 71, 73].

Dogs

As with studies in the rat, FK506 was found to be effective in controlling allograft rejection in dogs [36, 37]. Its side effects in dogs, however, including anorexia and vasculitis have caused considerable concern [33-34]. The vascular lesions were shown to be relatively species-specific and not strongly associated, if at all, with FK506 [38, 129]. At 1.0 mg/kg, p.o., and 0.16 mg/kg, i.m., FK506 induced long-term renal graft survival with healthy functioning grafts [33]. Other groups however, have reported a less significant improvement [36-38, 129-131]. Combinations of suboptimal, ineffective doses of FK506 and CsA resulted in significant prolongation of renal allograft survival [36, 38, 44], with reduction in the incidence of anorexia associated with FK506 and the toxicity attributed to CsA. Withdrawal of FK506 usually resulted in the reoccurrence of rejection [33]. FK506 rescue treatment could reverse 80 % of ongoing rejection in renal allografts [38, 131]. Apart from prolonging renal allograft survival, a short course of FK506 treatment can also prolong liver [38, 131, 132], pancreas [133] and pancreaticoduodenal [134] graft survival in dogs at dosages similar to those that prolong renal allograft survival.

Sub-human primates

Renal transplants performed on cynomolgus monkeys and baboons [38, 40, 130, 135] demonstrated that FK506 was effective in graft prolongation. Compared to the doses used to inhibit rejection in rats and dogs, a higher dose of FK506 (12-18 mg/kg/d, p.o.) is necessary to achieve renal graft prolongation in baboons [40]. This may be due to the difference in sensitivity to FK506 of lymphocytes from different species, since MLR reactivity of lymphocytes of baboons appears to be more resistant to the effect of FK506 [80, 135]. Induction of tolerance is not seen with respect to renal grafts, as termination of FK506-treatment leads to reoccurrence of rejection [40, 131]. However, a 3-day course of treatment with FK506 (1 to 2 mg/kg) can effectively overcome the rejection [40, 131, 136].

Apart from being effective in renal transplantation, FK506 at 10 mg/kg was also shown to inhibit rejection of liver [137] and pancreaticoduodenal transplants [136] in primates. Good liver function was obtained in long-graft survival recipients 200 days after termination of FK506-treatment, implying that tolerance may be developed in these liver-transplanted animals. Hyperglycemia, which was thought to be caused by early rejection following pancreatic transplantation, was overcome by a 2-day, short course of intramuscular injection of FK506 [136].

- *Autoimmunity*

Although the beneficial effect of FK506 in organ transplantation has been extensively studied in various animal models, its effects on autoimmune disorders, is as yet, less well understood. Using MRL/lpr and NZB x NZW (B/W Fl) mice, -animal models of human systemic lupus erythematosus (SLE), FK506 was shown to prolong the lifespan, to reduce proteinuria, and to prevent the progression of nephropathy [138, 139]. High dose (2 mg/kg/day) treatment suppressed serum anti-ssDNA, anti-dsDNA levels and the total amount of serum IgG. FK506 has also been shown to induce antigen-specific tolerance in active Heymann's nephritis and in the autologous phase of Masugi nephritis in the rat [140]. In addition to these observations on immune-mediated renal disease, FK506 has recently been shown to prevent the occurrence of diabetes in BB rats, an experimental analogue of human juvenile (type I) diabetes mellitus [141]. About 75 % of FK506-treated animals, which were diabetes-free by the end of the drug treatment period, remained in the non-diabetic state 45 to 75 days after stopping FK506. Additional studies, in non-obese diabetic mice, have shown that FK506 has a preventive effect on insulitis and diabetes by suppression of cell-mediated immunity [142]. FK506 also inhibits development of experimental autoimmune thyroiditis in PVG/r rats [143]. Development of type II collagen-induced arthritis was specifically inhibited in FK506-treated rats [144, 145] and mice [110]. More recently, Arita *et al.* [146], have shown that a single administration of FK506 after the clinical onset of arthritis in rats immunized with type II collagen is effective in suppressing the severity of the disease. This demonstrates an important curative action of FK506 when applied therapeutically. The effect of FK506 on experimental autoimmune uveoretinitis (EAU) and experimental allergic encephalomyelitis (EAE) has been investigated [147] and the drug has been shown to be effective if given during the afferent phase of the disease. Further studies of EAU by Mochizuki and colleagues have shown that FK506 treatment is effective in suppressing ongoing disease and that immune responses to the uveitogenic S-antigen are suppressed long after the cessation of drug administration [148]. Moreover, recent data indicate that FK506 markedly inhibits IL-2 receptor expression on T cells inside the eye [149] and induces antigen-specific Ts cells [150] that may contribute to the uniquely prolonged and intensive immunosuppression by FK506. The profound beneficial effect of FK506 in reducing disease pathogenesis and prolonging life in experimental animal models indicates its potential application in clinical autoimmune disorders. The effects of FK506 on experimental autoimmunity have been reviewed [151].

Clinical studies

Pharmacokinetics in patients

This topic has recently been reviewed [56]. Studies on the optimal route of administration and dosage of FK506 for clinical study were hampered by the severe toxic effects of the drug in dogs. Fortunately, the choice for the method of drug delivery in the first clinical trial, *i.e.* 0.15 mg/kg given intravenously over a hour soon after the liver was revascularized, followed by 0.075 mg/kg/12 hours until the patient could eat, then switched to oral doses at 0.15 mg/kg/12 hours, was found to be reasonably well-tolerated in humans [152] although the i.v. doses have required revision downward [63, 153]. Peak plasma concentration was observed at the end of infusion and then levels declined slowly over the next 24 hours [50, 154]. Plasma trough levels tended to be about 1 ng/ml, the effective immunosuppressive concentration *in vitro*. The half-life ranges from 5.5 to 16.6 hours, with a mean of 8.7 hours. Drug absorption following oral administration is highly variable. Peak plasma level of 0.4 to 3.7 ng/ml was reached after 1 to 4 hours of an oral dose at 0.15 mg/kg [50]. The half-life of CsA is prolonged in patients receiving FK506, from a normal 6 to 15 hours to ranges from 26 to 74 hours. This indicates FK506 may affect CsA metabolism, a phenomenon recently demonstrated *in vitro* [52].

Experience gained from studies in CsA-treated liver transplant patients indicates that alterations in the absorption and metabolism of CsA occur with changing liver function [155]. Because of its similar physical properties to CsA, the same issues are expected to arise for FK506. In 5 jaundiced patients with liver dysfunction, peak and trough FK506 levels were higher than in patients with good hepatic function [156]. Moreover, the half-life of FK506 was increased and its clearance was reduced in patients with hepatic dysfunction [156]. As a result, the overall bioavailability of FK506 was expected to increase because of the greatly reduced intrinsic clearance [50, 154].

The full impact of hepatic dysfunction on FK506 pharmacokinetics was not appreciated until clinical trials were far along [57, 153]. In liver transplant recipients, whose grafts do not function well initially and/or fail to recover quickly, the daily i.v. dose of 0.15 mg/kg leads quickly to enormously high trough plasma levels (> 100 ng/ml has been recorded), complete renal failure, and neurotoxicity which can progress to mutism, convulsions and coma. Prompt dose reduction is required and guidance for this is provided by rapid turn-around time in the plasma assays. Dose control of the i.v. FK506 is easier if the drug is given by constant infusion instead of the 2-hour bolus which was originally used.

Even with well functioning liver grafts, or in kidney and heart recipients whose hepatic function is normal, the University of Pittsburgh patients now are given a smaller i.v. dosage of 0.075 or 0.10 mg/kg/day instead of the 0.15 mg/kg originally employed. The larger doses cause unacceptable increases in plasma levels and can cause acute renal failure or neurotoxicity [57, 153]. Failure to make these revisions constitutes an unnecessary risk. Plasma levels of 3 to 5 ng/ml can be accepted during the perioperative period of constant drug infusion if there is no evidence of toxicity, but otherwise the doses should be reduced to < 3 ng/ml.

Clinical trials phase I

Studies of FK506 in human organ transplantation were first reported by Starzl *et al.* from the University of Pittsburgh. They first published their results in *The Lancet* in October, 1989 [23], and have since presented their data in more detail [61, 157-161]. A comprehensive account of the clinical experience up to August 1990 was presented at the 13th International Congress of the Transplantation Society (San Francisco, USA ; *Transplantation Proceedings* 1993 ; 23 (1) : 1732). Further experience up to June 1991 was reported in the Proceedings of the First International Congress on FK506, Pittsburgh, 1991 (*Transplantation Proceedings* 1991 ; 23 (6) : 2709-3380).

FK506 was first shown successfully to reverse rejection in 7/10 CsA-treated patients with liver allografts who were unresponsive to maximum therapy with conventional immunosuppressive drugs (including steroids and OKT-3) [22]. More recently, FK506 was used as primary immunosuppressive therapy in 110 adult recipients of liver transplants, 92 % of whom were alive 6-12 months after surgery, although 10 patients required a second or third graft [162]. Patient survival was significantly improved compared with results from CsA-treated historical controls, with fewer episodes of rejection and reduced steroid requirement [163]. Indeed, in some patients, steroids were successfully withdrawn. Recently, the results of multi-center prospective randomized trials componing FK506 to CsA after primary liver transplantation have been reported. The results of the US multi-center trial have shown that FK506 plus corticosteroids is more effective than CsA-based immunosuppressive regimens for prophylactic immunosuppression [164].

Of 65 renal transplant recipients treated with FK506, 51 (79 %) had satisfactory function of the first graft 2-11 months after transplantation [161]. Many centres using CsA, however, report that 80 % of recipients of a first kidney allograft have satisfactory graft function at 1 year, and further data are clearly required to determine whether FK506 is as effective as experience with previous immunosuppressive regimens. Eight out of the 65 patients acquired CMV infection that required treatment with gancyclovir. On the other hand, steroid therapy has been stopped in 50 % of patients with functioning grafts, which may indicate a valuable, steroid-sparing effect of FK506.

Early results also indicate that FK506 might be useful in cardiac and pulmonary transplantation [165, 166] and Tzakis and Starzl and their colleagues have also reported successful pancreatic-islet-cell transplantation and small-bowel transplantation in man where FK506 was the main immunosuppressant used [55, 63, 166].

A handful of patients with chronic GVHD long after bone marrow transplantation have been rescued with FK506 [57, 167]. These trials were based on the demonstration in rats that reversal and prevention of GVHD could be accomplished [127, 128].

Autoimmunity

With respect to human autoimmune disease, FK506 has also been used to treat patients with nephrotic syndrome caused by steroid-resistant focal sclerosing glomerulonephritis, as well as other renal diseases, with reduced proteinuria and no decline in renal function [63, 168, 169], and has had beneficial effects in all patients with severe, recalcitrant pyoderma gangrenosum and chronic plaque psoriasis [55]. Currently the drug is being evaluated in a wide variety of human autoimmune disorders at the University of Pittsburgh [151]. Appropriate, prospective randomized clinical trials are awaited to explore the potential of FK506 in treatment of a variety of human autoimmune disorders.

Pathology

Side-effects of FK506 and CsA are similar in humans, although hirsutism, gingival hyperplasia, and coarsening of facial features have not been reported in patients given FK506 [55, 63]. Initial results showed evidence of adverse effects of FK506 on renal function [23] or glucose tolerance [170], and more recent results indicate that FK506 may have similar effects to CsA in these respects [63, 159, 162, 171]. However, the therapeutic margin may be greater than with CsA. Hypertension is uncommonly seen with FK506 [172].

Neurological side-effects, including tremors, parasthesias and expressive dysphasia, have been reported [173] and serious neurotoxicity, probably caused by FK506 overdosage has been observed in 3 recipients of heart or liver allografts [153]. FK506 concentrations are greatly raised by hepatic impairment, which may predispose to nephrotoxicity, and potential drug interactions may have similar risks : an interaction between FK506 and CsA has already been reported [23], possibly caused by the capacity of FK506 to interfere with CsA metabolism by human liver microsomal cytochrome P450 isoenzymes [52].

Infections remain major problems for patients on any immunosuppressive regimen. The Pittsburgh group have reported a lower incidence of both bacterial and fungal infections in patients treated with FK506 compared with historical CsA controls, possibly because of a reduced requirement for additional immunosuppression but with a similar incidence of viral infections [174]. Twenty-three of 110 consecutive liver transplant recipients acquired CMV infection, and infection remains a common cause of death.

Conclusions

Preliminary clinical results indicate that FK506 is a promising addition to the rather narrow range of immunosuppressants now available. FK506 has substantial hepatotrophic properties, which may explain its particular success in liver transplant rescue ; a US prospective randomized study to compare FK506 with CsA immunosuppression in liver transplantation has shown that FK506 plus corticosteroids is more effective than CsA-based regimens for prophylactic immunosuppression. The limited data so far available do not indicate a survival benefit for renal transplants but more investigations into the relative efficacy of FK506 and CsA immunosuppression in recipients of renal allografts and other organs are underway to determine the toxicity, potential benefits, and most appropriate clinical applications of this very powerful new immunosuppressant.

References

1. Groth CG. Landmarks in clinical renal transplantation. *Surg Gynecol Obstet* 1972 ; 134 : 323-8.
2. Hau T. Kidney transplantation. In : Lances R, ed. Austin TX : Clio Chirurgica.
3. Starzl TE, Fung JJ, Jordan M, Shapiro R, Tzakis A, McCaulcy J, Johnston J, Iwaki Y, Jain A, Alessiani M, Todo S. Kidney transplantation under FK506. *JAMA* 1990 ; 264, 63-7.
4. Borel JF, Feurer C, Gubler HU, Stahelin H. Biological effects of Cyclosporin A : a ncw antilymphocytic agent. *Agents Actions* 1976 ; 6 : 468-75.
5. Borel JF. Pharmacology of Cyclosporine. Pharmacological effects on immune function : *in vivo* studies. *Pharmacol Rev* 1990 ; 41 : 304-72.
6. Kahan BD. *Cyclosporine. Therapeutic use in transplantation.* Orlando : Grune & Stratton, 1988
7. Thomson AW. *Cyclosporin. Mode of action and clinical application.* London : Kluyer Academic Press, 1989.
8. Kahan BD. Cyclosporine. *N Engl J Med* 1989 ; 321 : 1725-38.
9. Calne RY, Rolles K, White DJG, Thiru S, Evans DB, McMaster P, Dunn DC, Craddock CN, Henderson RG, Aziz S, Lewis P. Cyclosporin A initially as the only immunosuppressant in 34 recipients of cadaveric organs : 32 kidneys, 2 pancreases, 2 livers. *Lancet* 1979 : 2 : 1033-6.
10. Starzl TE, Weil R III, Iwatsuki S, Klintman G, Schroter GPJ, Koep LJ, Iwaki Y, Terasaki PI, Porter KA. The use of cyclosporin A and prednisone in cadaver kidney transplantation. *Surg Gynecol Obstet* 1980 ; 151 : 17-26.
11. Klintmalm GBG, Iwatsuki I, Starzl T. Nephrotoxicity of cyclosporin A in liver and kidney transplant patients. *Lancet* 1981 ; 1 : 470-1.
12. Myers BD, Ross J, Newton L, Leutscher J, Perloth M. Cyclosporine-associated chronic nephropathy. *N Engl J Med* 1984 ; 311 : 699-705.
13. Myers BD. Cyclosporine toxicity. *Kidney Int* 1986 ; 30 : 964-74.
14. Blair JT, Thomson AW, Whiting PH, Davidson RJL, Simpson JG. Toxicity of the immunosuppressive agent cyclosporin A in the rat. *J Pathol* 1982 ; 138 : 163-78.
15. Thiru S. Pathological effects of cyclosporin A in clinical practice. In : Thomson AW, ed. *Cyclosporin. Mode of action and clinical application.* London : Kluwer Academic Publishers, 1989 : 324.
16. Atkinson K, Biggs J, Darveniza P, Boland J, Concannon A, Dodds. A cyclosporine-associated central nervous system toxicity after allogeneic bone marrow transplantation. *Transplantation* 1984 ; 38 : 34-37.
17. Goto T, Kino T, Hatanaka H, Nishiyama M, Okuhara M, Kohsaka M, Aoki H, Im-

anaka H. Discovery of FK506, a novel immunosuppressant isolated from *Streptomyces tsukubaensis*. *Transplant Proc* 1987 ; 19, Suppl. 6 : 4-8.
18. Kino T, Hatanaka H, Hashimoto M, Nishiyama M, Goto T, Okuhara M, Kohsaka M, Aoki H, Imanaka H. FK506, a novel immunosuppressant isolated from a *Streptomyces*. I. Fermentation, isolation and physiochemical and biological characteristics. *J Antibiot* 1987 ; 40 : 1249-55.
19. Kino T, Hatanaka H, Miyata S, Inamura N, Nishiyama M, Yajima T, Goto T, Okuhara M, Kohsaka M, Aoki H, Ochiai T. FK506, a novel immunosuppressant isolated from a *Streptomyces*. II. Immunosuppressive effect of FK506 in vitro. *J Antibiot* 1987 ; 40 : 1256-65.
20. Ochiai T, Nakajima K, Nagata M, Suzuki T, Asano T, Uematsu T, Goto T, Hori S, Kenmachi T, Nakagori T, Isono K. Effect of a new immunosuppressive agent, FK506, on heterotopic allotransplantation in the rat. *Transplant Proc* 1987 ; 19 : 1284-6.
21. Sawada S, Suzuki G, Kawase Y, Takaku F. Novel immunosuppressive agent, FK506. *In vitro* effects on the cloned T cell activation. *J Immunol* 1987 ; 139 : 1797-803.
22. Thomson AW. FK506 : profile of an important new immunosuppressant. *Transplantation Rev* 1990 ; 4 : 1-13.
23. Starzl TE, Fung J, Venkataramman R, Todo S, Demetris AJ, Jain A. FK506 for liver, kidney and pancreas transplantation. *Lancet* 1989 ; ii : 1000-4.
24. Peters DH, Fitton A, Plosker GL, Faulds. Tacrolimus : a review of its pharmacology and therapeutic potential in hepatic and renal transplantation. *Drugs* 1993 ; 46 : 746-94.
25. Tanaka H, Kuroda A, Marusawa H, Hashimoto M, Hatanaka H, Kino T, Goto T, Okuhara M. Physiochemical properties of FK506, a novel immunosuppressant isolated from *Streptomyces tsukubaensis*. *Transplant Proc* 1987 ; 19, Suppl. 6 : 11-6.
26. Harding MW, Galat A, Uehling DE, Schreiber SL. A receptor for the immunosuppressant FK506 in a *cis-trans* peptidyl-prolyl isomerase. *Nature* 1989 ; 341 : 758-60.
27. Siekierka JJ, Staruch MJ, Hung SHY, Sigal NH. FK506, a potent novel immunosuppressive agent, binds to a cytosolic protein which is distinct from the cyclosporin A-binding protein, cyclophilin. *J Immunol* 1989 ; 143 : 1580-3.
28. Nalesnik MA, Todo S, Murase, Gryzan S, Lee PH, Makowka L, Starzl TE. Toxicology of FK506 in the Lewis rat. *Transplant Proc* 1987 ; 19, Suppl. 6 : 89-92.
29. Stephen M, Woo J, Hasan NU, Whiting PH, Thomson AW. Immunosuppressive activity, lymphocyte subset analysis, and acute toxicity of FK506 in the rat. *Transplantation* 1989 ; 47 : 60-5.
30. Pugh-Humphreys RGP, Ross CSK, Thomson AW. The influence of FK506 on the thymus : an immunophenotypic and structural analysis. *Immunology* 1990 ; 70 : 398-404.
31. Woo I, Ildstad ST, Thomson AW. FK506 inhibits thymocyte maturation but not negative selection of T cells receptor Vβb5+ and vβII+ T lymphocytes *in vivo*. *Transplant Immunology* 1994 (in press).
32. Takai K, Jojima K, Sakatoku J, Fukumoto T. Effects of FK506 on rat thymus : time-course analysis by immunoperoxidase technique and flow cytofluormetry. *Clin Exp Immunol* 1990 ; 82 : 445-9.
33. Ochiai T, Hamaguchi K, Isono K. Histological studies in renal transplant recipient dogs receiving treatment with FK506. *Transplant Proc* 1987 ; 19 (Suppl. 6) : 93-7.
34. Ochiai T, Nagata M, Nakajima K, *et al*. Studies of the effects of FK506 on renal allografting in the beagle dog. *Transplantation* 1987 ; 44 : 729.
35. Collier DStJ, Thiru S, Calne R. Kidney transplantation in the dog receiving FK506. *Transplant Proc* 1987 ; 19 (5), (Suppl. 6) : 62.
36. Todo S, Demetris A, Ueda Y, Imventarza O, Okuda K, *et al*. Canine kidney transplantation with FK506 alone or in combination with cyclosporin and steroids. *Transplant Proc* 1987 ; 19, Suppl. 6 : 57-61.
37. Todo S, Podesta L Chapchap P, Khan D Pan CE, Ueda Y, Okuda K, Inventarza O, Casavilla A, Demetris AJ, Makowka, Starzl TE. Orthotopic liver transplantation in dogs receiving FK506. *Transplant Proc* 1987 ; 19, Suppl. 6 : 64-7.
38. Todo S, Ueda Y, Demetris JA, Inventarza O, Nalesnik M, Venkataramanan R, Makowka L, Starzl TE. Immunosuppression of canine, monkey and baboon allografts by

FK506 : with special reference to synergism with other drugs and to tolerance induction. *Surgery* 1988 ; 104 : 239-49.
39. Calne R, Collier, Thiru S. Observations about FK506 in primates. *Transplant Proc* 1987 ; 19 (5), (Suppl.6) : 63.
40. Todo S, Demetris A, Ueda Y, Imventarza O, Cardoff E, Zeevi A, Starzl TE. Renal transplantation in baboons under FK506. *Surgery* 1989 ; 106 : 444-51.
41. O'Hara K, Billington R, James RW, Dean GA, Nishiyama M, Noguchi H. Toxicologic evulation of FK506. *Transplant Proc* 1990 ; 22 : 83-6.
42. Thiru S, Collier D.St.J., Calne R. Pathological studies in canine and baboon renal allograft recipients immunosuppressed with FK506. *Transplant Proc* 1987 ; 19 : 98-101
43. Starzl TE, Kaupp HA, Brock DR, Lazarus RE, Johnson RV. Reconstructive problems in canine liver homotransplantation with special reference to the postoperative role of hepatic venous flow. *Surg Gynecol Obstet* 1960 ; 111 : 733-41.
44. Ochiai T, Sakamoto K, Gunji Y, Hamaguchi K, Isegawa N, Suzuki A, Shimada H, Hayashi H, Yasumoto A, Asano T, Isono K. Effects of combination treatment with FK506 and cyclosporine on survival time and vascular changes in renal-allograft-recipient dogs. *Transplantation* 1989 ; 48 : 193-7.
45. Tamura K, Kobayashi M, Hashimoto K, Kojima K, Nagase K, Iwasaki K, Kaizu T, Tanaka H, Niwa M. A highly sensitive method to assay FK506 in plasma. *Transplant Proc* 1987 ; 19, Suppl. 6 : 23-9.
46. Cadoff EM, Venkataramanan R, Krajack A, Jain AS, Fung JJ, Todo S, Starzl TE. Assay of FK506 in plasma. *Transplant Proc* 1990 ; 22 : 50-1.
47. Ochiai T, Gunji Y, Sakamoto K, Suzuki T, Isegawa N, Asano T, Isono K. Optimum serum trough levels of FK506 in renal allotransplantation of the beagle dog. *Transplantation* 1989 ; 48 : 189-93.
48. Zeevi A, Duquesnoy R, Eiras G, Rabinowich H, Todo S, Makowka L, Starzl TE. Immunosuppressive effect of FK506 on *in vitro* lymphocyte alloactivation : synergism with cyclosporin A. *Transplant Proc* 1987 ; 19 : 40-4.
49. Murase N, Todo S, Lee PH, Lai HS, Chapman F, Nalesnik MA, Makowka L, Starzl TE. Heterotopic heart transplantation in the rat receiving FK506 alone or with cyclosporine. *Transplant Proc* 1987 ; 19, Suppl. 6 : 71-5.
50. Venkataramanan R, Jain A, Cadoff E, Warty V, Iwasaki K, Nagase K, Krajack A, Imventarza O, Todo S, Fung JJ, Starzl TE. Pharmacokinetics of FK506 : Preclinical and clinical studies. *Transplant Proc* 1990 ; 22, Suppl. 1 : 52-6.
51. Venkataramanan R, Jain A, Warty V, Abu-Elmagd K, Furukawa H, Imventarza O, Fung JJ, Todo S, Starzl TE. Pharmacocinetics of FK506 following oral administration. A comparison of FK506 and cyclosporine. *Transplant Proc* 1991 ; 23 : 931-3.
52. Burke MD, Omar G, Thomson AW, Whiting PH. Inhibition of the metabolism of cyclosporine by human liver microsomes by FK506. *Transplantation* 1990 ; 50 : 901-2.
53. Morris RE, Hoyt EG, Murphy MP, Shorthouse R. Immunopharmacology of FK506. *Transplant Proc* 1989 ; 21 : 1042-4.
54. Francavilla A, Barone M, Todo S, Zeng Q, Porter KA, Starzl TE. Augmentation of rat liver regeneration with FK506 compared with cyclosporine. *Lancet* 1989 ; ii : 1248-9.
55. Starzl TE, Abu-Elmagd K, Tzakis A, Fung JJ, Porter KA, Todo S. Selected topics on FK506 with special reference to rescue of extrahepatic whole organ grafts, transplantation of 'forbidden organs', side effects, mechanisms, and practical-pharmacokinetics. *Transplant Proc* 1991.
56. Venkataramanan R, Warty V. Pharmakokenetics and monitoring of FK506. In : Thomson AW, Starzl TE, eds. *New immunosuppressive drugs developments in anti rejection therapy*. London : Eduard Arnold, 1993.
57. Starzl TE, Thomson AW, Todo SN, Fung JJ. Proceedings of the First International Congress on FK506. *Transplant Proc* 1991 ; 23 : 2709-3380.
58. Francavilla A, Barone M, Starzl TE, Zeevi A, Scotti C, Carrieri G, Mazzaferro V, Prelich J, Todo S, Eiras, Fung J, Porter KA. FK506 as a growth control factor. *Transplant Proc* 1990 ; 22 : 90-2.
59. Francavilla A, Barone M, Van der Brink MRM, Markus P, Todo S, Zeng Q, Porter

KA, Starzl TE. Further studies on the stimulatory effect of FK506 on liver regeneration by using NHI-RNU nude rat model. *Hepatology* 1990 ; 12 : 942.
60. Mazzaferro V, Scott-Foglieni CL, Porter KA, Trejo Bellido J, Carrieri G, Todo S, Fung JJ, Francavilla A, Starzl TE. *Studies of the hepatotrophic qualities of FK506 and CsA* 1990 ; 22 : 93-5.
61. Fung Jl, Todo S, Jain A, McCauley J, Alessiani M, Scotti C, Starzl TE. Conversion from cyclosporine to FK506 in liver allograft recipients with cyclosporine-related complications. *Transplant Proc* 1990 ; 22 : 6-12.
62. Sakr MF, Zetti GM, Farghali H, Hassanein TH, Gavaler JS, Starzl TE, Van Thiel. Protective effect of FK506 against hepatic ischemia in rats. *Transplant Proc* 1991.
63. Starzl TE, Abu-Elmagd K, Fung JJ, Todo S, Tzakis A, McCauley J, Demetris AJ. Clinical experience with FK506. *Presse Med* 1991 ; 23 : 914-9.
64. Thomson AW. FK506. How much potential ? *Immunol Today* 1989 ; 10 : 6-9.
65. Propper DJ, Woo J, Thomson AW, Catto GRD, Macleod AM. FK506-influence on anti-class I MHC alloantibody responses to blood transfusions. *Transplantation* 1990 ; 50 : 267-71.
66. Woo J, Stephen M, Thomson AW. Spleen lymphocyte populations and expression of activation markers in rats treated with the potent new immunosuppressive agent FK506. *Immunology* 1988 ; 65 : 153-5.
67. Yoshimura N, Matsui S, Hamashima T, Oka T. Effect of a new immunosuppressive agent, FK506, on human lymphocyte responses *in vitro*. I. Inhibition of expression of alloantigen-activated suppressor cells, as well as induction of alloreactivity. *Transplantation* 1989 ; 47 : 351-6.
68. Murase N, Kim DG, Todo S, Cramer DV, Fung J, Starzl TE. FK 506 suppression of heart and liver allograft rejection. II. The induction of graft acceptance in rats. *Transplantation* 1990 ; 50 : 739-44.
69. Ochiai T, Nakajima K, Nagata M, Hori S, Asano T, Isono K. Studies of the induction and maintenance of long-term graft acceptance by treatment with FK506 in heterotopic cardiac allotransplantation in rats. *Transplantation* 1987 ; 44 : 734-8.
70. Jones MC, Power DA, Cummingham C, Catto GRD. The influence of repeated transfusions and cyclosporine on secondary alloantibody responses in inbred rat. *Transplantation* 1988 ; 45 : 1094-9.
71. Murase N, Kim DG, Todo S, Cramer DV, Fung J, Starzl TE. Suppression of allograft rejection with FK506. I. Prolonged cardiac and liver survival following short course therapy. *Transplantation* 1990 ; 50 : 186-9.
72. Murase N, Kim DG, Todo S, Cramer DV, Fung J, Starzl TE. Induction of liver, heart, and multivisceral graft acceptance with a short course of FK506. *Transplant Proc* 1990 ; 22 : 74-5.
73. Murase N, Demetris AJ, Matsuzaki T, Yagihashi A, Todo S, Drash AL, Starzl TE Long survival in rats after multivisceral versus isolated small bowel allotransplantation under FK506. *Surgery* 1991 ; 110 : 87.
74. Woo J, Ross CS, Milton JI, Thomson AW. Immunosuppressive activity of FK506 in rats : flow cytometric analysis of lymphocyte populations in blood, spleen and thymus during treatment and following drug withdrawal. *Clin Exp Immunol* 1990 ; 79 : 115-22.
75. Wicker LS, Boltz RC, Matt V, Nichols EA, Peterson LB, Sigal NH. Suppression of B cell activation by cyclosporin A, FK506 and rapamycin. *Eur J Immunol* 1990 ; 20 : 2277-83.
76. Thomson AW, Pugh-Humphreys RGP. Antilymphocytic activity of FK506 and its influence on the thymic microenvironment. *Thymus Update*. Vol. 4 (Ceds. MD Kendall and MA Rittes) : 93-127.
77. Metcalfe SM, Richards FM. Cyclosporine, FK506, and rapamycin. Some effects on early activation events in serum-free, mitogen-stimulated mouse spleen cells. *Transplantation* 1990 ; 49 : 798-802.
78. Walliser P, Benzie CR, Kay JE. Inhibition of B-lymphocyte proliferation by the novel immunosuppressive drug FK506. *Immunology* 1989 ; 68 : 434-5.

79. Suzuki W, Sakane T, Tsunematsu T. Effect of a novel immunosuppressive agent, FK506 on human B cell activation. *Clin Exp Immunol* 1990 ; 79 : 240-5.
80. Eiras G, Imventarza O, Murase N, Ueda Y, Todo S, Starzl T, Duquesnoy RJ, Zeevi A. Species differences in sensitivity of T lymphocytes to immunosuppressive effects of FK506. *Transplantation* 1990 ; 49 : 1170-2.
81. Woo J, Sewell HF, Thomson AW. The influence of FK506 on the expression of IL-2 receptors and MHC class II antigens on T cells following mitogen- or alloantigen-induced stimulation : a flow cytometric analysis. *Scand J Immunol* 1990 ; 31 : 297-304.
82. Zeevi A, Eiras G, Bach FH, Fung JJ, Todo S, Starzl T, Duquesnoy R. Functional differentiation of human cytotoxic T lymphocytes in the presence of FK506 and CyA. *Transplant Proc* 1990 ; 22 (6) : 106-9.
83. Zeevi A, Eiras G, Burckart G, Jain A, Kragack A, Venkataramanan R, Todo S, Fung JJ, Starzl T, Duquesnoy R. Bioassay of plasma specimens from liver transplant patients on FK506 immunosuppression. *Transplant Proc* 1990 ; 22 : 60-3.
84. Kay JE, Benzie CR. T lymphocyte activation through the CD28 pathway is insensitive to inhibition by the immunosuppressive drug FK506. *Immunol Lett* 1990 ; 23 : 155-60.
85. Kay JE, Benzie CR, Goodier MR, Wick CJ, Doe SEA. Inhibition of T-lymphocyte activation by the immunosuppressive drug FK506. *Immunology* 1989 ; 67 : 473-7.
86. Vathsala A, Chou TC, Kahan BD. Analysis of the interactions of immunosuppressive drugs with cyclosporine in inhibiting DNA proliferation. *Transplantation* 1990 ; 49 : 463-72.
87. Woo J, Propper DJ, Macleod AM, Thomson AW. Influence of FK506 and cyclosporin A on alloantibody production, lymphocyte activation antigen expression and lymphoproliferative responses following blood transfusion. *Clin Exp Immunol* 1990 ; 82 : 462-8.
88. Thomas J, Mattews C, Carroll R, Loreth R, Thomas F. The immunosuppressive action of FK506 : *in vitro* induction of allogeneic unresponsiveness in human CTL precursors. *Transplantation* 1990 ; 49 : 390-6.
89. Christians U, Kruse C, Kownatzki R, Schiebel HM, Schwinzer R, Sattler M, Schottmann R, Linck A, Almeida VMF, Braun F, Sewing K-Fr. Measurement of FK506 by HPLC and isolation and characterization of its metabolites. *Transplant Proc* 1991 ; 23 (1) : 940-1.
90. Zeevi A, Eiras G, Kaufman C, Alessiani M, Demetris AJ, AbuElmagd K, Jain A, Warty V, Venkataramanan R, Burckart G, Starzl T, Todo S, Fung JJ, Duquesnoy R. Correlation between bioassayed plasma levels of FK506 and lymphocyte growth from liver transplant biopsies with histological evidence of rejection. *Transplant Proc* 1991 ; 23 : 1406-8.
91. Yoshimura N, Matsui S, Hamashima T, Oka T. Effect of a new immunosuppressive agent, FK506, on human lymphocyte responses *in vitro*. II. Inhibition of the production of IL-2 and γ-IFN, but not B cell-stimulating factor 2. *Tranplantation* 1989 ; 47 : 36-9.
92. Tocci MJ, Matkovich DA, Collier KA, Kwok P, Dumont F, Lin S, Degudicibus S, Siekierka JJ, Chin J, Hutchinson NI. The immunosuppressant FK506 selectively inhibits expression of early T cell activation genes. *J Immunol* 1989 ; 143 : 718-26.
93. Dumont FJ, Staruch MJ, Koprak SL, Melino MR, Sigal NH. Distinct mechanisms of suppression of murine T cell activation by the related macrolides FK506 and rapamycin. *J Immunol* 1990 ; 144 : 251-8.
94. Bierer BE, Schreiber SL, Burakoff SJ. Mechanism of immunosuppression by FK506. Preservation of T cell transmembrane signal transduction. *Transplantation* 1990 ; 49 : 1168-202.
95. Fujii Y, Fujii S, Kaneko T. Effect of a novel immunosuppressive agent, FK506, on mitogen-induced inositol phospholipid degradation in rat thymocytes. *Transplantation* 1989 ; 47 : 1081-2.
96. Gschwendt M, Kittstein W, Marks F. The immunosuppressant FK506, like cyclosporins and didemnin B, inhibits calmodulin-dependent phosphorylation of the elongation

factor 2 *in vitro* and biological effects of the phorbol ester TPA on mouse skin in vivo. *Immunobiology* 1989 ; 179 : 1-7.
97. Siekierka JJ, Hung SHY, Poe M, Lin SC, Sigal NH. A cytosolic binding protein for the immunosuppressant FK506 has peptidyl-prolyl isomerase activity but is distinct from cyclophilin. *Nature* 1989 ; 341 : 755-7.
98. Standaert RF, Galat A, Verdine GL, Schreiber SL. Molecular cloning and overexpression of the human FK506-binding protein FKBP. *Nature* 1990 ; 346 : 671-4.
99. Tropschug M, Wachter E, Mayer S, Schonbrunner, Schmid FX. Isolation and sequence of an FK506-binding protein from *N. crassa* which catalyses protein folding. *Nature* 1990 ; 346 : 674-7.
100. Maki N, Sekiguchi F, Nishimaki J, Miwa K, Hayano T, Takahashi N, Suzuki M. Complementary DNA encoding the human T-cell FK506-binding protein, a peptidylprolyl cis-trans isomerase distinct from cyclophilin. *Proc Natl Acad Sci USA* 1990 ; 87 : 5440-3.
101. Takagishi K, Yamamoto M, Nishimura A, Yamasaki G, Kanazawa N, Hotokebuchi T, Kaibara N. Effects of FK506 on collagen arthritis in mice. *Transplant Proc* 1989 ; 21 : 1053-5.
102. Fischer G, Wittmann-Liebold B, Lang K, Kiefhaber T, Schmid FX. Cyclophilin and peptidyl-prolyl *cis-trans* isomerase are probably identical proteins. *Nature* 1989 ; 337 : 476-8.
103. Takahashi N, Hayano T, Suzuki M. Peptidyl-prolyl *cistrans* isomerase is the cyclosporin A-binding protein cyclophilin. *Nature* 1989 ; 337 : 473-5.
104. Rosen MK, Standaert RF, Galat A, Nakatsuka M, Schreiber SL. Inhibition of FKBP rotamase activity by immunosuppressant FK506 : twisted amide surrogate. *Science* 1990 ; 248 : 863-6.
105. Harrison RK, Stein RL. Substrate specificities of the peptidyl prolyl cis trans isomerase activities of cyclophilin and FK506 binding protein : evidence for the existence of a family of distinct enzymes. *Biochemistry* 1990 ; 29 : 3813-6.
106. Dumont FJ, Melino MR, Staruch MJ, Koprak SL, Fischer PA, Sigal NH. The immunosuppressive macrolides FK506 and rapamycin act as reciprocal antagonists in mature T cells. *J Immunol* 1990 ; 144 : 1418-24.
107. Schreiber SL. Chemistry and biology of the immunophilins and their immunosuppressive ligands. *Science* 1991 ; 251 : 283-7.
108. Durand DB, Bush MR, Morgan JG, Weiss A, Crabtree GR. A 275 basepair fragment at the 5' end of the interleukin 2 gene enhances expression from a heterologous promoter in response to signals from the T cell antigen receptor. *J Exp Med* 1987 ; 165 : 395.
109. Williams TM, Eisenberg L, Burlein JE, Norris CA, Pancer S, Yao D, Burger S, Kamoun M, Kant JA. Two regions within the human IL-2 gene promoter are important for inducible IL-2 expression. *J Immunol* 1988 ; 141 : 662-6.
110. Muegge K, Durum SK. Cytokines and transcription factors. *Cytokines* 1990 ; 2 : 1-8.
111. Shaw J, Utz P, Durand D, Toole J, Emmel E, Crabtree G. Identification of a putative regulator of early T-cell activation genes. *Science* 1988 ; 241 : 202.
112. Bierer BE, Mattila PS, Standaert RF, Herzenberg LA, Burakoff SJ, Crabtree G, Schreiber SL. Two distinct signal transmission pathways in T lymphocytes are inhibited by complexes formed between immunophilin and either FK506 or rapamycin. *Proc Natl Acad Sci USA* 1990 ; 87 : 9231-5.
113. Randak C, Brabletz T, Hergenrother M, Sobtta I, Serfling E. Cyclosporin A suppresses the expression of the interleukin 2 gene by inhibiting the binding of the lymphocyte-specific factors to the IL-2 enhancer. *EMBO J* 1990 ; 9 : 2529-36.
114. Liv J, Farmer JD, Lane WS, Friedman J, Weissman L, Schreiber SL. Calcineunin in a common target of cyclophilin. Cyclosporin A and FKBP-FK 506 complexes. *Cell* 1991 ; 66 : 807-15.
115. Flanagan WM, Corthesy B, Bram RJ, of Crabtree GR.. Nuclear association of a T-cell transcription factor blocked by FK 506 and cyclosporin. *Nature* 1991 ; 352 : 803-7.
116. Schreider SL, Crabtree GR. The mechanism of action of cyclosporin A and FK506. *Immunol Today* 1992 ; 13 : 136.

117. Sigal NH, Dumont FJ.. Cyclosporin A, FK506, and rapamycin pharmacologic probes of lymphocyte signal transduction. *Annu Rev Immunol* 1992 ; 10 : 519-60.
118. Liv J. FK506 and cyclosporin, molecular probes for studying intracellular signal transduction. *Immunol Today* 1973 ; 14 : 290-5.
119. Inamura N, Nakahara K, Kino T, Goto T, Aoki H, Yamaguchi I, Kohsaka M, Ochiai T. Prolongation of skin allograft survival in rats by a novel immunosuppressive agent, FK506. *Transplantation* 1988 ; 45 : 206-9.
120. Ochiai T, Sakamoto K, Nagata M, Nakajima K, Goto T, Hori S, Kenmochi T, Nakagori T, Asano T, Isono K. Studies on FK506 in experimental organ transplantation. *Transplant Proc* 1988 ; 20, Suppl. 1 : 209-14.
121. Lim SML, Thiru S, White DJG. Heterotopic heart transplantation in the rat receiving FK506. *Transplant Proc* 1987 ; 19, Suppl. 6 : 68-70.
122. Inagaki K, Fukuda Y, Sumimoto K, Matsuno K, Ito H, Takahashi M, Dohi K. Effects of FK506 and 15-deoxyspergualin in rat orthotopic liver transplantation. *Transplant Proc* 1989 ; 21 : 1069-71.
123. Arai K, Hotokebuchi T, Miyahara H, Arita C, Mohtai M, Sugioka Y, Kaibara N. Prolonged limb allograft survival with short-term treatment with FK506 in rats. *Transplant Proc* 1989 ; 21 : 3191-3.
124. Kuroki H, Ikuta Y, Akiyama M. Experimental studies of vascularized allogeneic limb transplantation in the rat using a new immunosuppressive agent, FK506 : morphological and immunological analysis. *Transplant Proc* 1989 ; 21 : 3187-90.
125. Yasunami Y, Ryu S, Kamei T, Konomi K. Effects of a novel immunosuppressive agent, FK506, on islet allograft survival in the rat. *Transplant Proc* 1989 ; 21 : 2720.
126. Hoffman AL, Makowka L, Banner B, Cai X, Cramer DV, Pascualone A, Todo S, Starzl TE. The use of FK506 for small intestine allotransplantation : Inhibition of acute rejection and prevention of fetal graft-*versus*-host disease. *Transplantation* 1990 ; 49 : 483-90.
127. Markus PM, Van den Brink MRM, Luchs BA, Fung JJ, Starzl TE, Hiserodt JC. Effects of *in vivo* treatment with FK506 on natural killer cells in rats *Transplantation* 1991 ; 51 : 913-5.
128. Markus PM, Cai X, Ming W, Demetris AJ, Fung JJ, Starzl TE. FK506 reverses acute graft-versus-host disease following allogenic bone marrow transplantation in rats. *Surgery* 1991 ; 110 : 357.
129. Todo S, Murase N, Ueda Y, Podesta L, Chapchap P, Kahn D, Okuda K, Imventarza O, Casavilla A, Demetris J, Makowka L, Starzl TE. Effect of FK506 in experimental organ transplantation. *Transplant Proc* 1988 ; 20, Suppl. 1 : 215-9.
130. Collier DStJ, Calne R, Thiru S, Friend PJ, Lim S, White DJG, Kohno H, Levickis J. FK506 in experimental renal allografts in dogs and primates. *Transpl Proc* 1988 ; 20, Suppl. 1 : 226-8.
131. Ueda Y, Todo S, Eiras G, Furukawa H, Imventarza O, Wu YM, Oks A, Zeevi A, Oguma S, Starzl TE. Induction of graft acceptance after dog kidney or liver transplantation. *Transplant Proc* 1990 ; 22 : 80-2.
132. Yokota K, Takishima T, Sato K, Osakabe T, Nakayama Y, Uchida H, Aso K, Masaki Y, Ohbu M, Okudaira M. Comparative studies of FK506 and cyclosporine in canine orthotopic hepatic allograft survival. *Transplant Proc* 1989 ; 21 : 1066-8.
133. Kenmochi T, Asano T, Enomoto K, Goto T, Nakagori T, Sakamoto K, Horie H, Ochiai T, Isono K. The effect of FK506 on sequental pancreas allografts in mongrel dogs. *Transplant Proc* 1988 ; 20, Suppl. 1 : 223-5.
134. Sato K, Yamagishi K, Nakayama Y, Yokota K, Uchida H, Masaki Y, Watanabe K, Aso K. Pancreaticoduodenal allotransplantation with cyclosporine and FK506. *Transplant Proc* 1989 ; 21 : 1074-5.
135. Imventarza 0, Todo S, Eiras G, Ueda Y, Furukawa H, Wu YM. Zhu Y, Oks A, Demetris J, Starzl TE. Renal transplantation in baboons under FK506. *Transplant Proc* 1990 ; 22 : 64-5.
136. Ericzon BG, Kubota K, Groth CG, Wijnen R, Tiebosch T, Buurman W, Kootstra G.

Pancreaticoduodenal allotransplantation with FK506 in the cynomolgus monkey. *Transplant Proc* 1990 ; 22 : 72-3.
137. Monden M, Gotoh M, Kanai T, Valdivia LA, Umeshita K, Endoh W, Nakano Y, Kawai M, Ohzato H, Ukei T, Dono K, Tono T, Murata M, Wang KS, Okamura J, Tanimoto Y, Hashimoto M, Mori T. A potent immunosuppressive effect of FK506 in orthotopic liver transplantation in primates. *Transplant Proc* 1990 ; 22, Suppl. 1 : 66-71.
138. Takabayashi K, Koike T, Kurasawa K, Matsumura R, Sato T, Tomioka H, Ito I, Yoshiki T, Toshida S. Effect of FK506, a novel immunosuppressive drug on murine systemic lupus erythematosus. *Clin Immunol Immunopathol* 1989 ; 51 : 110-7.
139. Yamamoto K, Mori A, Nakahama T, Ito M, Okudaira H, Miyamoto T. Experimental treatment of autoimmune MRL-lpr/lpr mice with immunosuppressive compound FK506. *Immunology* 1990 ; 69 : 222-7.
140. Okuba Y, Tsukada Y, Maezawa A, Ono K, Yano S, Naruse T. FK506, a novel immunosuppressive agent, induces antigenspecific immunotolerance in active Heymann's nephritis and in the autologous phase of Masugi nephritis. *Clin Exp Immunol* 1990 ; 82 : 450-5.
141. Murase N, Lieberman I, Nalesnik M, Mintz D, Todo S, Drash AL, Starzl TE. FK506 prevents spontaneous diabetes in the BB rat. *Lancet* 1990 ; ii, 373-4.
142. Miyagawa J, Yamamoto K, Hanafusa T, Itoh N, Nakagawa C, Otsuka A, Katsura H, Yamagata K, Miyazaki A, Kono N, Tarui S. Preventive effect of a new immunosuppressant FK506 on insulinitis and diabetes in non-obese diabetic mice. *Diabetologia* 1990 ; 33 : 503-5.
143. Tamura K, Woo J, Murase N, Carrieri G, Nalesnik MA, Thomson AW. Suppression of autoimmune thymoid disease by FK506 : influence of thymoid infiltrating cells, adhesion molecule expression and anti-thyroglobulin autoantibody production. *Clin Exp Immunol* 1993 ; 91 : 368-75.
144. Inamura N, Hashimoto M, Nakahara K, Aoki H, Yamaguchi I, Kohsaka M. Immunosuppressive effect of FK506 on collagen-induced arthritis in rats. *Clin Immunol Immunopathol* 1988 ; 46 : 82-90.
145. Arita C, Hotokebuchi T, Miyahara H, Arai K, Sugioka Y, Takagishi K, Kaibara N. Effect of FK506 (FR900506) on collagen arthritis in rats : a preliminary report. *Transplant Proc* 1989 ; 21 : 1056-8.
146. Arita C, Hotokebuchi T, Miyahara H, Arai K, Sugioka Y, Takagishi K, Kaibara N. Inhibition by FK506 of established lesions of collagen-induced arthritis in rats. *Clin Exp Immunol* 1990 ; 82 : 456-61.
147. Kawashima H, Fujino Y, Mochizuki M. Effects of a new immunosuppressive agent, FK506, on experimental autoimmune uveoretinitis in rats. *Invest Ophthalmol Vis Sci* 1988 ; 29 : 1265.
148. Mochizuki M Kawashima H. Effects of FK506, 15-deoxyspergualin and cyclosporine on experimental autoimmune uveoretinitis in the rat. *Autoimmunity* 1990 ; 8 : 37-41.
149. Ni M, Chan C-C, Nussenblatt RB, Mochizuki M. FR900506 (FK506) and 15-deoxyspergualine (15-DSG) modulate the kinetics of infiltrating cells in eyes with experimental autoimmune uveoretinitis. *Autoimmunity* 1990 ; 8 : 43-51.
150. Kawashima H, Fujino Y, Mochizuki M. Antigen-specific suppressor cells induced by FK506 in experimental autoimmune uveoretinitis in the rat. *Invest Ophthalmol Vis Sci* 1990 ; 31 : 31-8.
151. Thomson AW, Starzl TE. FK506 and autoimmune disease : perspective and prospects. *Autoimmunity* 1992 ; 12 : 303-13.
152. Todo S, Fung JJ, Starzl TE, Tsakis A, Demetris AJ, Kormos R, Jain A, Alessiani M, Takaya S. Liver, kidney, and thoracic organ transplantation under FK506. *Ann Surg* 1990 ; 212 (3) : 295-307.
153. Abu-Elmagd K, Fung lJ, Alessiani M, Jain A, Venkataramanan R, Warty VS, *et al.* The effect of graft function on FK506 plasma levels, doses and renal function : with particular reference to the liver. *Transplantation* 1991 ; 52 : 71-7.

154. Venkataramanan R, Jain A, Warty V, Abu-Elmagd K, Furukawa H, Imventarza O, Fung JJ, Todo S, Starzl TE. Pharmokinetics of FK506 following oral administration. A comparison of FK506 and cyclosporine. *Transplant Proc* 1991 ; 23 : 931-3.
155. Grevel J, Kahan BD. Pharmacokinetics of cyclosporin A. In : Thomson AW, ed. *Cyclosporine. Mode of action and clinical application*. London : Kluwer Academic Publishers, 1989 : 252-66.
156. Jain AB, Venkataraman R, Cadoff E, Fung JJ, Todo S, Krajack A, Starzl TE. Effect of hepatic dysfunction and T tube clamping on FK506 pharmacokinetics and trough concentrations. *Transplant Proc* 1990 ; 22 : 57-9.
157. Starzl TE, Fung JJ, Todo S. Comtempo 90 : Transplantation. *JAMA* 1990 ; 263 : 2686-7.
158. Starzl TE. The development of clinical renal transplantation. *Am J Kidney Dis* 1990 ; 26 : 548-56.
159. Fung JJ, Todo S, Tsakis A, Demetris A, Jain A, et al. Conversion of live allograft recipients from ciclosporine to FK-506-based immunosuppression : benefits and pitfalls. *Transplant Proc* 1991 ; 23 : 14-15.
160. Todo S, Fung JJ, Demetris AJ, Jain A, Venkataramanan R, Starzl TE. Early trials with FK506 as primary treatment in liver transplantation. *Transplant Proc* 1990 ; 22 : 13-6.
161. Shapiro R, Jordan M, Fung J, McCaulay J, Johnston J, Iwaki, et al. Kidney transplantation under FK506 immunosuppression. *Transplant Proc* 1990 ; 23 (1) : 920-3.
162. Todo S, Fung JJ, Tzakis A, Demetris AJ, Jain A, Alessiani M, Takaya S, Starzl TE. 110 consecutive primary orthopic liver transplants under FK506 in adults. *Transplant Proc* 1991 ; 23 : 1347-402.
163. Jain AB, Fung JJ, Todo S, Alessiani M, Takaya S, Abu-Elmagd K, et al. Incidence and treatment of rejection episodes in primary orthotopic liver transplantation under FK506. *Transplant Proc* 1991 ; 23 (1) : 928-30.
164. Mc Diarmid S and the US Multi-Center FK506 Liver Study Group. A multi-center prospective randomized trial componing FK506 to ciclosporine (CsA) after liver transplantation : comparison of efficacy based on incidence severity and treatment of rejection. Am Assoc Transplant *Physicians*, 12th Annual Meeting, Houston, 1993. Abstract.
165. Armitage JM, Kormes RL, Fung J, Lavee J, Fricker FJ, Griffith B, et al. Preliminary experience with FK506 in thoracic transplantation. *Transplant Proc* 1991 ; 52 : 164-7.
166. Armitage JM, Kormes RL, Griffith BP, Hardesty Rl, Frickes FJ, Stuart RS, et al. A clinical trial of FK 506 is primary and rescue immunosuppression in cardiac transplantation. *Transplant Proc* 1991 ; 23 : 1149-52.
167. Tzakis AG, Ricodi C, Alejandro R, Zeng Y, Fung JJ, Todo S, et al. Pancreatic islet transplantation after upper abdominal exenteration and liver replacement. *Lancet* 1991 ; ii ; 402.
168. McCauley J, Bronster O, Fung JJ, Todo S, Starzl TE. Treatment of cyclosporin induced haemolytic uraemic syndrome with FK506. *Lancet* 1990 ; ii ; 1516.
169. McCauley J, Tzakis AG, Fung JJ, Todo S, Starzl TE. FK506 in steroid-resistant focal sclerosing glomerulonephritis of childhood. *Lancet* 1990 ; i : 674.
170. Mieles L, Todo S, Fung JJ, Jain A, Furukawa H, Susuki M, et al. Oral glucose tolerance test in liver recipients treated with FK506. *Transplant Proc* 1990 ; 22 : 41-3.
171. Mieles L, Gordon RD, Mintz D, Toussaint RM, Imvartarza O, Starzl TE. Glycemia and insulin need following FK506 rescue therapy in liver transplant recipients. *Transplant Proc* 1991 ; 23 (1) : 949-53.
172. McCauley J, Takaya S, Fung JJ, Abu-Elmagd K, Jain A, Todo S, Starzl TE. The question of FK506 nephrotoxicity after lives transplantation. *Transplant Proc* 1991 ; 23 (1) : 1444-7.
173. Reyes J, Gayoiski T, Fung J, Todo s, Alessiani M, Starzl TE. Expressive dysphasia possibly related to FK506 in 2 liver transplantation recipients. *Transplantation* 1990 ; 5 : 1043-5.
174. Alessiani M, Kusne S, Martin M, Jain A, Abu-Elmagd K, Mooser J, et al. Infection

in adult liver transplantation under FK506 immunosuppression. *Transplant Proc* 1991 ; 23 : 1501-3.

13

Antisense oligonucleotides as tools for immune regulation

S. ESNAULT, N. BENBERNOU, M. GUENOUNOU

Laboratoire d'immunologie, Institut de Recherche médicale André Demonchy, Université de Reims, Reims, France.

The concept of antisense inhibition of gene expression represents an elegant approach to inhibit protein synthesis. Oligonucleotides that bind to the targeted mRNA or the double-stranded DNA (antigene) interfere with the intracellular protein production [1]. Zamecnick and Stephenson [2] showed for the first time that oligonucleotides complementary to a segment of reiterated terminal sequence of Rous sarcoma virus inhibit viral replication. Synthetic oligonucleotides have been used as antisense inhibitors of mRNA translation *in vitro* [3-6] and *in vivo* [7].

Production of antisense RNA may be a naturally occurring genetic control mechanism in prokaryotes. Also, antisense RNA was shown to induce sequence specific inhibition of target gene expression when introduced artificially into eukaryotic cells, either by microinjection of performed antisense molecules, or through transfection with DNA plasmid constructs carrying genes inverted relative to an appropriate transcriptional promoter.

It has become clear that antisense oligonucleotides can be used not only to investigate normal and pathological mammalian gene functions, but also to serve as the future therapeutic agents in a spectrum of pathologic processes ranging from viral infections to physiological disorders. The feasability of the approach has been documented in numerous *in vitro* experiments [5, 8]. This new technology has lead to the proliferation of several antisense pharmaceutical companies. However, the potential role of antisense oligonucleotides in combating completely viruses and cancer where it is desirable in many instances to eliminate targeted proteins completely remains somewhat controversial. Antisense strategy would be most satisfied in immune regulation when certain degrees of protein synthesis inhibition were achieved, thus leading to re-establish the homeostasis in the immune system. Furthermore, oligodeoxynucleotides are especially useful when a conventional inhibitor or antagonist is unavailable or shows limited selectivity, particularly when autocrine mechanisms are involved.

Cytokines are produced by many cell types in response to different stimuli and have important functions in cell to cell communication in the immune system, thus regulating cellular growth, differentiation and biological function [9]. It becomes clear that cytokines are involved in several physiological dysregulation, and in several cases as autocrine factors. One of the deal of these pathologies is to regulate such mediators in a specific manner. Several studies have proved that antisense strategy could represent a useful tool for immune regulation.

This paper presents the antisense RNA techniques that offer at present interesting possibilities to manipulate various genes specifically.

Selection of antisense oligonucleotides

Standard computer programs for optimizing oligonucleotide sequences (relating to duplex formation energy) were used for the selection of antisense oligonucleotides. It is imperative to check any similarities with other sequences present in gene databases. Several investigations, including those performed in our laboratory, have shown the efficiency of ODNs that have been designed to bind to the region surrounding the translation initiation AUG codon. Other sites corresponding to 5'- or 3'- untranslated regions (capping region) can be targeted with different efficiencies. Our recent studies have shown the importance of the choice of target sites for antisense effect [10].

It appeared that a minimum length of ODN sequence (11-15 nucleotides) is required in order to have only one target site in the genome. This also corresponds to the minimum length for effective hybridization with the target to form a duplex. On the other hand, ODN length would not exceed 20-25 nucleotides for an efficient cellular uptake. Oligonucleotides of 15-20 nucleotides have often been used [1]. Furthermore, it is essential to test the optimal concentrations of ODNs that lead to the desired effect without toxicity.

Mechanisms of action of antisense oligonucleotides

The actual mechanism(s) of action of oligonucleotides on intact cells remained to be more elucidated. The antisense strategy interfere with the information flow from the gene to protein. Several hypothesis for antisense way of action are suggested.

(a) Inhibition of translation : steric hindrance can prevent translation progression. Initiation region seems to be the best target [11].

(b) RNase H activation by the formation of heteroduplex ODN/preRNA in the nucleus area ; thus leading to an enzymatic lysis of RNA. No mature RNA can produce functional protein. RNA splicing can also be blocked by targeting around splicing site [12, 13].

(c) Downregulation of endogenous genes through authentic triple helix formation. Formation of triple helix (DNA/ODN) prevent RNA synthesis. By a hoogsten type appariement, ODN goes in the major groove of double helix. Thymidine is associated with a AT pair, and guanidine with GC pair. Only purine (A and G) rich on one strand (TC rich on the other hand) can be targeted [14, 15]. This hypothesis has not been formally demonstrated in intact cells, although promising data have been obtained [16, 17].

(d) Ribozymes are small oligoribonucleotides that have a specific base sequence that confers upon them natural self-splicing activity [18]. This activity can be directed against any RNA by flanking the catalytic domain with sequences antisense to the target RNA.

Synthesis of ODN

In the last decay, oligonucleotide synthesis has been very improved. For the common form, synthesis is automatized (phosphodiester, phosphorothioate, methylphosphonate...) [19, 20] and followed usually the phosphoramidite method.

The chemistry of oligonucleotides implicates the attachment of deoxynucleoside containing a 3'-p-nitrophenylsuccinate group to a silicat-based support through an ester linkage. The addition of one deoxynucleotide to the support-bound deoxynucleoside is completed in four steps : (1) removal of the dimethoxytrityl protecting group with acid ; (2) condensation with a deoxynucleotide 3'-phosphoramidite to yield the deoxynucleoside phosphite triester ; (3) acylation or capping of unreacted 5'-hydroxyl groups ; (4) oxidation of the phosphite triester to the phosphite triester. The oxidation step can be replaced with a sulfurization to make phosphorothioates. Further multiple repetitions of this sequence can lead to the synthesis of DNA segments containing up to 150 deoxynucleotides. Purification of ODN could be performed by polyacrilamide electrophoresis (PAGE) or by high performance liquid chromatography (HPLC).

Stable oligonucleotide analogs

The principal difficulties with using oligonucleotides to inhibit gene expression concern their biological stability, solubility or cellular uptake. Consequently, novel oligonucleotide analogues are high-piority targets for medicinal chemistry [19-21]. Oligonucleotides are susceptible to degradation by nucleases present *in vivo*. The presence of exonuclease or endonuclease activities would dramatically decrease the specificity of an antisense oligonucleotide.

A number of chemistry modifications have been studied to improve antisense efficiency and to overcome the problem of degradation by nucleases. The most common are phosphorothioates, methylphosphonates which are modified at the phosphodiester group by substitution of a methyl group or a sulfure atom for one of the non-bridging oxygens, and α-oligodeoxynucleotides derivatives which have an unnatural glycosidic configuration. These three analogs are nuclease-resistant but display different properties. Phosphorothioates are able to induce RNase H activity, whereas the α-oligonucleotides and methylphosphonates are not inducers of RNase H [22, 23].

Phosphorothioates oligonucleotides have been shown to block the *de novo* infection of susceptible cells by the human immunodeficiency virus (HIV-1) and to inhibit viral expression and proliferation in already infected cells [24, 25].

Other chemical modifications applied to oligonucleotides that inhibit expression of specific genes include 2-modified oliogdeoxynucleotides, oligodeoxynucleotides conjugated at 5' to cholesterol [26], polylysine [27], psoralen [28], and acridine [22]. Further development of new generations of oligodeoxynucleotides with improved properties are expected in the next years.

Cellular uptake

The plasma membrane is a natural barrier to many large and negatively charged molecules. However, the cellular uptake of oligonucleotides takes place better than it has been expected from a polyanionic compound of this size. The study of Zamecnik *et al.* [29] has demonstrated that ODNs penetrate into the cells in 15 min to few hours. The time course of cellular uptake is linear in the initial phase and then reaches a plateau that usually lasts from 2 to 3 hours [21, 29].

The existence of cell membrane-bound DNA has long been recognized. Studies of Bennett *et al.* [30] showed the existence of a 30 kDa protein on peripheral blood lymphocytes that binds double-stranded DNA with Kd = 1 nM. Loke *et al.* [31] have isolated a 80 kDa cell-surface protein (p80) which appeared to be responsible for specific oligonucleotide binding to the HL60 cell line. Yakubov *et al.* [32] also identified cell-surface proteins (79 and 90 kDa) in L929 cells that could bind to oligonucleotides. However, these authors have shown that the majority of oligonucleotide internalization was not due to receptor-mediated endocytosis, but was rather due to pinocytosis (fluid-phase endocytosis).

Other types of studies, particularly those performed by Loke *et al.*, have shown that intracellular accumulation of ODN in leukemia HL60 cell line was observed as from 16 hours of culture with a maximum after 50 hours, thus supporting the hypothesis that cellular uptake is variable with the nature of cell type. The cellular uptake process of ODNs appeared to be energy-dependent [3]. More recently, there appeared evidence that the ODN uptake is mediated by endocytosis/pinocytosis [26], and certain studies suggested that this phenomenon required a receptor-like recognition [32].

Phosphorothioate ODNs have been shown to present a slower uptake rate than did their native phosphodiester analogs or the methylphosphonate derivatives [33, 34]. This could be explained by the fact that the phosphorothioates are negatively charged, and are water soluble, whereas the methylphosphonates, because they are uncharged, are more lipophilic.

Other types of ODNs modifications have been recently developed to improve the cellular uptake. Poly-L-lysine allows the efficient delivery of small oligonucleotides to various cell lines and could conceivably be used to promote the internalization of antisense oligonucleotides [35]. Oligonucleotide conjugated to poly-L-lysine, and targeted to the HIV-1 *tat* mRNA translation initiation site were approximately 100 times more efficient and much more selective than non-conjugated material [24]. Likewise, liposomes targeted with anti-CD3 antibodies and containing an antisense RNA to the HIV *env* region inhibited viral protein expression [36].

Liposomes and nanoparticles are also proved to constitute usefull ODNs derivative molecules [37, 38].

Studies with antisense ODNs and analogs

A growing attention has been attracted to the antisense application. Several studies have described the anti-viral properties of antisense oligonucleotides [39]. Antisense oligonucleotides were also used to determine the role of oncogenes [40-42], and more recently to the selective inhibition of cytokines [43-50].

The first use of synthetic antisense for therapeutic purposes was from Zamecnik and Stephenson in 1978 who showed the inhibitory effects of antisense oligonucleotide (13 mer) in the inhibition of the growth of Rous Sarcoma virus in cell culture. The application of antisense to viruses is still topical. Other viruses have also been studied, in particular, vesicular stomatitis virus, herpes simplex virus, influenza virus, B hepatitis virus [51] and human immunodeficiency virus (HIV) [52]. In competitive investigations on HIV studies, phosphorothioate ODNs inhibited HIV replication *in vitro* in both acutely and chronically infected T cell assays.

The other main field of antisense application is cancer. Several oncogene or proto-oncogene activities have been studied by using antisense oligonucleotides. Additionnally, antisense were also used to study the role of growth factors including cytokines in the proliferation of tumor cells. Modulation of neoplastic cell growth by cytokines is well documented for different cells and cell lines of tumorigenic origin ; IL-6 acts as autocrine factor of non-Hodgkin's B lymphoma, and of multiple myeloma cells [53-57]. Growth of EBV-infected cell lines, furthermore, is reported to be sustained by cell-secreted TNF-β [58] and by IL-1-like factors [59, 60]. B cells of chronic lymphocytic leukemia secrete IL-β and IL-6, and DNA synthesis of these cells is stimulated by both TNF-α and TNF-β. Approximately half of the B lymphoma lines analyzed were reported to secrete autocrine factors. Tumor cells *in vivo* are thought to escape from growth restriction of normal cells by secretion and reinternalization of autocrine factors [61]. Autonomous growth of tumor cell lines *in vitro* is assumed to reflect this capability. Alterations in retro-control of physiologic B cell proliferation may lead to the development of lymphomas. In this concept, several studies have shown the growth-stimulatory activities of the cytokine network in neoplastic B cells *in vitro* using antisense approach, and these results have led to great interests in this strategy as potential anti-tumor agents resulting to a re-establishment of the normal physiologic mechanisms of cell proliferation and differentiation [46, 62].

The antisense oligonucleotides could also represent a useful approach to investigate immunological mechanisms. Kawasaki *et al.* [63] was the first author demonstrating the inhibition of cytokine production in xenopus oocytes. Human IL-2 single strand complementary DNA (SScDNA) or synthetic complementary ODN were hybridized with mRNA and coinjected in oocyte. Antisense oligonucleotides injected before or after mRNA injection inhibit IL-2 expression.

The recent study of Witsell et al. [64] of murine bone marrow-derived macrophages differenciation has shown the involvement of an autocrine mechanism in which TNF expression in macrophage cultures signals the onset of differentiation and the cessation of proliferation.

Research in our own group has shown that antisense oligonucleotides targeted to specific cytokines were able to regulate efficiently immunoglobulin production. We recently showed that antisense to IL-4 was able to regulate Ig production in cultures of spleen cells from *Nippostrongylus brasiliensis* infected rats. Antisense to IL-4 selected near the AUG initiation codon of the murine IL-4 mRNA inhibited IgG2a and IgE synthesis and increased IgM production [10, 65]. Both the Ig secretion in culture supernatants and the number of Ig secreting cells were influenced by the presence of antisense IL-4 ODNs. The use of antisense oligonucleotides show the involvement of IL-2 and IL-4 in the regulation of isotype selection during antibody synthesis and that IL-2 and IL-4 do operate differently on IgE production. A selective inhibition of Th-cell derived cytokines by antisense oligonucleotides was also shown in murine T cell lines by Harel-Bellan, and results showed a specific inhibition through the degradation of mRNA by RNAseH activity.

Controls

It is obviously necessary to rule out any non-specific effect of oligodeoxynucleotides on proteins other than the targeted one. Most studies involved the use of sense sequences of the corresponding active oligodeoxynucleotide molecules or irrelevant analogues as controls. Stringent mismatched analogues maintaining the same base composition as the antisense molecule should also be used as controls. The specificity of an antisense approach is a critical issue when dealing with modified oligonucleotides. Antisense effects could be masked by non-sequence-specific interference as it was described in cells infected with HIV [52, 66]. As the degradation of mRNA by RNase H seems to be the most important mechanism of protein inhibition, the quantitative analysis of the targeted mRNA and other irrelevant mRNA, by Northern blotting or by RT-PCR could be informative. It is also necessary to test the possible toxicity of oligonucleotides in cultured cells *in vitro*.

Conclusion

The inhibition induced by antisense oligonucleotides in studies performed *in vitro* could serve as a basis for strategies to reduce the aberrant expression of mediators involved in physiological dysregulations. There is an immediate question. Can the technology be applied *in vivo* ? Recent *in vivo* studies have shown promizing results. A major problem of pharmacology is the difficulty in designing agents that act specifically on a particular target cell. Thus, it remains to be seen whether the problems of getting antisense oligonucleotides in patients can be overcome by use of modified probes with novel delivery systems.

References

1. Degols G, Leonetti JP, Mechti N, Lebleu B. Antiproliferative effects of antisense oligonucleotides directed to the RNA of c-myc oncogene. *Nucleic Acid Res* 1991 ; 19 : 945-7.
2. Stephenson ML, Zamecnik PC. Inhibition of Rous sarcoma viral RNA translation be a specific oligodeoxnucleoide. *Proc Natl Acad Sci USA* 1978 ; 75 : 285-8.
3. Stein C, Cohen J. Oligodeoxy nucleotides as inhibitors of gene expression : a review. *Cancer Res* 1988 ; 48 : 2659-68.
4. Zon G. Oligonucleotide analogues as potential chemotherapeutic agents. *Pharm Res* 1988 ; 5 : 539-49.
5. Helene C, Toulme JJ. Specific regulation of gene expression by antisense, sense and antigene nucleic acids. *Biochim Biophys Acta* 1990 ; 1049 : 99-125.
6. Calabretta B. Inhibition of proto-oncogene expression by antisense oligodeoxynucleotides : biological and therapeutic implications. *Cancer Res* 1991 ; 51 : 4505-10.
7. Burch RM, Mahan LC. Oligonucleotides antisense to interleukin 1 receptor mRNA block the effects of interleukin 1 in cultured murine and human fibroblasts and in mice. *J Clin Invest* 1991 ; 88 : 1190-6.
8. Degols G, Leonetti JP, Lebleu B. Antisense oligonucleotides as pharmacological modulators of gene expression in targeted drug delivery. In : Juliano RL, ed. *Handbook for experimental pharmacology*. Heidelberg : Springer Verlag, 1991 : 329.
9. Paul WE. Piking holes in the network. *Nature* 1992 ; 357 : 16-8.
10. Benbernou N, Matsiota-Bernard P, Guenounou M. Antisense oligonucleotides to interleukin 4 regulate IgE and IgG2a production by spleen cells from Nippostrongylus brasiliensis-infected rats. *Eur J Immunol* 1993 ; 23 : 659-63.
11. Boiziau C, Kufusts R, Cazenave C, Roig V, Thyong NT, Toulme JJ. Inhibition of translation initiation by antisense oligonucleotides via an RNase-H independent mechanism. *Nucleic Acids Res* 1991 ; 19 : 1113-9.
12. Furdon PJ, Kole R. Inhibition of splicines but not cleavage at the 5' splice side by truncating human beta-globine pre-mRNA. *Proc Natl Acad Sci USA* 1986 ; 83 (4) : 927-31.
13. Dash P, Lotan I, Knapp M, Kandel ER, Goelet P. Selective elimination of mRNAs *in vivo* : Complementary oligodeoxynucleotides promote RNA degradation by an RNase H-like activity. *Proc Natl Acad Sci USA* 1987 ; 84 : 7896-900.
14. Baran N, Lapidot A, Manor H. Formation of triple helixs accounts for arrests of DNA synthesis at d(TC)n and d(GA)n tracts. *Proc Natl Acad Sci USA* 1991 ; 88 : 507-11.
15. Maher LJ, Wold B, Dervan PB. Inhibition of DNA binding proteins by oligonucleotide-directed triple helix formation. *Science* 1989 : 245 : 725-30.
16. Cooney M, Czernuszewicz G, Postel EH, Flint SJ, Hogan ME. Site-specific oligonucleotide binding represses transcription of the human c-myc gene *in vitro*. *Science* 1988 ; 241 : 456.
17. Grigoriev M, Praseuth D, Robin P, Hemar A, Saison-Behmoraras J, Dautry-Varsat A, Thuong NT, Hélène C, Harel-Bellan A. A triple helix forming oligonucleotide intercalator conjugate acts as transcriptional repressor *via* inhibition of NFκB binding to interleukin 2 receptor α-regulatory sequence. *J Biol Chem* 1992 ; 267 : 3389.
18. Haseloff J, Gerlach WL. Simple RNA enzymes with new and highly specific endoribonuclease activities. *Nature* 1988 ; 334 (6183) : 585-91.
19. Goodchild J. Conjugates of oligonucleotides and modified oligonucleotides. A review of their synthesis and properties. *Bioconjugate Chemistry* 1990 ; 1 : 165.
20. Carathers MH. Synthesis of oligonucleotides and oligonucleotide analogues 7-22. In : Cohen JS, ed. *Topics in structural and molecular biology : oligodeoxynucleotides : antisense inhibitors of gene expression*. Boca Raton, Florida : CRC Press, 1989.
21. Uhlmann E, Peyman A. Antisense oligonucleotides. A new therapeutic principle. *Chemical Rev* 1990 ; 90 : 544.
22. Cazenave C, Chevrier M, Thuong NT, Helene C. Rate of degradation of alpha and beta oligodeoxynucleotides in xenopus oocytes. Implications for anti-messager strategies. *Nucleic Acids Res* 1987 ; 15 : 10507-21.

23. Miller PS. Oligonucleotide methylphosphonates as antisense reagents. *Bio/Technology* 1991 ; 9 : 358-62.
24. Degols G, Leonetti JP, Milhaud P, Mechti N, Lebleu B. Antisense inhibitors of HIV : problems and perspective. *Antiviral Res* 1992 ; 17 : 279.
25. Matsukura M, Zon G, Shinozuka K, Robert-Guroff M, Shimada T, Stein CA, Mitsuya H, Wong-Staal F, Cohen JS, Broder S. Regulation of viral expression of human immundeficiency virus *in vitro* by antisense phosphorothioate oligodeoxynucleotide against rev (art/trs) in chronically infected cells. *Proc Natl Acad Sci* 1989 ; 86 : 4244-8.
26. Krieg AM, Thonkinson J, Matson S, Zhao Q, Saxon M, Zhang LM, Bhanja U, Yakubov L, Stein CA. Modification of antisense phosphodiester oligodeoxynucleotides by a 5'cholesteryl moiety increases cellular association and improves efficacy. *Proc Natl Acad Sci USA* 1993 ; 90 : 1048-52.
27. Lemaitre M, Bayard B, Lebleu B. Specific antiviral activity of a poly (L-lysine) — conjugated oligodeoxyribonucleotide sequence complementary to vesicular stomatitis N protein mRNA initiation site. *Proc Natl Acad Sci USA* 1987 ; 84 : 648-52.
28. Keean JM, Murakami A, Blake KR, Cushman CD, Miller PS. *Biochemistry* 1988 ; 27 : 9113-21.
29. Zamecnik PC, Goodchild J, Taguchi Y, Sarin PS. Inhibition of replication and expression of human T cell lymphotropic virus type III in cultured cells by exogenous synthetic oligonucleotides complementary to viral RNA. *Proc Natl Acad Sci USA* 1986 ; 83 : 4143-6.
30. Bennett R, Gabor G, Merritt M. *J Clin Invest* 1985 ; 76 : 2182-90.
31. Loke S, Stein C, Zhang X, et al. *Proc Natl Acad Sci USA* 1989 ; 86 : 3474-8.
32. Yakubov L, Deeva E, Zarytova V, et al. *Proc Natl Acad Sci USA* 1989 ; 86 : 6454-8.
33. Thierry AR, Dritshilo A. Intracellular availability of unmodified phopshorothiated and liposomally encapsulated oligodeoxynucleotides for antisense activity. *Nucleic Acids Res* 1992 ; 20 : 5691-8.
34. Zhao Q, Matson S, Herrera CJ, Fisher E, Yu H, Krieg AM. Comparison of cellular binding and uptake of antisense phosphodiester, phosphorothioate, and mixed phosphorothioate and methyl phosphorate oligonucleotides. *Antisense Rev Dev* 1993 ; Spring 3 : 53-6.
35. Clarenc JP, Degols G, Leonetti JP, Milhaud P, Lebleu B. Delivery of antisense oligonucleotides by poly-L-lysine conjugation and liposome encapsulation. *Anti-cancer Drug Design* 1993 ; 8 : 81-94.
36. Renneisen K, Leserman L, Matthes E, Schroder HC, Muller WEG. Inhibition of expression of human immunodeficiency virus-1 *in vitro* by antibody-targeted liposomes containing RNA to the *env* region. *J Biol Chem* 1990 ; 265 : 16337.
37. Bayard B, Lesserman LD, Bisbal C, Lebleu B. *EJB* 1985 ; 151 : 319.
38. Chavany C, Le Doan T, Couvreur P, Puisieux F, Hélène C. Polyalkylcyanoacrylate nanoparticles as polymeric carriers for antisense oligonucleotides. *Pharmaceutical Res* 1992 ; 9 : 441-9.
39. Goodchild J, Agrawal S, Civeira MP, Sarin PS, Sun D, Zamecnik PC. Inhibition of human immunodeficiency virus replication by antisense oligonucleotides. *Proc Natl Acad Sci* 1988 ; 85 : 5507-11.
40. Holt JT, Redner RL, Nienhuis AW. An oligomer complementary to c-myc mRNA inhibits proliferation of HL-60 promyelocytic cells and induce differentiation. *Mol Cell Biol* 1988 ; 8 : 963-73.
41. Anfossi G, Gewirtz AM, Calabretta B. An oligomer complementary to c-myb-encoded mRNA inhibits proliferation of human myeloid leukemia cell lines. *Proc Natl Acad Sci USA* 1989 ; 86 : 3379-83.
42. Redd JC, Stein C, Subasinghe C, Haldar S, Croce CM, Yum S, Cohen J. Antisense-mediated inhibition of bcl2 protooncogene expression and leukemic cell growth and survival : Comparisons of phosphodiester and phosphorothioate oligodeoxynucleotides. *Cancer Res* 1990 ; 50 : 6565-70.
43. Manson J, Brown T, Duff G. Modulation of interleukin 1 beta gene expression using antisense phosphorothioate oligonucleotides. *Lymphokine Res* 1990 ; 9 : 35-42.

44. Fujiwara T, Grimm EA. Specific inhibition of interleukin 1 β gene expression by an antisense oligonucleotide : obligatory role of interleukin 1 in the generation of lymphokine-activated killer cells. *Cancer Res* 1992 ; 52 : 4954-9.
45. Maier JAM, Voulalas P, Roeder D, Maciag T. Extension of the life-span of human endothelial cells by an interleukin 1 alpha antisense oligomer. *Science* 1990 ; 249 : 1570-4.
46. Levy Y, Tsapis A, Brouet JC. Interleukin 6 antisense oligonucleotides inhibits the growth of human myeloma cell lines. *J Clin Invest* 1991 ; 88 : 696-9.
47. Birchenall-Roberts MC, Ferrer C, Ferris D, Falk LA, Kasper J, White G, Ruscetti FW. Inhibition of murine monocyte proliferation by a colony-stimulating factor-1 antisense oligodeoxynucleotiude. Evidence for autocrine regulation. *J Immunol* 1990 ; 154 : 3290-6.
48. Kobayashi S, Teramura M, Sugawara I, Oshimi K, Mizoguchi H. Interleukin 11 acts as an autocrine growth factor for human megakaryoblastis cell lines. *Blood* 1993 ; 81 : 889-93.
49. Louie SW, Ramirez LM, Krieg AM, Maliszewski CR, Bishop GA. Endogenous secretion of IL-4 maintains growth and Thy-1 expression of a transformed B cell clone. *J Immunol* 1993 ; 150 : 399-406.
50. Segal GM, Smith TD, Heinrich MC, Ey FS, Bagby GC. Specific repression of granulocyte-macrophage and granulocyte colony-stimulating factor gene expression in interleukin-1-stimulated endothelial cells with antisense oligonucleotides. *Blood* 80 : 609-16.
51. Blum HE, Galun E, Weizsacker FV, Wands JR. Inhibition of hepatitis B virus by antisense oligodeoxynucleotides. *Lancet* 337 : 1230.
52. Stein CA, Matsukura M, Subasinghe C, Broder S, Cohen JS. Phosphorothioate oligodeoxynucleotides are potent sequence non specific inhibitors of de novo infection by HIV. *AIDS Res Hum Retrovir* 1989 ; 5 : 639.
53. Yee C, Biondi A, Wang XH, Iscove NN, De Soussa J, Aarden LA, Wong GG, Clark SC, Messner HA, Minden MD. A possible autocrine role of interleukin-6 in two lymphoma lines. *Blood* 1989 ; 74 : 798.
54. Brouet JC, Levis Y. IL-6 and lymphoproliferative disorders. *Nouv Rev Fr Hematol* 1991 ; 33 : 433-6.
55. Lu C, Kerbel RS. Interleukin 6 undergoes transition from paracrine growth inhibitor to autocrine stimulator during human melanoma progression. *J Cell Biol* 1993 ; 120 : 1281-8.
56. Schwarb G, Siegall CB, Aarden LA, Neckers LM, Nordan LP. Characterization of an interleukin-6-mediated autocrine growth loop in the human multiple myeloma cell line, U-266. *Blood* 1991 ; 77 : 587-93.
57. Kawano M, Hirano T, Matsuda T, Tada T, Horii Y, Iwato K, Asaoku H, Tnag B, Tanabe O, Tanaka H, Kuramoto A, Kishimoto T. Autocrine generation and requirement of BSF/IL-6 for human multiple myelomas. *Nature* 332 : 83.
58. Seregina TM, Mekshenkov MI, Turetskaya RL, Nedospavov SA. An autocrine growth factor constitutively produced by a human lymphoblastoid B cell line is serogically related to lymphotoxin (TNF-β). *Mol Immunol* 1989 ; 26 : 339.
59. Vandenabeele PB, Jayara B, Devos R, Shaw A, Fiers W. Interleukin 1α acts as an autocrine growth factor for RPMI 1788, an Epstein-Barr virus-transformed human B cell line. *Eur J Immunol* 1988 ; 18 : 1027.
60. Gordon J, Guy G, Walker L. Autocrine models of B lymphocyte growth. *Immunology* 1986 ; 57 : 419.
61. Sporn M, Roberts A. Autocrine growth factors and cancer. *Nature* 1985 ; 313 : 745.
62. Abken H, Fluck J, Willecke K. Four cell-secreted cytokines act synergistically to maintain long term proliferation of human B cell lines *in vitro*. *J Immunol* 1992 ; 149 : 2785-94.
63. Kawasaki ES. Quantitative hybridization-arrest of mRNA in Xenopus oocytes using single-stranded comlementary DNA or oligonucleotide probes. *Nucleic Acid Res* 1985 ; 13 : 4991-5003.
64. Witsell AL, Schook LB. Tumor necrosis factor alpha is an autocrine growth regulator during macrophage differentiation. *Proc Natl Acad Sci USA* 1992 ; 89 : 4754-8.

65. Benbernou N, Matsiota-Bernard P, Guenounou M. Effect of cytokine-specific antisense oligonucleotides on the immunoglobulin production by rat spleen cells *in vitro*. *Biochimie* 1993 ; 75 : 55-65.
66. Majumdar C, Stein CA, Cohen JS, Broder S, Wilson SH. Stepwise mechanism of HIV reverse transcriptase : primer function of phosphorothioate oligodeoxynucleotide. *Biochemistry* 1989 ; 28 : 1340.

14

Interferons

Christian BILLARD

INSERM U 365, Institut Curie, Section de Biologie,
26, rue d'Ulm, 75231 Paris Cedex 05, France.

Presentation of interferons

Historical background

Interferon (IFN) was discovered in 1957 by Isaacs and Lindenmann who observed that virus-infected cells released a factor capable of « viral interference », rendering other cells resistant to any viral infection.

Thereafter, IFNs proved to be a family of proteins and glycoproteins exhibiting multiple biological effects. At first, IFNs were found to inhibit cell growth *in vitro* as well as tumor development in animals. Further, a study by Gresser et al. [1] provided evidence for stimulatory effects of IFNs on immune defense : mice inoculated with tumor cells made resistant to IFN *in vitro* were protected from tumor development when treated with the same IFN. Afterwards, a wide number of works demonstrated that IFNs are strong immunomodulating agents. IFNs are now considered as a class of cytokines. In the following, the different types of IFN and their properties are presented. For a complete information, the reader can refer to the book of De Maeyer and De Maeyer-Guignard [2].

Types and properties of interferons

All cells of vertebrates are capable of producing IFN, whose activity is species specific. There are three types of IFN : alpha (IFN-α), beta (IFN-β) and gamma (IFN-γ), which are different in cell origin and way of induction. IFN-α and IFN-β are produced after viral infection by leucocytes and fibroblasts, respectively. Double-stranded RNA are also inducers of IFN-α and IFN-β, likely by mimicing viral replicative forms. On the other hand, IFN-γ is induced during activation of T lymphocytes (Table I).

Table I. Main types of human interferons.

Interferon	Cell origin	Induction	Proteins	Genes	Localisation	Receptors
α	Macrophages B cells T and NK cells	Virus dsRNA B mitogens	166 amino acids 20 kDa about 20 subtypes with 80 % homology	About 20 with 10 % homology No intron	Chromosome 9	Similar binding sites
β	Fibroblasts Epithelial cells	Virus dsRNA	166 amino acids 20 kDa only one protein with 30 % homology with IFN-α	1 gene No intron	Chromosome 9	
γ	Activated T lymphocytes NK cells	T mitogens Specific antigens IL-2	146 amino acids 17 kDa No homology with IFN-α and -β	1 gene 4 exons 3 introns	Chromosome 12	Independent binding sites

ds : double-stranded.

All three types of IFN also differ in a number of properties : antigenicity, physicochemical characteristics (molecular weight, isoelectric point, acid-lability) and biochemical properties (polypeptide sequence, degree of glycosylation). Recombinant DNA technology allowed to determine the structures of IFN genes and proteins. Nearly twenty subtypes of IFN-α, but only one IFN-β and one IFN-γ were identified. Polypeptide sequence of IFN-β shows about 30 % of homology with IFN-α. By contrast, IFN-γ shows no homology with IFN-α and -β.

In this connection, IFN-α and -β share a number of properties, whereas IFN-γ is clearly distinguishable from the two other IFN types, regarding the structure, organization and localization of the genes (Table II), induced proteins, various biological properties, as well as specific cell surface receptors. Indeed, IFN-α and -β compete for the same binding sites, contrarily to IFN-γ which recognizes other receptors. In addition, the cloned cDNA sequences encoding for IFN-α and IFN-γ receptors do not show any homology [3, 4].

Finally, a second type of fibroblast IFN was identified. Initially called IFN-β2, this molecule turned out to be another cytokine produced by monocytes, activated T lymphocytes and other cell types. Its antiviral activity is controversial and its range of activity exceeds widely that of IFN family : B cell differentiation factor (BCDF, BSF-2), hepatocyte stimulating factor, acute phase protein stimulating factor, B cell hybridoma growth factor, tumoral growth factor in multiple myeloma, T cell activating factor, etc. This cytokine mediates communication between injured tissues and hepatocytes. IFN-β2 is now named interleukin 6 [5].

Biological effects

The IFNs possess a vast number of biological properties which are reviewed below and summarized in Table II. In addition to their antiviral activity, IFNs regulate major cellular functions : immune responses, cell growth and differentiation.

Furthermore, they modulate gene and oncogene expression. All these data suggested early that IFNs are potential antitumoral agents.

Table II. Biological effects of interferons.

Induction of genes
- Enzymes : 2-5A synthetase, p68 kinase
- Transcription factors : IRF1/ISGF2, IRF2
- MHC class I and class II
- Fcγ receptors
- β2-microglobulin
- Mx family

Inhibition of genes
- Oncogenes (c-myc, c-fos, c-abl, c-Ha-ras)
- Ornithine decarboxylase

Antiviral effects

Inhibition of cell growth

Effects on cell differentiation

Antitumor effects
- Murine tumors
- Human tumors transplanted in *nude* mice
- Reversion of « transformed » phenotype
- Decrease in tumorigenicity

Antagonism with growth factor
- Inhibition of PDGF, EGF and BCGF activities
- Inhibition of growth factors receptor expression (EGF, transferrine)

Modulation of immune functions
- Increase of T cell cytotoxicity and NK cell activity
- Increase in antitumoral cytotoxicity by macrophages
- Modulation of Ig production
- Activation of macrophages
- Enhancement of HLA-A, B, C and DR antigen expression

Other effects
- Elevation of cGMP and cAMP concentrations
- Augmentation of collagenase IV synthesis (invasiveness)

- *Antiviral activity*

The IFNs are able to establish a typical « antiviral state » in cells by protecting them against any virus. The mechanism of the antiviral action will be described below. The antiviral activity is measured by checking the capacity to protect cell cultures using serial dilutions of IFN. One antiviral unit corresponds to the dilution which allows 50 % of cells to be protected against an infection with a challenge virus. Specific activities of IFN-α and -β are around 2×10^8 U/mg, whereas that of IFN-γ is lower (2 to 4×10^7 U/mg). It is noticeable that retroviruses are also sensitive to IFNs.

- *Modulation of gene expression*

About a hundred of genes are specifically induced by IFNs, and only a few of them are identified. Among these genes are enzymes such as 2'-5' oligoadenylate synthetase (2-5A S) and 68 kDa protein kinase (p68), antigens of the major histocompatibility complex (class I and class II), Fcγ receptors for IgG. IFNs can also inhibit the expression of some genes such as ornithine decarboxylase (a metabolic pathway likely involved in the control of cell division).

- *Modulation of oncogene expression*

Oncogene expression plays an important role in cell cycle regulation and tumor development. Numerous works showed the inhibition of some oncogenes by IFNs. Among these oncogenes are *c-myc*, *c-abl*, *c-Ha-ras* and *c-fos*, which is known to be a transcription factor.

- *Antagonism with growth factor*

The IFNs can inhibit the activity of certain growth factors such as platelet-derived growth factor (PDGF), epidermal growth factor (EGF) or B cell growth factor of low molecular weight ($BCGF_{low}$). They can also inhibit the expression of cell surface receptors for EGF, insuline and transferrine, for instance.

- *Antiproliferative effects*

Inhibition of cell growth by IFNs was extensively described in various types of normal and tumoral cell lines. This effect is dose-dependent, with a variability according to the type of cell and even to each cell line for a given cell type. Moreover, the inhibitory effect is sometimes specific for the type of IFN. For example, 1 U/ml of IFN-α induces 50 % of growth inhibition in the Daudi cell line (Burkitt's lymphoma), while 10^4 U/ml of IFN-γ have no effect on cell density. Inhibition of cell growth by IFNs results from a cytostatic effect associated with lengthening of all phases of the cell cycle by unknown mechanisms.

- *Antitumoral effects*

In vivo antitumoral activity of IFNs was shown using murine tumors and human tumors transplanted in *nude* mice. Other antitumoral effects were described, such as reversion of the malignant phenotype in cell culture or loss of tumorigenicity in animals.

- *Differentiating effects*

Certain human and murine tumoral cell lines which are blocked at an immature stage of differentiation, can undergo maturation when treated with chemical agents (dimethyl sulfoxide, hexamethylen bis-acetamide, phorbol ester) or physiological compounds (vitamin D3, retinoic acid). These cell lines are considered as models of myeloid differentiation (monocyte, granulocyte, megacaryocyte and red cells). Their study enabled to show that IFNs are capable of enhancing the effects of the differentiating agents, and even in some instances to induce themselves maturation events. These effects depend on the type of IFN and can be different according to the concentration used (induction by low concentrations and inhibition by high concentrations of IFN).

- *Modulation of immune functions*

All three types of IFN are regulators of immune responses by their effects on immunocompetent cells (monocytes, B and T lymphocytes, particularly). IFNs stimulate the cytotoxic activity of T lymphocytes and natural killer (NK) cells and the tumoricidal activity of macrophages (phagocytosis mediated by enhanced expression of Fcγ receptors).

Regarding T cells, IFN-α can either enhance or suppress some functions ; IFN-α increases the production of IL-2 which is the main factor in generating cytotoxic T cell clones ; finally, IFN-α stimulates lymphokine activated killer (LAK) cells. Regarding monocytes, it is now clear that IFN-γ is a strong macrophage activator, as shown by *in vitro* and *in vivo* stimulation of peroxide generation, killing of microorganisms as well as antitumoral cytotoxicity [6].

IFNs increase the expression of HLA class I and class II antigens. The effect on class II antigens seems specific for IFN-γ, which is also able to induce these antigens on tumor cells, when they are not expressed spontaneously.

The effects of IFNs on B cell functions are very complex. They are active on all three phases of B cell maturation : activation, proliferation and production of Ig. The latter can be either enhanced or inhibited by IFN-α, depending on its concentration (low or high, respectively), the duration and order of treatment (before or after the mitogen). Effects on Ig production also depend on the activating agent (*Staphylococcus aureus*, anti-Ig antibody, specific antibodies), mitogenic agent (IL-2, PMA, BCGF) and the type of IFN. IFN-γ is a stronger regulator of Ig production than IFN-α or -β, on the basis of antiviral units.

Clinical studies

The pleiotropic properties of IFNs found during the sixties and seventies suggested their potential use in the treatment of not only viral diseases but also malignancies. Due to species specificity, there was no pre-clinical studies in animals. The first trials with natural IFN-α, partially purified from human cells, were carried out at the end of the seventies [7]. They were performed on malignant tumors refractory to classical chemotherapy, such as : renal cancer, malignant melanoma, osteosarcoma, breast cancer, chronic lymphocytic leukemia (CLL) or multiple myeloma. The initial euphoric period was followed by a period of septicism, because the first results were not confirmed. This was partly due to the heterogeneity of the partially purified preparations, which contained sometimes less than 5 % of the active compound and therefore a number of contaminating proteins depending on each preparation. Moreover, IFNs were used empirically regarding the choice of the IFN type, dosage and schedule of administration. Protocols were based on those of chemotherapy, *i.e.* the use of maximal tolerable doses. It is now evident that protocols have to be established on the basis of minimal biologically active doses.

The irruption during the eighties of pure molecules of IFN derived from recombinant bacteria enabled to demonstrate that IFNs are actually antitumoral agents. The first clinical results were not always confirmed, but new indications were found. A similar efficacy was reported for the various subtypes of recombinant IFN-α and for natural IFN-α which are a mixture of several subtypes. Trials with recombinant IFN-β and IFN-γ were initated later because of difficulties during molecular cloning and for the obtention of stable molecules. It is now clear that IFN-α has numerous indications in oncology and virology, as well as in some benign and malignant tumors of viral origin, with regard to fiels as different as hematology, dermatology and hepatology. This chapter summarizes the main informations provided by the clinical trials. For more details, excellent reviews are available [8, 9].

Phase I trials

- *Toxicology*

The flu-like syndrome is the most important effect observed following IFN administration: fever, chills, myalgias, headache, malaise. A marked leukopenia also occurs. These side effects are dose-dependent, peak by 12 to 24 h after injection and revert thereafter. They are qualitatively similar for all three IFNs. Low dosage (3-5 MU) and medium dosages (10-15 MU) are generally well tolerated. High doses of IFN-β are better tolerated than with IFN-α. Other side effects result from chronic treatment (Table III).

Table III. Side-effects of interferons.

Initial injections
- Fever
- Chills
- Headache
- Myalgias
- Malaise
- Leukopenia

Chronic administration
- Mental fatigue
- Anorexia
- Mild neutropenia
- Transaminase elevation
- Diarrhea

Less common effects
- Mental confusion
- Nausea
- Vomiting
- Alopecia
- Thrombocytopenia

- *Pharmacology*

Pharmacokinetics of IFN-α are different from those of IFN-β and IFN-γ. Intravenous injection of 10 MU of IFN-α is followed within 30 min by a peak of serum IFN levels of about 1,000 U/ml while the serum IFN levels are around 100 U/ml after IFN-β or IFN-γ injection. Parallely, intramuscular or subcutaneous injection of 10 MU results in serum levels of 100 U/ml with IFN-α, but no IFN level is detected with IFN-β or IFN-γ. However, in the latter cases, 2-5A S activity (as a marker of IFN action) is induced to a similar extent than after intravenous injection of IFN-β or IFN-γ. It is now known that maximal tolerable doses based on serum IFN levels are not required to obtain optimal biological effects.

Phase II trials

Several thousands of patients were enrolled into the numerous trials performed in the world with IFN-α. The best results were obtained in hematology (Table IV). A number of leukemias and lymphomas as well as other hematologic disorders appeared to show high response rates. This antitumoral activity of IFN-α is not specific for the cell type since it is exerted in myeloproliferative as well as lymphoproliferative disorders. It has yet to be noted that several B cell but only one T cell malignancies are sensitive to IFN-α therapy [10].

Table IV. Therapeutic activity of interferon-α.

B cell malignancies	
• Hairy cell leukemia	3
• Low-grade lymphomas	2
• Multiple myeloma	1
• Chronic lymphocytic leukemia (early stages)	3*
• Essential mixed cryoglobulinemia	3
T cell malignancies	
• Cutaneous T lymphomas	3
Myeloid malignancies	
• Chronic myelogenous leukemia	3
• Essential thrombocythemia	3
• *Polycythemia vera*	3
Solid tumors	
• Kaposi's sarcoma in AIDS	2
• Basal cell carcinoma	3
• Squamous cell carcinoma (skin, cervix)	2/3*
• Carcinoids	2*
• Malignant melanoma	1
• Renal cell carcinoma	±
• Condyloma acuminatum	3
• Laryngeal papillomatosis	3
• Ovarian carcinoma (intraperitoneal)	2
• Glioma (intrathecal)	2
• Superficial bladder carcinoma (intravesicular)	2

Response rate < 33 % = 1 ; between 33 % and 66 % = 2 ; > 66 % = 3.
* Studies enrolling more patients are required.

• *Lymphoid malignancies*

— **Hairy cell leukemia :** The most impressive results were recorded in this chronic leukemia of low malignancy, which affects the pre-plasmocyte stage of B cell differentiation. This leukemia, which was refractory to any chemotherapy, had a median survival of 4 to 5 years. IFN-α administered at low dosage (3 MU daily of three times weekly) induces 80 % to 90 % of complete and partial responses. The presence of less than 5 % of residual tumoral cells was chosen as a criteria of complete response, due to the difficulty to identify hairy cells. This caused a controversy regarding the complete response rate ranging from 0 to 40 % (mean around 10 %). Nevertheless, the quality of life is similar for all the responders, including minor responders (about 10 %), evaluated in terms of correction of cytopenias, hemoglobin levels and disappearance of severe infections. An interesting observation is that relapses occur only after discontinuation of the therapy. Relapse frequencies are about 1/3 of complete responders and 2/3 of partial responders. Patients who relapsed respond again when treatment was reinitiated, with the same quality of response [11].

— **Non-Hodgkin's lymphomas** : Response rate is around 45 % (11 % of complete responses) in low grade, but 15 % or less in high grade B cell lymphomas. The median duration of response to IFN-α given at low or medium doses is approximately 8 months.

— **Multiple myeloma** : In this disease characterized by the proliferation in the marrow of a malignant plasma cell clone, the first results were not confirmed by using recombinant IFN. Response rates are now less than 20 % for advanced diseases and 30 % for early stage diseases. However, interesting results with this tumor, which remains incurable, were observed in maintenance treatment of patients in remission or stabilized by chemotherapy : IFN-α administered at low dosage (3 to 5 MU three times weekly) induces a marked augmentation in the median durations of response and survival, compared to patients remained untreated [12].

— **Chronic lymphocytic leukemia (CLL)** : Trials with natural IFN-α were not confirmed with recombinant IFN-α. Response rates to low or high doses in advanced B-CLL are very low. Two publications indicate that early stage B-CLL (stages A and B) show a 50 % response rate to 1.5 to 5 MU of IFN-α [13], which has to be confirmed in more complete studies.

— **Cryoglobulinemia** : Mixed essential cryoglobulinemia of type II is characterized by the hyperproduction of IgM, resulting in the formation of immune complexes with polyclonal IgG. One recent publication seems to show that this B cell tumor is sensitive to IFN-α therapy : 77 % of responses with 50 % of complete responses [14].

— **Cutaneous T cell lymphomas** : IFN-α appeared efficient in the treatment of these malignant proliferations of helper T lymphocytes, presenting skin infiltration and an indolent clinical development (mycosis fungoides and Sezary's syndromes). From 45 % to 75 % of responses including high rates of complete remission were found after treatment with IFN-α given at high doses ($>$ 25 MU). A 92 % response rate was recorded with early stage patients. It seems now that lower dosage (6-9 MU) is capable of similar results (40 % of complete responses). The association with retinoic acid seems promising [15].

— **Other lymphoid malignancies** : In a trial performed with a small number of patients with acute lymphocytic leukemia, it was found 30 % of partial responses of short duration, using very high doses of IFN-α. Low dosage was not tested and no other trial has been reported. Hodgkin's lymphoma does not seem to be sensitive to IFN-α therapy, but very few trials were carried out.

- *Myeloid malignancies*

The observation that IFN-α treatment induces myelosuppression has led to the development of successful trials in chronic myeloid leukemia and more recently in other myeloproliferative disorders such as essential thrombocythemia and polycythemia vera [16].

— **Chronic myelogenous leukemia (CML)** : This leukemia, characterized by the accumulation of mature and immature granulocytes, shows high rate of complete hematologic responses (60-80 %) to treatment with doses of 5 MU. These results are similar to those obtained after busulfan or hydroxyurea treatment. However, IFN-α therapy induces a strong proportion of complete cytogenetic remissions (disparition of the chromosome Ph1 resulting from the translocation t[9,22] in 15 to 35 % of cases), whereas chemotherapies do not produce this result. The bcr-abl gene rearrangement associated with the translocation is sometimes no more detectable using PCR, but is often persisting, even in case of cytogenetic remission. The available data cannot answer the question whether IFN-α therapy can prolong the chronic phase of the disease or prevent the blastic crisis. It seems that the best results are achieved when treatment starts soon after diagnosis and prior to any other therapy. It is recommended to treat the responding patients without discontinuation. Associations with hydroxyurea, busulfan, IFN-γ or cytosine arabinoside are under study.

— **Essential thrombocythemia and polycythemia vera** : Recent studies demonstrated the strong efficacy of IFN-α in myeloproliferative disorders other than CML : diseases characterized by high levels of circulating platelets such as essential thrombocythemia, CML-associated thrombocytosis, as well as polycythemia vera, which show complete response rates of about 75 %. Although the number of patients enrolled into the trials is still low, long-term results indicate that relapses occur after dicontinuation of treatment and that remission occurs again when patients are retreated, as in hairy cell leukemia.

- *Solid tumors*

The efficacy of IFN-α in the treatment of solid malignancies is less impressive than in hematologic disorders. Despite interesting results in cancer which are insensitive to established therapies, it is clear that IFN-α does not show any efficacy in current cancers of the adult, such as lung, breast, colon, prostate or the hepatocellular carcinoma. The best results are observed in dermatology. Furthermore, the development of intralesional therapy allowed to find out better effects that IFN-α given by systemic route [17-19].

— **Malignant melanoma and renal cancer** : These two metastatic malignancies are refractory to any therapy. The initial results obtained with natural IFN-α were not confirmed with recombinant IFN-α. Response rates are 16 % to 18 % for melanoma, that is nevertheless similar to interleukin 2 (IL-2) treatment. Results are lower in renal carcinoma (12 %), but long duration remissions are recorded. A large number of trials combining IFN-α and chemotherapy or IL-2 are in progress.

— **Carcinoid tumors** : Recent results which have to be confirmed by long term studies with a large number of patients seem to show a new indication for IFN-α in the malignant carcinoid syndromes such as mid-gut carcinoids and other neuroendocrine tumors (endocrine pancreatic tumors). These uncommon indolent malignancies are serious because of clinical symptoms, such as hormone hypersecretion and liver metastases. About 50 % of objective responses to IFN-α therapy were reported [20].

— **Kaposi's sarcoma** : This tumor, which is associated with AIDS (30 % of cases), shows a 30-40 % response rate, with about 20 % of complete regression of the cutaneous lesions. High dosage (at least 20 MU) appears to be required, while low doses are without effect. More responders are found in patients not presenting with opportunistic infections. Patients with low CD4 counts do not respond. Some studies suggest that IFN-α therapy prolongs the lifespan of HIV-infected patients. The antitumoral effect is associated with inhibition of HIV replication. The combination therapy with AZT seems interesting.

— **Other virus-associated tumors** : IFN-α shows a regular efficacy in the treatment of several benign tumors known for their viral etiology, such as tumors involving papilloma virus (HPV). Laryngeal papillomatosis and condyloma acuminatum (anogenital warts) show high response rates (50-90 %). For condyloma, IFN-α used at very low doses (1 MU given in s.c. or i.m. injections, or 0.1 MU administered intralesionaly) are efficient. Results, yet less impressive, were also reported in cervix cancer (squamous cell carcinoma) which is also related to HPV-16 and -18 infections. The association with retinoic acid seems to induce about 50 % of responses. Finally, some results were obtained in naso-pharyngeal carcinoma related to Epstein-Barr virus (EBV).

— **Cutaneous cancers** : In addition to cutaneous T cell lymphomas and Kaposi's sarcoma, other antitumoral activities were recently found in two frequent cancers of the skin : basal-cell carcinoma and squamous cell carcinoma. In both diseases, the activity of IFN-α is spectacular : more than 90 % of responses to IFN-α given in low dosage (generally 1.5 MU).

- *Intralesional therapy*

An important potential for IFN therapy has been revealed by trials using intratumoral injection of IFN-α, allowing local IFN concentrations higher than those obtained with systemic administration, and a virtual absence of systemic symptoms. Results are encouraging with intraperitoneal use in metastatic ovarian carcinoma, intravesicular injection in superficial bladder cancer and intrathecal administration in glioblastoma (about 50 % of objective responses).

- *Chronic hepatitis*

A number of viral infections (herpes, rhinovirus, influenza, zona, etc.) were tested for a long time for their sensitivity of IFN-α treatment. Although the results have confirmed the potential use of IFN in viral diseases, no indication justifies its therapeutic use, except in the case of active chronic hepatitis. Indeed, hepatitis B and C, which are involved in the development of hepatocellular carcinoma and liver cirrhosis, as well as chronic hepatitis δ show a 40 % response rate. This effect is associated with inhibition of HBV virus replication and disappearance of HBV antigens. However, permanent responses were observed in only 10 % of cases. Doses of 3 MU are efficient. It seems that the effects of IFN-α depend on the immune status of patients, and that re-treatment of relapsing patients induces again responses [20, 21].

- **Approved indications for IFN-α**

IFN-α has been approved for 13 indications in 49 countries. Among the most approved indications are hairy cell leukemia, chronic hepatitis, Kaposi's sarcoma and condyloma acuminatum.

IFN-β and IFN-γ

Clinical trials with IFN-β and -γ were started later than studies with IFN-α, due to above mentioned reasons. It appeared that IFN-β has similar effects that IFN-α (only one approved indication in intraepithelial cancer of the cervix). Note that IFN-β showed a regular efficacy in viral infections, and a potential efficacy in EBV-related nasopharyngeal carcinoma and in glioblastoma.

The case of IFN-γ is different since very few results are obtained in oncology (ovarian cancer, mesothelioma, for instance). Results are often lower than with IFN-α (*e.g.* CML) and no greater efficacy was observed in combining IFN-α and IFN-γ, compared to IFN-α alone (one FDA-approved indication for IFN-γ in chronic granulomatous disease).

However, IFN-γ appears of great interest in parasitology. Very impressive results were obtained in visceral and muco-cutaneous leishmaniasis [22], likely due to the fact that IFN-γ is a strong macrophage activator. Promising results seem to occur in infectious diseases due to other intracellular parasites or to mycobacteria (leprosis).

Antibody formation

Long-term treatment with recombinant IFN-α induces the formation of antibodies. The IFN-α2a subtype appeared more immunogenic than IFN-α2b subtype. Only a fraction of these antibodies have neutralizing properties, and clinical response is abolished in only a few proportion of patients presenting neutralizing antibodies. Finally, it is now well demonstrated that those patients who lost responsiveness to recombinant IFN-α respond again when treated with natural IFN-α (which does not induce antibody formation).

Comments

A number of conclusions can be drawn from more than 10 years of therapy with recombinant IFN-α :
(a) IFN-α shows antitumoral activity in diseases affecting a various range of cell types.
(b) This activity is particularly strong in indolent tumors, of low malignancies, in which no efficient treatment was known (*e.g.* hairy cell leukemia, cutaneous T lymphomas, thrombocythemia, carcinoids). It is striking that low grade but not high grade B cell lymphomas are sensitive to IFN-α.
(c) IFN-α appears more active when the tumor load is low, either if it is a characteristic of the disease (basal cell carcinoma, condyloma), or in case of residual disease (melanoma or renal cancer after surgery, myeloma after chemotherapy). IFN-α, therefore, can be an adjuvant agent.

(d) Early stage disease and early intervention are factors favorable to IFN-α responsiveness (*e.g.* myeloma, cutaneous T lymphoma, B-CLL, CML)
(e) IFN-α is more efficient when immune status is maximal (Kaposi's sarcoma).
(f) Long-term therapy with low dosage (3 MU three times weekly for 12 months) is recommended for a number of indications, except for Kaposi's sarcoma and certain solid tumors requiring high concentrations achieved by intralesional administration.
(g) Data harvested until now do not allow to conclude whether IFN-α therapy may induce cures.

Mechanisms of action

The first step in IFN action is the interaction with specific cell surface receptors. This step is followed by down-regulation of IFN-α receptor expression, which was shown not only in cultured cell lines, but also *in vivo*, during treatment of patients. Although lack of receptor down-regulation was correlated with absence of patient's response to IFN-α, its role in signal transduction is not known. The investigations on second messengers have suggested several possible signalling pathways (rapid changes in lipid metabolism, activation of protein kinase C isoforms specific for IFN α and β, etc.) but their role in the control of gene activation is not ascertained. Recent works clearly show that signal transmission from membrane receptor to the genes is very direct, at least in some cell types. After IFN-α binding to its receptor, the tyk-2 tyrosine kinase is activated, leading to the phosphorylation of three proteins residing in the cytoplasm, which form the complex ISGF3α (IFN-stimulated gene factor). This complex is then translocated to the nucleus where it interacts with the transcription factor ISGF3γ. The latter can bind a sequence of DNA called ISRE (IFN-stimulated responsive element) whithin the promoter, that triggers the transcriptional activation of inducible genes [23, 24]. In spite of this crucial advance in the knowledge of signalling pathways leading to induction of genes by IFN-α, very few data are available for the understanding of cellular mechanisms which are specifically involved in the various biological effects of IFN, with the exception of the antiviral effect.

Antiviral mechanisms

Antiviral resistance is not due to a direct inhibition of virus replication, but to indirect effects resulting from the induction of two enzyme genes: first, the 2-5A synthetase, which catalyzes the polymerization of (2'-5') oligoadenylates, capable of activating the RNAse L which, in turn, degrades the viral RNA. The other IFN-induced enzyme is the p68 kinase, which phosphorylates the initiation factor of translation (eIF-2). The formation of the initiation complex is thereby prevented, resulting in inhibition of viral protein translation [25].

Antitumoral actions

The therapeutic effects of IFNs can be mediated through two different types of mechanisms. First, a direct action on tumor cells by antiproliferative, differentiating or antiviral mechanisms. Second, an indirect action on host cells by immune defense stimulation or by changes in interactions between non-immune host cells and tumor cells.

Each of these mechanisms might theoretically induces tumor regression, perhaps with a specificity for the tumor type. Tumor regression might also results from several simultaneous mechanisms.

- *Direct effects*

Recent advances have been done on the knowledge of the molecular mechanisms controlling the cell cycle and some of the involved factors (transcription factors, oncogenes, kinases). Data suggest that antiproliferative effects of IFN may be explained by interferences with some of these factors, implying a role of the anti-oncogene effects of IFNs. The antagonism with growth factors and their receptors are also thought to play an important role. Some authors have suggested the 2-5A system as a possible mediator of the antiproliferative action *via* activation of RNAse L, which would degrade mRNA for certain transcription or growth factors.

No strong evidence has been provided so far to extrapolate the differentiating effects of IFN observed in cultured cells to the *in vivo* setting. It has yet to be noted that cell division and differentiation are closely related, suggesting that an antiproliferative event is likely differentiating and reversely, at least in cells of hematopoietic origin.

Although the antiviral activity alone may explain the effects of IFN in some virus-related tumors (condyloma, papillomatosis), this does not seem to be the case of Kaposi's sarcoma. Indeed, regression of cutaneous lesions requires minimal levels of $CD4^+$ cells, suggesting the occurrence of immune mechanisms. Interestingly, this seems also to be the case for chronic hepatitis, since inhibition of virus replication is not sufficient for induction of permanent remissions [21].

- *Indirect effects*

The fact that a number of immune functions are modulated by IFN suggests a potential role of immune defense stimulation in the antitumor action of IFN. The activation of cytotoxic functions of various leukocyte populations together with the enhanced expression of MHC antigens on tumor cells should be of particular importance. Regarding the activation of NK cells, too divergent results do not favor a close relationship with therapeutic action.

Other indirect effects involving non-immune cells play probably a major role, at least in some tumors. For instance, IFN can antagonize a tumoral growth factor produced by stromal cells, or inhibit angiogenesis as shown for TNF.

Specific mechanisms

Convergent data favor the major role of direct effects of IFN-α in hematologic malignancies which are amoung the most sensitive to IFN-α therapy. Studies on hairy cells isolated during the treatment of HCL patients showed down-regulation of IFN-α receptors, induction of 2-5A S and inhibition of *c-fos* oncogene expression, that was not observed in unresponsive patients ; furthermore, these *in vivo* studies also showed that IFN-α treatment of the patients results in antagonism on the activity of B cell growth factor (of low molecular weight), which induces the proliferation of hairy cells and is thought to be a tumoral growth factor in this leukemia [26, 27]. Therefore, IFN-α acts, at least partly, by an antiproliferative effect mediated through its antagonistic properties on a growth factor. Differentiating effects have also been suggested by *in vitro* studies. However, indirect mechanisms are unlikely : the role of the induction of cytotoxic T cell clones was never shown and the role of NK cell activation can be excluded.

Antigrowth factor properties of IFN-α may also play a major role in other B cell neoplasias, such as non-Hodgkin's lymphoma (autocrine B cell growth factors) and multiple myeloma in which IL-6 is the main tumoral growth factor. In multiple myeloma, it is not known at present whether IFN-α acts directly on the malignant plasma cell clone or indirectly on bone marrow stromal cells. The autocrine or paracrine production of IL-6 is indeed a question subject to controversy.

It is possible that the effects of IFN-α in B lymphoproliferations may be specific for the stage of differentiation characterizing the malignant cells, and that responses to some growth factors are also specific for some discrete stage of differentiation.

Experimental data on CML also favor direct effects of IFN-α on stem cells at the origin of the malignant clone (chromosome Ph1 positive), by inhibiting their self renewal capacities. The mechanism of IFN-α action in thrombocytosis is unknown ; a decrease in the number of circulating megakaryocytes during therapy has been reported, suggesting interactions of IFN-α with cytokines controlling megakaryocyte maturation.

It is interesting to note that IFN-α is an inhibitor of platelet production in thrombocytosis, whereas, by contrast, it induces a correction of thrombocytopenia in hairy cell leukemia, for example.

Another interesting feature comes from the observation that IFN-α is active in the treatment of two malignancies which are so different in that one is characterized by an excess of $CD4^+$ T lymphocytes (cutaneous T lymphoma), whereas the other one is related to a lack of $CD4^+$ T lymphocytes (Kaposi's sarcoma). These data suggest that one of the pathways mediating the antitumoral activity of IFN-α involves interactions of IFN-α with cytokines regulating cells of the immune system.

Antiproliferative effects of IFNs seem also to be involved in some solid tumors, as suggested by the successful use of IFN in local injections which allow very high concentrations of IFN at the tumor site. However, stimulation of immune defense probably plays an important role in diseases of viral origin (Kaposi's sarcoma, chronic hepatitis) and in metastatic renal cancer or melanoma after surgery.

In conclusion, the antitumoral activity of IFNs is thought to be mainly exerted by their growth-regulatory properties [28], except in case of adjuvant therapy.

Perspectives and new directions

The study of the role of IFN as a therapeutic agent is only at the beginning. At present, it is clear that IFNs are able to improve the quality of life of patients and to prolong their lifespan. The next step will be to determine whether IFNs have also curative capacities. Experiments should be performed in the three following directions.

Optimization of therapeutic protocols

Phase III trials are required for evaluating optimal dosage specific for each tumor, as well as treatment duration. Biological tests for prediction of patient's responsiveness to IFN therapy should be established, as suggested for IFN-α receptor down-regulation and 2-5A synthetase induction [29, 30].

Increased knowledge of modes of action

Some observations suggest that IFN may act partly through restoration of physiologic regulatory mechanisms within the cytokine network. The study of interactions of IFNs with other cytokines appears therefore crucial for the full understanding of specific mechanisms of action [31, 32]. Such studies should not only improve the clinical use of IFN but also facilitate the development of combinations with other cytokines.

Combination with other therapies

Based on a wide body of experimental evidences, trials combining IFNs and other antitumoral treatments are currently developed and should be amplified. Of particular interest are trials associating IFNs with chemotherapy (5-FU in solid cancers, DTIC in melanoma, 2 CdA or pentostatin in HCL, busulfan, hydroxyurea or cytosine-arabinosin in CML). Associations with other cytokines (IFN-γ, TNF or IL-2) or with other biological therapies (LAK cells, tumor-infiltrating lymphocytes, tumor-specific monoclonal antibodies) seem of great potentiality.

In addition to post-surgery adjuvant therapy (renal cancer, melanoma), maintenance treatment after chemotherapy appears very promising. Based on the excellent results obtained in multiple myeloma, trials are developing in non-Hodgkin's lymphoma.

Acknowledgements

I thank the Ligue Nationale Française Contre le Cancer (Comité de Paris) for its financial support. I gratefully acknowledge Mrs Agnès Birot for her excellent secretarial assistance.

References

1. Gresser I. Antitumor effects of interferons. *Adv Cancer Res* 1972 ; 16 : 97-140.
2. De Maeyer E, De Maeyer-Guignard J. *Interferons and other regulatory cytokines.* New York : Wiley J. and Sons, eds, Wiley Interscience, 1988.
3. Aguet M, Dembic Z, Merlin G. Molecular cloning and expression of the human interferon-γ receptor. *Cell* 1988 ; 55 : 273-80.
4. Uzé G, Lutfalla G, Gresser I. Genetic transfer of a functional human interferon-α receptor into mouse cells : cloning and expression of its cDNA. *Cell* 1990 ; 60 : 225-34.
5. Kishimoto T. The biology of interleukin 6. *Blood* 1989 ; 74 : 1-10.
6. Nathan CF, Murray HW, Wiebe ME, *et al.* Identification of interferon gamma as the lymphokine which activates human macrophages oxidative metabolism and antimicrobial activity. *J Exp Med* 1983 ; 158 : 670-89.

7. Strander H, Cantell K, Inginarison S, *et al.* Interferon treatment of osteogenic sarcoma : a clinical trial. In : Conference on modulation of host immune resistance in the prevention and treatment of induced neoplasms'. Washington DC : United States Government Printing Office, 1980 ; 28 : 377-81.
8. Hersey P. The evolving role of alpha interferon in the treatment of malignancies. *Aust NZ J Med* 1986 ; 16 : 425-37.
9. Borden EC. Effects of interferons in neoplastic diseases in man. *Pharmacol Ther* 1988 ; 37 : 213-29.
10. Roth MS, Foon KA (1986) Alpha interferon in the treatment of hematologic malignancies. *Am J Med* 1986 ; 81 : 871-82.
11. Platanias LC, Ratain MJ. Hairy cell leukemia : the role of alpha interferon. *Eur J Cancer* 1991 : 27 ; S53-S57.
12. Mandelli F, Avvisati G, Amadori S, Boccadoro M, Gernone A, Lauta VM, Marmont F, Petrucci MT, Tribalto M, Vegna ML, Dammacco F, Pileri A. Maintenance treatment with recombinant interferon alpha-2b in patients with multiple myeloma responding to conventional induction chemotherapy. *N Engl J Med* 1990 ; 322 : 1430-4.
13. Pangalis GA, Griva E. Recombinant alpha-2β-interferon therapy in untreated, stages A and B chronic lymphocytic leukemia. A preliminary report. *Cancer* 1988 ; 61 : 869-72.
14. Casato M, Lagana B, Antonelli G, Dianziani F, Bonomo L. Long-term results of therapy with interferon-α for type II essential mixed cryogobulinemia. *Blood* 1991 ; 78 : 3142-7.
15. Dréno B, Claudy A, Meynardier J, Verret JL, Souteyrand P, Ortonne JP, Kalis B, Godefroy WY, Beerblock J, Thill L. The treatment of 45 patients with cutaneous T-cell lymphoma with low doses of interferon-α2a and etretinate. *Br J Dermatol* 1991 ; 125 : 456-9.
16. Schiffer CA. Interferon studies in the treatment of patients with leukemia. *Semin Oncol* 1991 ; B : 1-6.
17. Spiegel RJ. Clinical overview of alpha interferon. Studies and future directions. *Cancer* 1987 ; 59 : 626-31.
18. Figlin RA. Biotherapy with interferon. *Semin Oncol* 1988 ; 15 : 3-9.
19. Bonnem EM. Alpha interferon : the potential drug of adjuvant therapy : past achievement and future challenges. *Eur J Cancer* 1991 ; 27 : S1-S6.
20. Spiegel RJ. Additional indications for interferon therapy : basal cell carcinoma, carcinoid, and chronic active hepatitis. *Semin Oncol* 1988 ; 15 : 41-5.
21. Daniels HM, Meager A, Eddleston ALW, Alexander GJM, Williams R. Spontaneous production of tumour necrosis factor-α and interleukin-1β during interferon-α treatment of chronic HBV infection. *Lancet* 1990 ; 335 : 875-6.
22. Badaro R, Falcoff E, Badaro FS, Carvalho EM, Pedral-Sampaio D, Barral A, Carvalho JS, Barral-Netto M, Silva L, Bina JC, Teixeira R, Falcoff R, Brandely M, Rocha H, Ho JL, Johnson WJ. Use of recombinant interferon-gamma combined with pentavalent antimony (Sb^v) in the therapy of visceral leishmaniasis. *N Engl J Med* 1990 ; 322 : 16-21.
23. Marx J. Taking a direct path to the genes. *Science* 1992 ; 257 : 744-5.
24. Velasquez L, Fellous M, Stark GR, Pellegrini S. A protein tyrosine kinase in the interferon α/β signaling pathway. *Cell* 1992 ; 70, 313-22.
25. Hovanessian AG. Interferon-induced and double-stranded RNA-activated enzymes : a specific protein kinase and 2',5' oligoadenylate synthetases. *J Interferon Res* 1991 ; 11 : 199-205.
26. Billard C, Sigaux F, Castaigne S, Valensi F, Flandrin G, Degos L, Falcoff E, Aguet M. Treatment of hairy cell leukemia with recombinant alpha interferon. II. *In vivo* down-regulation of alpha interferon receptors on tumor cells. *Blood* 1986 ; 67 : 821-6.
27. Génot E, Billard C, Sigaux F, Mathiot C, Degos L, Falcoff E, Kolb JP. Proliferative response of hairy cells to B cell growth factor (BCGF) : *In vivo* inhibition by interferon-α and *in vitro* effects of interferon-α, -β and -γ. *Leukemia* 1987 ; 1 : 590-6.
28. Balkwill FR, Smyth JF. Interferon in cancer therapy : a reappraisal. *Lancet* 1987 ; ii : 317-9.
29. Billard C, Ferbus D. Predicting responses to interferon. *Lancet* 1990 ; 336 : 1388-9.

30. Billard C, Ferbus D, Diez RA, Kolb JP, Mathiot C, Belanger C, Auzanneau G, Varet B, Falcoff E, Dumont J. Correlation between the biological and therapeutic effects of interferon-alpha in low-grade nodular non-Hodgkin's lymphoma : lack of *in vivo* downregulation and reduduced affinity of IFN-α receptors in unresponsive patients. *Leukemia Res* 1991 ; 15 : 121-8.
31. Billard C, Wietzerbin J. On the mechanism of action of interferon-alpha on hairy cell leukemia. *Eur J Cancer* 1990 ; 26 : 67-9.
32. Billard C, Sigaux F, Wietzerbin J. IFN-α *in vivo* enhances tumor necrosis factor receptor levels on hairy cells. *J Immunol* 1990 ; 145 : 1713-8.

15

Tumor necrosis factor and its inhibitors

Warren S. LIAO, Bharat B. AGGARWAL

Department of Biochemistry and Molecular Biology and Department of Clinical Immunology and Biological Therapy, University of Texas, MD Anderson Cancer Center, Houston, Texas 77030, USA.

The biology of tumor necrosis factor (TNF) is closely linked with that of endotoxin or lipopolysaccharides (LPS). This link has been known since the report more than a century ago that infection of patients with gram-negative bacteria could lead to tumor regression [1]. It was demonstrated in 1961 that the serum of animals injected with endotoxin can cause the necrosis of tumors [2]. The confirmation of these observations in 1975 led to naming this activity of the serum tumor necrosis factor [3]. In spite of major advances in recent years in the understanding of TNF and LPS made since then, the precise mechanism of tumor regression by these agents remains an enigma.

The hyperplasia of macrophages in endotoxin-injected animals led to the suggestion that macrophages play a role in the production of TNF [3]. Now it is also known that besides macrophages TNF is produced by a wide variety of cell types including T and B lymphocytes, natural killer cells, neutrophils, mast cells, granulosa cells, keratinocytes, vascular smooth muscle cells, epidermal cells, Kupffer cells, astrocytes, and synovial fibroblasts [4]. Besides normal cells, certain tumors such as breast tumors, ovarian tumors, and fibrosarcoma have also been shown to express TNF [5]. In fact, a role for TNF in the induction of self-resistance has been proposed [6].

High levels of TNF mRNA expression have been found in several diseases. For instance, this cytokine has been detected in the kidneys of MRL-1pr mice with lupus nephritis, in the serum of patients with Reye's syndrome, in the serum of cancer patients, and in patients with parasitic or bacterial infections. Autologous bone marrow transplantation patients and AIDS patients also have elevated TNF levels. Interestingly, TNF was discovered independently as cachectin, *i.e.* a factor responsible for induction of cachexia during parasitic infection [7].

Even though it was initially shown that endotoxin can induce TNF, it is now obvious that a wide variety of agents can trigger the expression of this cytokine, including bacteria, viruses, and protozoa, certain parasites, cytokines, immune complexes, hormones, complements (Table I). The specific agents responsible for inhibiting the production can be suppressed by steroids, prostaglandins, lipooxygenase inhibitors, cyclosporin A, vitamin D3, TGF-β, PAF antagonists, IL-4, and IL-6 (Table II).

Table I. A list of agents responsible for induction of human tumor necrosis factor.

Micro-organisms and its products
    Gram Negative bacteria
    Listeria monocytogenes
    Mycobacterial proteins
    Lipopolysaccharides
    Toxic Shock Syndrome Toxin-1
    Sendai Virus
    Neurotropic paramyxovirus
    Mycoplasma orale
    Lipid A
    Gram Negative bacteria
    GLA-60

Cytokines
    Interferons
    Interleukin-1
    Interleukin-2
    Granulocyte-Macrophage Colony Stimulating Factor
    Neuropeptides
    Bradykinins

Others
    Lithium chloride, Phorbol esters
    Soluble malarial antigens
    Glucose modified proteins
    Complements (C5a)
    Tumor cells
    Chineese herbal drugs
    Platelet activating factor
    Anti CD-3 antibodies
    Retinoic acid

Table II. A partial list of agents which inhibit TNF production.

Cyclosporin A
Transforming growth factor beta
Inhibitors of cyclooxygenase and lipooxygenase pathway
Polyunsaturated fatty acids
Prostaglandins
Interleukin-4
Interleukin-6
Interleukin-10
Anti-inflammatory drugs

The methods for detection of TNF are either immunoassay or bioassay. TNF's cytotoxic effects against certain tumor cells treated with a protein synthesis inhibitors has become the classical *in vitro* bioassay for TNF. There is no international standard on unit for TNF, but usually 50 % inhibition of cell viability is considered one unit.

Physicochemical characteristics of TNF

Mature human TNFα, mainly produced by macrophages in response to endotoxin, is secreted as a 157-amino-acid protein [8]. It is initially synthesized with an unusually long propeptide segment of 76 amino acids [8], whose functional importance is not clear. While the mature TNFα is highly conserved between human and mouse (79 %), the propeptide segment is even more conserved (86 %) [9]. It has been shown that this propeptide segment is excised to yield the mature 17-kDa hormone [10, 11]. However, Kriegler *et al.* [12] described a cell membrane-bound form of TNFα (26 kDa) containing the propeptide segment, suggesting that this segment may serve as a membrane-anchoring domain for TNFα. The 17-kDa mature protein is derived from the 26-kDa membrane form by proteolytic cleavage [12, 13].

In addition to serving as a precursor to mature hormone, the transmembrane form of TNFα may also interact with membrane receptor on neighboring cells and thereby mediate intercellular communication [12]. Moreover, when expressed on the surface of monocytes and/or macrophages, the membrane-anchored TNFα may mediate other immunomodulatory actions of the mature hormone.

In contrast to the molecular mass of 17 kDa as determined by denaturing sodium dodecylsulfate polyacrylamide gel electrophoresis, human TNFα exhibits an apparent molecular size of 45 kDa under native conditions [8]. These observations suggest that under native conditions TNFα aggregates *in vitro* to yield a trimer. In fact, dimers, trimers, pentamers, and perhaps higher-order multimers have been reported. However, X-ray crystallographic studies indicate that human TNFα is a trimeric structure arranged in an extensive antiparallel β-sheet form [13, 14]. Under native conditions, TNFα from all species exist as oligomeric structures. Such oligomerization, which is dependent on protein concentration, can be dissociated into monomeric form by a lower pH or by chaotropic agents [15].

Human TNFα has an isoelectric point between 5 and 6 [8]. There is no methionine residue in the mature protein, but it contains two cysteine residues at positions 69 and 101. While the murine TNFα has one N-linked glycosylation site, the human TNFα has none. In contrast to TNFβ, TNFα is highly susceptible to proteases. Treatment with trypsin, chymotrypsin, and V8 protease [8] results in rapid loss of all biological activities.

TNF gene and its regulation

The TNF locus is located on the short arm of human chromosome 6 [16] and murine chromosome 17 [17] at the boundary of the class III and class I regions of the major histocompatibility genes [18]. It comprises two genes coding for TNFα and TNFβ that are closely linked [19]. In human, mouse, and rabbit, the TNFβ

gene is always 5' to the TNFα gene and the genes are transcribed in the same direction. Each gene is approximately 3 kilobase pairs long and consists of four exons and three introns (Figure 1) [20, 21]. More than 80 % of the coding sequence contributing to the mature TNFα is encoded in the fourth exon, while exons 1 and 2 contain almost entirely leader peptide sequence. The amino acid sequence for TNFα is highly conserved between species, with 77 % homology between humans and mice and greater than 70 % homology between humans and rabbits [22, 23]. This high degree of sequence conservation is consistent with the lack of species specificity in response to TNF. In human and mouse, TNFα is approximately 30 % homologous to TNFβ [10, 24, 25]. The greatest homology occurs in the carboxyl terminal amino acids encoded by exon 4, where they share over 50 % homology at the nucleotide level [26]. Similarities in their gene organization, close linkage, and common biological properties strongly suggest that the two genes are evolutionarily related and arose from a common ancestral gene by gene duplication.

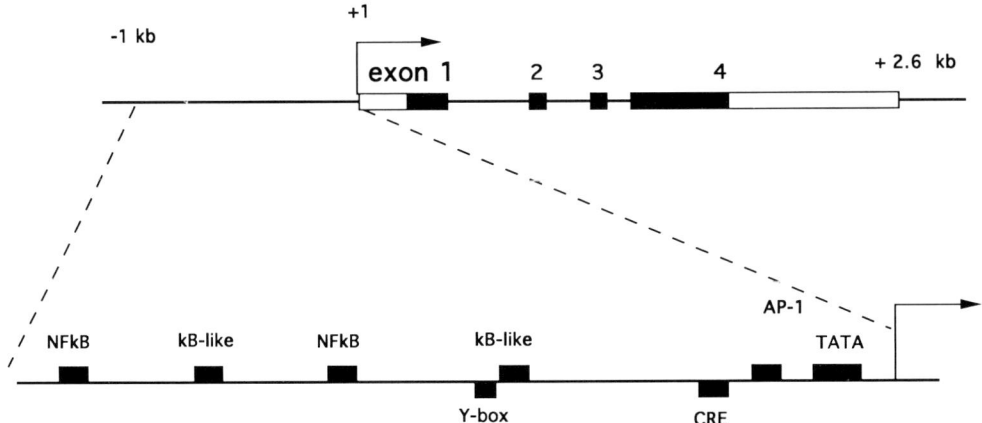

Figure 1. TNF-α gene structure and its regulatory elements. *Top line.* The four exons of the TNF-α gene are represented by the boxes with the coding portions of the exons shaded. The *inset* shows locations of regulatory elements identified in the 5'-flanking region important for the transcriptional regulation of TNF-α expression. The arrow indicates the transcription start site and the direction of transcription.

The high degree of sequence homology between TNFα and TNFβ coding regions does not extend to the 5'-flanking regions, which contain most of the *cis*-acting elements important for transcriptional regulation [26-28]. Sequence divergence of the regulatory regions has resulted in the differential regulation of TNFα and TNFβ. Appropriate stimulation induces the expression of TNFα in a wide variety of cells. For example, lipopolysaccharide (LPS) induces TNFα expression primarly in the macrophage. TNFα is produced by all types of macrophages, including macrophages of pulmonary, hepatic, peritoneal, and bone marrow origin [29]. Several other cell types have also been reported to produce TNFα. These include T- and B-lymphocytes [30], NK cells [30], neutrophils [31], astrocytes [32], endothelial cells [33], and smooth muscle cells [34]. In contrast, TNFβ expression is much more restricted. It is expressed in T- and B-lymphocytes [35-37] and astrocytes [32]. Some cells (astrocytes and T- and B-lymphocytes) can be stimulated to make both TNFα and TNFβ. However, different inducers and different signal transduction pathways may account for their induction in a single cell suggesting different mechanisms of regulation.

Sequence comparison of the 5'-flanking regions of rabbit, mouse, and human TNF genes [27] revealed that the 200 bp flanking the transcription start site is highly homologous, implying the presence of important regulatory elements. In addition to the highly conserved TATA and GC boxes in the proximal regions of the TNF promoter, several putative regulatory elements have been identified (Figure 1). Approximately 40 bp upstream from the TATA box is a sequence that may participate in the induction of TNF by phorbol ester; it resembles the c-*jun*/AP-1 binding site consensus sequence. In addition, a TPA-responsive element was localized to a region 90 to 165 bp 5' of the TATA box [38] and a potential cyclic AMP response element was found 80 bp upstream from the TATA box [39]. Further upstream, Jongeneel *et al.* [40] have identified several regulatory elements in the mouse TNF gene associated with induction by LPS. These include two sequences similar to the NFκB enhancers found in the immunoglobulin genes, located 480 bp and 820 bp 5' of the TATA box, and two other variant sequences of the NFκB enhancer at 230 bp and 650 bp from the TATA box. Finally, a decanucleotide resembling the « Y-box » of the MHC class II promoter is located 240 bp 5' from the TATA box (Figure 1). A 5'-flanking region containing these regulatory regions was responsive to LPS when transfected into cultured bone marrow macrophages [27]. Furthermore, sequential deletions of portions of the 5' flanking regions, including the NFκB enhancer-like sequences, reduced the LPS response. When the Y-box sequence was deleted, inducibility was further reduced. Taken together, these results suggest a functional importance for these conserved sequences in the regulation of TNF gene expression by LPS in the mouse [27].

In addition to transcriptional activation, TNF gene expression is also regulated at the posttranscriptional level through a conserved sequence element in the 3' untranslated region. An AU-rich sequence, conserved in the 3' untranslated region of many cytokine genes, was identified in the human and murine TNF [41]. This sequence is implicated in the regulation of gene expression by controlling mRNA stability, in as much as mRNAs possessing this AU-rich sequence are selectively degraded by ribonucleases [42, 43].

Receptors and signal transduction

TNF, IL-1, and IL-6 are multifunctional cytokines that have emerged as important mediators of host defense. They induce a wide spectrum of biological activities by a variety of cell types, including the regulation of the immune response, hematopoiesis, and inflammation. Their functions are widely overlapping and are often biologically indistinguishable, and yet these cytokines are structurally distinct and each interacts with its own membrane receptors.

The receptors for TNF are highly ubiquitous. TNF binds to virtually all cell types with the exception of red blood cells. Most cells interact with TNF through a single class of high affinity receptors. Usually, 500-5,000 receptor sites per cell with an affinity of 0.1-1 nM have been found [44]. Some cells show a heterogeneous population of receptors. Both low and high-affinity TNF receptors have been identified on some cells. Several different molecular masses for the TNF receptor have been demonstrated. Most receptor-ligand cross-linking studies with bifunctional reagents have indicated a molecular mass of approximately 100 kDa for the complex [45]. However, there are also some reports of somewhat higher molecular sizes.

Though gel filtration studies of detergent-solubilized cells have indicated a molecular size greater than 300 kDa for the TNF receptor [46], the latter most likely represents the polymeric structure of the receptor.

Using recombinant DNA techniques, two different cDNAs for the TNF receptor have been cloned [47-49]. The cDNA for TNF-RI codes for 455 amino acid residues with a protein mass of 47 kDa. Its mRNA is approximately 3 kb in size. It consists of an extracellular domain (182 amino acid residues), a single transmembrane domain (21 amino acid residues), and a cytoplasmic domain (223 residues). The extracellular domain of the receptor is organized into four cysteine-rich domains. In contrast, TNF-RII cDNA codes for 461 amino acid residues with a protein mass of 46 kDa, and the extracellular, transmembrane, and intracellular domains are 235, 30, and 174 amino acid residues in length, respectively [49]. Even though there is significant sequence homology in the extracellular domains of TNF-RI and TNF-RII, they are distinct in the intracellular domain structure. The TNF-R extracellular domains also show a significant homology to nerve growth factor receptor, B-cell surface antigen CD-40 and T2 antigen on Shope fibroma virus. When expressed on the cell surface, TNF-RI gene produces a protein with a molecular mass of 60 kDa, whereas a protein with a molecular mass of 80 kDa is synthesized from the TNF-RII gene. Therefore, TNF-RI and TNF-RII are also referred to as p60 and p80, respectively. From the deduced amino acid sequence, TNF-RI has three potential N-linked glycosylation sites, whereas TNF-RII has two potential N-linked and some O-linked carbohydrate attachment sites. Both types of receptor have been shown to bind to TNF with essentially equal affinity. At present, the biological significance for the presence of two distinct receptors for TNF is not clear. Whether all cells express both kinds of receptors or transduce signals differently is not known. At present, it is also not clear if the genes for these two receptors are differentially regulated. However, it is clear that the expression of TNF receptor alone is not sufficient to transduce the signal.

The mechanisms involved in signal transduction for TNFα are largely unknown. TNF receptors, unlike several other growth factor receptors, do not possess intrinsic protein kinase activities. However, it has been reported that within minutes after exposure of cells to TNF several proteins are phosphorylated [50-52]. Recent studies suggest that TNF may function through at least two different signal transduction pathways, one involving adenylate cyclase and the other requiring protein kinase C (PKC) activation. Zhang et al. [53] reported that induction of IL-6 by TNFα in a human fibroblast cell line is preceded by a rapid activation of adenylate cyclase and an increase in intracellular cAMP levels, leading to protein kinase A activation. However, Sehgal et al. [54] suggested that IL-6 induction by TNF involves activation of the PKC pathway rather than the cAMP-dependent pathway. Recent studies suggest that alternate signal transduction pathways also may be activated by TNF. Treatment with TNF enhanced autophosphorylation of tyrosine in the EGF receptor [55], an autophosphorylation that occurs independently of PKC. In fibroblasts, both TNF and IL-l induce rapid phosphorylation of three distinct 27-kDa cytosolic proteins [56]. In addition, Shiroo and Matsushima [57] observed that early signal transduction in response to TNF involves rapid phosphorylation of a 26-kDa cytosolic protein at the serine residues. The identity of the protein kinase responsible for TNF induced serine phosphorylation remains to be determined.

TNF exerts pleiotropic effects through its ability to activate a wide variety of genes in numerous biological systems. Among the genes activated by TNF are transcription factors (NFkB [58-60], c-*fos* [61], c-*jun* [62] IRF-1 and 2 [63, 64] and NFIL-6 [65], cytokines (IL-l [66, 67]), IL-6 [68], IL-8 [69], TNFα [70], and IFNβ [71], and growth factors (PDGF [72]), GM-CSF [73], and M-CSF [74] — all of which contribute to the pleiotropic nature of TNF action by eliciting a multitude of biological actions. A case in point is the transcription factor NFκB. Its expression was initially thought to be specific to B cells. However, it was subsequently found in essentially all cell types examined, but usually in an inactive state. Stimulation by TNF, IL-l, and phorbol ester causes a rapid conversion of the inactive cytosolic form of NFκB to an active form, which translocates to the nucleus, binds to a specific DNA sequence, and *trans*-activates the transcription of target genes. Activation of NFκB, which is independent of protein synthesis, is due to phosphorylation of an inhibitor of NFκB, IκB, mediated by cAMP-dependent protein kinase and PKC [75, 76]. NFκB has been shown to be an important transcription factor in the regulation of genes with a wide spectrum of biological activities. These include, but are not limited to, the regulation of cytokines (IL-l, IL-6, IL-8, TNF), receptor (IL-2 receptor), virus (HIV-l), and acute-phase proteins (angiotensinogen, serum amyloid A).

Biological effects *in vitro* and *in vivo*

Because TNF mediates many biological activities (Figure 2) in most tissues and alters the immune function of leukocytes, it plays a central role as a general mediator of the inflammatory response.

Inflammation

It has become increasingly evident that TNF, along with IL-l and IL-6, is an important inflammatory mediator in eliciting the acute-phase response in the liver. Among the proteins induced by TNF are a_1-antichymotrypsin, serum amyloid A, and complement proteins C3 and factor B [77-79]. In contrast, albumin and transferrin expression *in vitro* are inhibited by TNF. These changes in hepatic protein synthesis are thought to serve as a host defense mechanism against infectious agents and trauma.

Effects on adipocyte

Another well-studied system for TNF action is the adipose tissue, where it enhances glycerol release, prevents or reverses adipocyte differentiation *in vitro* [80], and suppresses the expression of lipoprotein lipase and a variety of adipose-tissue specific proteins. Similar effects were observed when TNF was administered *in vivo*.

Neutrophil activation

One of the major biological activities of TNF is its action on neutrophils. Neutrophils activated by TNF have enhanced phagocytic activity, increased cytotoxicity, and elevated production of superoxide and H_2O_2. Furthermore, TNF stimulates neutrophil degranulation, inhibits migration, and causes adhesion to endothelial cells [81-84].

Immunomodulatory

Among other functions, TNF is a potent immunoregulatory cytokine. It can mediate severe inflammatory reactions, stimulate collagenase and prostaglandins, stimulate fibroblasts and endothelial cells, regulate T- and B-cell immune responses, induce class I and class II MHC molecules, and regulate the expression of other cytokines [85-88].

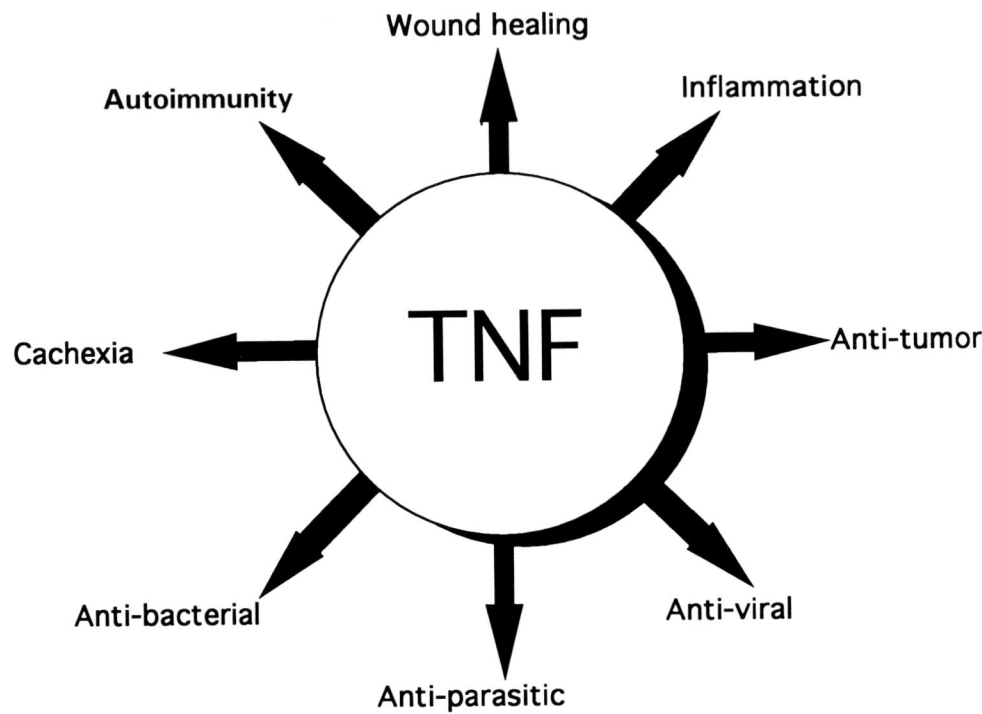

Figure 2. The diverse biological effects of TNF-α.

Antiproliferative and antitumor activities

Initial studies with the murine L929 fibroblasts by Carswell *et al.* [3] demonstrated that TNF had selective toxicity for tumor cells and transformed cell lines. Selective antiproliferative effects of TNF were also reported by Sugarman *et al.* [89], where an antiproliferative response of TNF was observed in 16 out of 34 tumor cell lines, while the growth of normal human cell lines from the colon, fetal skin, and lung was not inhibited. TNF can have either growth stimulatory or antiproliferative actions on normal cells and tumor cells, depending on the *in vitro* conditions [90]. TNF has antiproliferative effects on normal cells such as endothelial and smooth muscle cells [91, 92], adipocytes [93], fibroblasts [94], keratinocytes [95], and hemopoietic progenitor cells [96]. The antiproliferative effects of TNF on tumor cell lines *in vitro* can be modulated by other growth factors (EGF, TGFα, TGFβ, and PDGF) [94, 97].

In addition to direct antiproliferative effects on tumor cells, TNF can activate other antitumor mechanisms such as tumoricidal macrophages [98], cytotoxic T cells [99], natural killer cells [100], and neutrophils [81]. Furthermore, TNF can affect the interaction of the host and tumor through its effects on host stromal cell populations and by inducing the release of other cytokines (IL-l and IL-6) that may have antitumor effects.

Bone resorption

In vitro, TNF can stimulate osteoclastic bone resorption. It increases the formation of osteoclasts, enhances the differentiation of committed osteoclast progenitors, and activates preformed osteoclastic cells to form lacunae on bone surfaces. It also increases osteoblast-like cell replication and inhibits differentiated function. The effects of TNF on bone organ cultures can be potentiated by other factors. For example, IL-1 has synergistic effects with TNF on bone resorption in fetal rat long-bone culture [101].

In vivo studies with normal mice injected locally with TNF showed an increase in osteoclast activity on endosteal surfaces and an increase in whole-blood ionized calcium concentrations [102, 103]. Johnson *et al.* [103] showed that mice bearing TNF-producing tumors became hypercalcemic and their calvarial bones showed increases in osteoclastic bone resorption, with increased numbers of osteoclasts, increased active resorption surfaces, and increased total resorption surfaces.

TNF antagonists

Because of the role of TNF in a wide variety of diseases (*see* Table III), there has been a great deal of emphasis on seeking potential down-modulators of either

Table III. A list of diseases/conditions associated with production of TNF.

Disease/Condition	Source	Reference
Cancer	Serum	[117]
Hairy cell leukemia	Bone marrow, PBL	[118]
AIDS	Monocytes	[119]
Multiple myeloma	Bone marrow	[120]
Rhematoid arthritis	Synovial fluids	[121]
Lupus nephritis	Kidney	[122]
Multiple sclerosis (demyelination)	Astrocytes and macrophages	[123]
Reye's syndrome	Macrophages	[124]
Septic shock	Serum	[125]
Cachexia	Serum	[126]
Resorption of bone and cartilage	Bone cells	[127]
Bone marrow	Serum	[128]
Transplantation	Decidua	[129]
Preterm labor		

TNF production or TNF activity. These approaches mainly fall into four distinct categories, soluble receptors, antisense oligonucleotides, other cytokines, and antibodies. One of the major problems with any of these approaches, however, is specificity. Besides inhibiting the harmful effects, a single agent might also inhibit all the beneficial effects of TNF. The mode of administration of the inhibitor, *i.e.* prophylactic *vs* anaphylactic, has also to be taken into consideration. Since multiple cytokines have been associated with the same disease, it is not clear if the use of a single cytokine antagonist would be sufficient. Following is a general description of each approach and its potential advantages and disadvantages.

Soluble receptors

It has been shown that the urine of febrile patients and the urine and serum of cancer patients can inhibit certain biological effects of TNF. Purification of this TNF inhibitory activity and determination of its structure revealed that it is the soluble form of the extracellular domain of the TNF receptor with a molecular mass of 25-30 kDa [104, 105]. Both TNF-RI and TNF-RII forms of the receptor have been identified in the urine. Precisely why the cellular receptors are shed in certain diseases is not understood, but it is conceivable that this is the body's response to neutralize excess ligand. Interestingly, the soluble form of the TNF receptors binds to its ligand with almost the same affinity as the cellular receptors. Cloning of the TNF receptor cDNA has made it possible to prepare sufficient quantities of the soluble receptor. Since most of the biological effects of TNF *in vitro* can be inhibited by the soluble receptor [106], it is being explored as a TNF antagonist *in vivo*. The fate of the ligand-receptor complex after the soluble receptors sequester all the TNF remains to be determined.

Other cytokines

Another approach relevant to designing TNF antagonists involves down-modulation of TNF production by cytokines and various cellular metabolites (*see* Table II). The conditioned cell supernatants of human tumor cells and of diploid fibroblasts can inhibit TNF production [107]. It has been shown *in vitro* that the production of TNF from macrophages can be suppressed by treatment with either IL-4 or IL-6 [108]. Since fibroblasts and tumor cells are known to secrete IL-6, it is possible that activities described earlier were due to IL-6. Whether these cytokines will also down-regulate the production of TNF *in vivo* is, however, not known. Since IL-1 is also known to up-regulate the production of TNF, it is possible that IL-1R antagonists can suppress TNF production as well. The production of TNF can also be inhibited by well-known immunosuppressive agents such as cyclosporin A. Natural immunosuppressive agents such as TGF-β are also capable of inhibiting TNF production *in vitro*. Its ability to inhibit TNF *in vivo*, however, is not known. Inhibitors of the cyclooxygenase and lipooxygenase pathways and antiinflammatory drugs have also been implicated in the suppression of TNF production. Most of these agents lack the specificity and thus exhibit major side effects.

Antisense approach

With the recent development of recombinant DNA technology, it is now possible to selectively turn off or modify the activity of any given gene. One of the methods involves creating antisense RNA or DNA molecules that hybridize specifically with a targeted gene's RNA message, thus interrupting the machinery that expresses a gene. An antisense oligonucleotide is synthesized from the sense strand of the mRNA of the given ligand and used to inhibit the production of the cytokine in question. This kind of approach is currently being investigated for both *in vitro* and *in vivo* studies [109]. It has been shown that the expression of certain oncogenes such as *myc, mos*, and *fos* can be inhibited by their respective antisense oligonucleotides [110]. The synthesis of certain cytokines such as fibroblast growth factor, IL-1, TGFα, and IL-2 has also been shown to be inhibited by their antisense oligonucleotides [111]. Thus, it may be possible to block the production of TNF by using antisense oligonucleotides to TNF. However, for reasons not yet clear, high concentrations of the agent are usually needed to block the expression of the given gene.

At present, this technology has several limitations for which one must find a solution. This includes the type and length of antisense oligonucleotide, the instability of the oligonucleotide in circulation, the inability of the oligonucleotide to enter the cell, and the short half-life of the agent in the cell. Since this approach is simple, highly specific, and apparently effective, it should be possible to inhibit the synthesis of macromolecules and the growth of virus, bacteria, etc.

Antibodies

Antibodies against TNF are being used first to determine the involvement of the cytokine in the pathology of the disease and second, to treat the disease itself. It was demonstrated several years ago that the passive immunization of mice with polyclonal antibodies to murine TNF six hours before administration of lethal doses of endotoxin protected them from death [112]. Since then, the antibody approach has become another tool to investigate TNF antagonists. For instance, it has been shown that the blocking antibodies to TNF can protect mice from cerebral malaria [113]. These antibodies have also been exploited to resolve graft *vs* host disease and to treat bacterial granulomas [114]. Both monoclonal and polyclonal antibodies are being tested in these model systems. As these are nonhuman antibodies against the human ligand, they may be recognized by the human body as foreign and thus lead to production of antiidiotypes. One must « humanize » these antibodies before they can be used clinically [115, 116]. It may also be desirable to use monoclonal antibodies rather than polyclonal ones given the specificity of monoclonal antibodies for a single defined epitope. However, more than one epitope of TNF may be involved in the pathology of the disease.

Conclusion

TNF was originally discovered as a cytokine with antitumor properties. It is clear that it is a highly pleiotropic cytokine with an important role in autoimmune diseases, septic shock, cachexia, inflammation, bone resorption, and perhaps also tumorigenesis. Therefore, the development of antagonists to TNF would be highly useful. Several approaches are being explored to design TNF inhibitors.

Acknowledgement

This research was conducted, in part, by The Clayton Foundation for Research and was supported, in part, by new program development funds from The University of Texas MD Anderson Cancer Center and by a grant from NIH AR38858. The expert secretarial assistance of San Juanita De La Cerda and Harriette Young is greatly appreciated.

References

1. Brunes P. Die Heilwirkung des Erysipels auf Geschwulste. *Beitr Klin Chir* 1868 ; 3 : 443.
2. O'Malley WE, Achinstein B, Shear MJ. Action of bacterial polysaccharide on tumors. II. Damage of sarcoma 37 by serum of mice treated with Serratia marcescens polysaccharide, and induced tolerance. *J Natl Cancer Inst* 1962 ; 29 : 1169-75.
3. Carswell EA, Old LJ, Kassel RJ, Green S, Fiore N, Williamson B. An endotoxin-induced serum factor that causes necrosis of tumors. *Proc Natl Acad Sci USA* 1975 ; 72 : 3666-70.
4. Aggarwal BB. Tumor necrosis factor. In : Aggarwal BB, Gutterman J, ed. *Human cytokines : handbook for basic and clinical researchers*. Cambridge, MA : Blackwell Press, 1991.
5. Spriggs DR, Deutsch S, Kufe DW. Genomic structure, induction and production of TNF-α. In : Aggarwal BB, Vilcek J, eds. *Tumor necrosis factor : structure, function and mechanism of action*. New York : Marcel Dekker Press, 1991 : 3.
6. Himeno T, Watanabe N, Yamauchi N, Maeda M, Tsuji Y, Okamoto T, Neda H, Niitsu Y. Expression of endogenous tumor necrosis factor as a protective protein against the cytotoxicity of exogenous tumor necrosis factor. *Cancer Res* 1990 ; 50 : 4941-5.
7. Beutler B, Cerami A. Tumor necrosis, cachexia, shock, and inflammation : a common mediator. *Annu Rev Biochem* 1988 ; 57 : 505-18.
8. Aggarwal BB, Kohr WJ, Hass PE, Moffat B, Spencer SA, Henzel WJ, Bringman TS, Nedwin GE, Goeddel DV, Harkins RN. Human tumor necrosis factor : production, purification, and characterization. *J Biol Chem* 1985 ; 260 : 2345-54.
9. Fiers W. Precursor structures and structure-function analysis of TNF and lymphotoxin. In : Aggarwal BB, Vilcek J, eds. *Tumor necrosis factors : structure, function and mechanism of action*. New York : Marcel Dekker Press, 1991 : 79-92.
10. Pennica D, Nedwin GE, Hayflick JF, Seeburg PH, Palladino MA, Kohr WJ, Aggarwal BB, Goeddel DV. Human tumor necrosis factor : Precursor structure, expression and homology to lymphotoxin. *Nature* 1984 ; 312 : 724-9.
11. Beutler B, Cerami A. Cachetin and tumor necrosis factor as two sides of the same biological coin. *Nature* 1986 ; 320 : 584-8.
12. Kriegler M, Perez C, DeFay K, Albert I, Lu SD. A novel form of TNF/cachectin is a cell surface cytotoxic transmembrane protein : Ramifications for the complex physiology of TNF. *Cell* 1988 ; 53 : 45-53.
13. Jones EY, Stuart DI, Walker NPC. Structure of tumor necrosis factor. *Nature* 1989 ; 338 : 225-8.
14. Eck MJ, Sprang SR. The structure of tumor necrosis factor-α at 2.6 Å resolution : implications for receptor binding. *J Biol Chem* 1989 ; 264 : 17595-605.
15. Smith RA, Baglioni C. The active form of tumor necrosis factor is a trimer. *J Biol Chem* 1987 ; 262 : 6951-4.
16. Spies T, Blanck G, Bresnahan M, Sands J, Strominger JL. A new cluster of genes within the human major histocompatability complex. *Science* 1989 ; 243 : 214-7.
17. Nedospasor SA, Hirt B, Shakhov AN, Dobrynin VN, Kawashima E, Accolla RS, Jongeneel CV. The genes for tumor necrosis factor (TNF-α) and lymphotoxin (TNF-β) are tandemly arranged on chromosome 17 of the mouse. *Nucleic Acids Res* 1986 ; 14 : 7713-25.
18. Muller U, Jongeneel CV, Nedospasov SA, Lindahl KF, Steinmetz, M. Tumor necrosis factor and lymphotoxin genes map close to H-2D in the mouse major histocompatibility complex. *Nature* 1987 ; 325 : 265-7.

19. Gardner SM, Mock BA, Hilgers J, Huppi KE, Roeder WD. Mouse lymphotoxin and tumor necrosis factor : structural analysis of the cloned genes, physical linkage, and chromosomal position. *J Immunol* 1987 ; 139 : 476-83.
20. Goeddel DV, Aggarwal BB, Gray PW, Leung DW, Nedwin GE, Palladino MA, Patton JS, Pennica D, Shepard HM, Sugarman BJ, Wong GHW. Tumor necrosis factor : gene structure and biological activities. *Cold Spring Harbor Symp Quant Biol* 1986 ; 51 : 597-609.
21. Gray PW, Chen E, Li CB, Tang WL, Ruddle NH. The murine tumor necrosis factor-beta (lymphotoxin) gene sequence. *Nucleic Acids Res* 1987 ; 15 : 3937.
22. Ito H, Shirai T, Yamamoto S, Akira S, Kawahara S, Todd CW, Wallace RB. Molecular cloning of the gene encoding rabbit tumor necrosis factor. *DNA* 1986 ; 5 : 157-65.
23. Marmenout A, Fransen L, Tavernier J, Van DHJ, Tizard R, Kawashima E, Shaw A, Johnson MJ, Semon D, Muller R. Molecular cloning and expression of human tumor necrosis factor and comparison with mouse tumor necrosis factor. *Eur J Biochem* 1985 ; 152 : 515-22.
24. Gray PW, Aggarwal BB, Benton CV, Bringman TS, Henzel WJ, Jarret JA, Leung DW, Moffat B, Ng, P, Svedersky, LP, Palladino NA, Nedwin G. Cloning and expression of cDNA for human lymphotoxin, a lymphokine with tumour necrosis activity. *Nature* 1984 ; 312 : 721-4.
25. Li CB, Gray PW, Lin PF, McGrath KM, Ruddle, FH, Ruddle NH. Cloning and expression of murine lymphotoxin cDNA. *J Immunol* 1987 ; 138 : 4496-501.
26. Nedwin GE, Naylor SL, Sakaguchi AY, Smith D, Jarret Nedwin J, Pennica D, Goeddel DV, Gray PW. Human lymphotoxin and tumor necrosis factor genes : structure, homology and chromosomal localization. *Nucleic Acids Res* 1985 ; 13 : 6361-73.
27. Shakhov AN, Collart MA, Vassalli P, Nedospasov SA, Jongeneel CV. Kappa B-type enhancers are involved in lipopolysaccharide-mediated transcriptional activation of the tumor necrosis factor alpha gene in primary macrophages. *J Exp Med* 1990 ; 171 : 35-47.
28. Goldfeld AE, Doyle C, Maniatis T. Human tumor necrosis factor a gene regulation by virus and lipopoly-saccharide. *Proc Natl Acad Sci USA* 1990 ; 87 : 9769-73.
29. Decker T, Lohmann-Matthes ML, Gifford GE. Cell associated tumor necrosis factor (TNF) as a killing mechanism of activated cytotoxic macrophages. *J Immunol* 1987 ; 138 : 957-62.
30. Cuturi MC, Murphy M, Costa-Giomi MP, Weinmann R, Perussia B, Trinchieri G. Independent regulation of tumor necrosis factor and lymphotoxin production by human peripheral blood lymphocytes. *J Exp Med* 1987 ; 165 : 1581-94.
31. Lindemann A, Riedel D, Oster W, Ziegler-Heitbrock HWL, Mertelsmann R, Herrmann F. Granulocyte-macrophage colony-stimulating factor induces cytokine secretion by human polymorphonuclear leukocytes. *J Clin Invest* 1989 ; 83 : 1308-12.
32. Lieberman AP, Pitha PM, Shin HS, Shin ML. Production of tumor necrosis factor and other cytokines by astrocytes stimulated with lipopolysaccharide or a neurotropic virus. *Proc Natl Acad Sci USA* 1989 ; 86 : 6348-52.
33. Libby P, Ordovas JM, Auger KR, Robbins AH, Birinyi LK, Dinarello CA. Endotoxin and tumor necrosis factor induce interleukin-l gene expression in adult human vascular endothelial cells. *Am J Pathol* 1986 ; 124 : 179-85.
34. Warner SJC, Libby P. Human vascular smooth muscle cells. Target for and source of tumor necrosis factor. *J Immunol* 1989 ; 142 : 100-9.
35. Eardley DD, Shen FW, Gershon RK, Ruddle NH. Lymphotoxin production by subsets of T cells. *J Immunol* 1980 ; 124 : 1199-202.
36. Jongeneel CV, Nedospasov SA, Plaetinck G, Naquet P, Cerottini JC. Expression of the tumor necrosis factor locus is not necessary for the cytolytic activity of T lymphocytes. *J Immunol* 1988 ; 140 : 1916-22.
37. Sung SS, Jung LKL, Walters JA, Jeffes EWB, Granger GA, Fu SM. Production of lymphotoxin by isolated human tonsillar B lymphocytes and B lymphocyte cell lines. *J Clin Invest* 1989 ; 84 : 236-43.
38. Hensel G, Meichle A, Pfizenmaier K, Kronke M. PMA-responsive 5'-flanking sequences of the human TNF gene. *Lymphokine Res* 1989 ; 8 : 347-51.

39. Economou JS, Rhoades K, Essner R, McBride WH, Gasson JC, Morton DL. Genetic analysis of the human tumor necrosis factor alpha/cachectin promoter region in a macrophage cell line. *J Exp Med* 1989 ; 170 : 321-6.
40. Jongeneel CV, Shakhov AN, Nedospasov SA, Cerottini JC. Molecular control of tissue-specific expression at the mouse TNF locus. *Eur J Immunol* 1989 ; 19 : 549-52.
41. Caput D, Beutler B, Hartog K, Thayer R, Brown SS, Cerami A. Identification of a common nucleotide sequence in the 3'-untranslated region of mRNA molecules specifying inflammatory mediators. *Proc Natl Acad Sci USA* 1986 ; 83 : 1670-4
42. Shaw G, Kamen, R. A conserved AU sequence from the 3' untranslated region of GM-CSF mRNA mediates selective mRNA degradation. *Cell* 1986 ; 46 : 659-67.
43. Han J, Brown T, Beutler B. Endotoxin-responsive sequences control cachectin/tumor necrosis factor biosynthesis at the translational level. *J Exp Med* 1990 ; 171 : 465-75.
44. Aiyer RA, Aggarwal BB. Tumor necrosis factors. In : Podack ER, ed. *Cytolytic lymphocytes and complement effectors of the immune system*, Vol. II. Boca Raton, Florida : CRC Press, 1988 : 105-32.
45. Stauber GB, Aiyer RA, Aggarwal BB. Human tumor necrosis factor receptor : purification by immunoaffinity chromatography and initial characterization. *J Biol Chem* 1989 ; 263 : 19098-104.
46. Aiyer RA, Aggarwal BB. Characterization of receptors for recombinant human tumor necrosis factor-α from human placental membranes. *Lymphokine Res* 1990, 9 : 333-44.
47. Schall TJ, Lewis M, Koller KJ, Lee A, Rice GC, Wong GHW, Gatanaga T, Granger GA, Lentz R, Raab H, Kohr WJ, Goeddel DV. Molecular cloning and expression of a receptor for human tumor necrosis factor. *Cell* 1990 ; 61 : 361-70.
48. Loetscher H, Pan YCE, Lahm HW, Gentz R, Brockhaus M, Tabuchi H, Lesslauer W. Molecular cloning and expression of the human 55 kd tumor necrosis factor receptor. *Cell* 1990 ; 61 : 351-9.
49. Smith CA, Davis T, Anderson D, Solam L, Beckmann MP, Jerzy R, Dower SK, Cosman D, Goodwin RG. A receptor for tumor necrosis factor defines an unusual family of cellular and viral proteins. *Science* 1990 ; 248 : 1019-23.
50. Schutze S, Scheurich P, Pfizenmaier K, Kronke M. Tumor necrosis factor signal transduction. Tissue-specific serine phosphorylation of a 26-kDa cytosolic protein. *J Biol Chem* 1989 ; 264 : 3562-7.
51. Robaye B, Hepburn A, Lecocq R, Fiers W, Boeynaems JM, Dumont JE. (1989). Tumor necrosis factor-alpha induces the phosphorylation of 28-kDa stress proteins in endothelial cells : Possible role in protection against cytotoxicity ? *Biochem Biophys Res Commun* 1989 ; 163 : 301-8.
52. Marino MW, Pfeffer LM, Guidon PT Jr, Donner DB. Tumor necrosis factor induces phosphorylation of a 28-kDa mRNA CAP-binding protein in human cervical carcinoma cells. *Proc Natl Acad Sci USA* 1989 ; 86 : 8417-21.
53. Zhang Y, Lin J, Vilcek J. Synthesis of interleukin 6 (interferon-β2/β-cell stimulatory factor 2) in human fibroblasts is triggered by an increase in intracellular cyclic AMP. *J Biol Chem* 1988 ; 263 : 6177-82.
54. Sehgal PB, Walther Z, Tamm I. Rapid enhancement of β2-interferon/β-cell differentiation factor BSF-2 gene expression in human fibroblasts by diacylglycerols and the calcium ionophore A23187. *Proc Natl Acad Sci USA* 1987 ; 84 : 3663-7.
55. Donato NJ, Gallick GE, Steck PA, Rosenblum MG. Tumor necrosis factor modulates epidermal growth factor receptor phosphorylation and kinase activity in human tumor cells. Correlation with cytotoxicity. *J Biol Chem* 1989 ; 264 : 20474-81.
56. Kaur P, Saklatvala J. IL-l and TNF increase phosphorylation of fibroblast protein. *FEBS Lett* 1989 ; 241 : 6-10.
57. Shiroo M, Matsushima K. *Cytokine* 1990 ; 2 : 13-20.
58. Lowenthal JW, Ballard DW, Bohnlein E, Greene WC. Tumor necrosis factor α induces proteins that bind specifically to Kappa B-like enhancer elements and regulate interleukin 2 receptor α-chain gene expression in primary human T lymphocytes. *Proc Natl Acad Sci USA* 1989 ; 86 : 2331-5.

59. Osborn L, Kunkel S, Nabel GJ. Tumor necrosis factor α and interleukin-1 stimulate the human immunodeficiency virus enhancer by activation of the nuclear factor kappa B. *Proc Natl Acad Sci USA* 1989 ; 86 : 2336-40.
60. Zhang Y, Lin JX, Vilcek J. Interleukin-6 induction by tumor necrosis factor and interleukin-1 in human fibroblasts involves activation of a nuclear factor binding to a KB-like sequence. *Mol Cell Biol* 1990 ; 10 : 3818-23.
61. Lin JX, Vilcek J. Tumor necrosis factor and interleukin-1 cause a rapid and transient stimulation of c-*fos* and c-*myc* mRNA levels in human fibroblasts. *J Biol Chem* 1987 ; 262 : 11908-11.
62. Brenner DA, O'Hara M, Angel P, Chojkier M, Karin M. Prolonged activation of Jun and collagenase genes by tumor necrosis factor-α. *Nature* 1989 ; 337 : 661-3.
63. Fujita T, Reis LFL, Watanabe N, Kimura Y, Taniguchi T, Vilcek J. Induction of the transcription factor IRF1 and interferon-β mRNAs by cytokines and activators of second-messenger pathways. *Proc Natl Acad Sci USA* 1989 ; 86 : 9936-40
64. Reis LFL, Fujita T, Lee TH, Taniguchi T, Vilcek J. In : Oppenheim JJ, Powanda MC, Kluger MJ, Dinarello CA, eds. *Molecular and cellular biology of cytokines*. New York : Wiley-Liss, 1990 : 1-6.
65. Akira S, Isshiki H, Sugita T, Tanabe O, Kinoshita S, Nishio Y, Nakajima T, Hirano T, Kishimoto T. A nuclear factor for IL-6 expression (NF IL-6) is a member of a C/EBP family. *EMBO J* 1990 ; 2 : 1897-906.
66. Turner M, Chantry D, Buchan G, Barrett K, Feldmann M. Regulation of expression of human IL-1 ~ and IL-1 ~ genes. *J Immunol* 1989 ; 143 : 3556-61.
67. Le J, Vilcek J. Tumor necrosis factor and interleukin-1 : cytokines with multiple overlapping biological activities. *Lab Invest* 1987 ; 56 : 234-48.
68. Kohase M, Henriksen-DeStefano D, May LT, Vilcek J, Sehgal PB. Induction of β 2-interferon by tumor necrosis factor : a homeostatic mechanism in the control of cell proliferation. *Cell* 1986 ; 45 : 659-66.
69. Mukaida N, Mahe Y, Matsushima K. Cooperative interaction of nuclear factor-kappa B- and *cis*-regulatory enhancer binding protein-like factor binding elements in activating the interleukin-8 gene by pro-inflammatory cytokines. *J Biol Chem* 1990 ; 265 : 21128-33.
70. Krönke M, Schutze S, Scheurich P, Pfizenmaier K. In : Aggarwal BB, Vilcek J, eds. *Tumor necrosis factor : structure, function and mechanism of action*. Marcel Dekker, Inc., 1991 : 189-216.
71. Jacobsen H, Mestan J, Mittnacht S, Diffenbach CW. β-interferon subtype 1 induction by tumor necrosis factor. *Mol Cell Biol* 1989 ; 9 : 3037-42.
72. Hajjar KA, Hajjar DP, Silverstein RL, Nachman RL. Tumor necrosis factor-mediated release of platelet-derived growth factor from cultured endothelial cells. *J Exp Med* 1987 ; 166 : 235-45.
73. Broudy VC, Kaushansky K, Segal GM, Harlan JM, Adamson JW. Tumor necrosis factor type α stimulates human endothelial cells to produce granulocyte/macrophage colony stimulating factor. *Proc Natl Acad Sci USA* 1986 ; 83 : 7467-71.
74. Oster W, Lindemann A, Horn S, Mertelsmann R, Herrmann F. Tumor necrosis factor (TNF)-α but not TNF-β induces secretion of colony stimulating factor for macrophages (CSF-1) by human monocytes. *Blood* 1987 ; 70 : 1700-3.
75. Ghosh S, Baltimore D. Activation *in vitro* of NFκB by phosphorylation of its inhibitor IKB. *Nature* 1990 ; 344 ; 678-82.
76. Shirakawa F, Mizel S. *In vitro* activation and nuclear translocation of NFκB catalyzed by cyclic AMP-dependent protein kinase and protein kinase C. *Mol Cell Biol* 1989 ; 9 : 2424-30.
77. Perlmutter DH, Dinarello CA, Punsal PI, Colten HR. Cachetin/tumor necrosis factor regulates hepatic acute phase gene expression. *J Clin Invest* 1986 ; 78 : 1349-54.
78. Sipe JD, Vogel SN, Douches S, Neta R. Tumor necrosis factor/cachetin is a less potent inducer of serum amyloid A synthesis than interleukin 1. *Lymphokine Res* 1987 ; 4 : 93-101.

79. Li X, Liao WSL. Expression of rat serum amyloid Al gene involves both C/EBP-like and NFκB-like transcription factors. *J Biol Chem*, 1991.
80. Torti FM, Dieckmann B, Beutler B, Cerami A, Ringold GM. A macrophage factor inhibits adipocyte gene expression : an *in vitro* model of cachexia. *Science* 1985 ; 229 : 867-9.
81. Shalaby MR, Aggarwal BB, Rinderknecht L, Svedersky B, Finkle S, Palladino MA. Activation of human polymorphonuclear neutrophils by gamma interferon and tumor necrosis factors. *J Immunol* 1985 ; 135 : 2069-74.
82. Gamble JR, Harlan JM, Klebanoff SJ, Vadas MA. Stimulation of the adherence of neutrophils to umbilical vein endothelium by human recombinant tumor necrosis factor. *Proc Natl Acad Sci USA* 1985 ; 82 : 8667-71.
83. Ming WJ, Bersani L, Mantovani A. *J Immunol* 1987 ; 138 : 1469-74.
84. Shalaby MR, Palladino MA Jr, Hirabayashi SE, Eessalu TE, Lewis GD, et al. *J Leuk Biol* 1987 ; 41 : 196-204.
85. Old LJ. Tumor necrosis factor (TNF). *Science* 1985 ; 230 : 630.
86. Bock G, March J *Tumor necrosis factor and related cytotoxins*. Ciba Foundation Symposium 131 : Symposium on tumor necrosis factor and related cytokines, Ciba Foundation, London, Jan. 20-22, Chichester, England : Wiley, 1987.
87. Bonavida B, Gifford GE, Kirchner H. *Tumor necrosis factor/cachectin and related cytokines*. Basel : Karger S, 1988.
88. Bonavida B, Granger G. *Tumor necrosis factor : structure, mechanism of action. Role in disease and therapy*. Basel : Karger S, 1990.
89. Sugarman BJ, Aggarwal BB, Hass PE. Recombinant human tumor necrosis factor alpha : effects of proliferation on normal and transformed cells *in vitro*. *Science* 1985 ; 230 : 943-5.
90. Lewis GD, Aggarwal BB, Eessalu TE, Sugarman BJ, Shepard HM. Modulation of the growth of transformed cells by human tumor necrosis factor-alpha and interferon-gamma. *Cancer Res* 1987 ; 47 : 5382-5.
91. Sato N, Goto T, Haranaka K, Satomi N, Nariuchi H, Mano-Hirano Y, Sawasaki Y. Actions of tumor necrosis factor on cultured vascular endolthial cells : morphologic modulation, growth inhibition, and cytotoxicity. *J Natl Cancer Inst* 1986 ; 76 : 1113-9.
92. Schuger L, Varani J, Marks RM, Kunkel SL, Johnson KJ, Ward PA. Cytotoxicity of tumor necrosis factor alpha for human umbilical vein endothelial cells. *Lab Invest* 1989 ; 61 : 6268.
93. Kawakami M, Watanabe N, Ogawa H, Kato A, Sandom H, Yamada N, Murase T, Takaku F, Shibata S, Oda T. Cachetin/TNF kills or inhibits the differentiation of 3T3Li cells according to developmental stage. *J Cell Physiol* 1989 ; 138 : 1-7.
94. Palombella VJ, Vilcek J. Mitogenic and cytotoxic actions of tumor necrosis factor in BALB/c 3T3 cells : role of phospholipase activation. *J Biol Chem* 1989 ; 264 : 18128-36.
95. Pillai S, Bilke DD, Eessalu TE, Aggarwal BB, Elias PM. Binding and biological effects of tumor necrosis factor alpha on cultured human neonatal foreskin keratinocytes. *J Clin Invest* 1989 ; 83 : 816-21.
96. Broxmeyer H, Willaims DE, Lu L, Cooper S, Anderson SL, Beyer GS, Hoffman R, Rubin BY. The suppressive influences of human tumor necrosis factors on bone marrow hematopoietic progenitor cells from normal donors and patients with acute leukaemia : synergism of tumor necrosis factor and interferon-γ. *J Immunol* 1986 ; 136 : 4487-95.
97. Sugarman BJ, Lewis GD, Eessalu TE, Aggarwal BB, Shepard HM. Effects of growth factors on the antiproliferative activity of tumor necrosis factors. *Cancer Res* 1987 ; 47 : 780-6.
98. Talmadge JE, Phillips H, Schneider M, Rowe T, Pennington R, Bowersox O, Lenz B. Immunomodulatory properties of recombinant murine and human necrosis factor. *Cancer Res* 1987 ; 48 : 544-50.

99. Nakano K, Okugawa K, Furuichi H, Matsui Y, Sohmura Y. Augmentation of the generation of cytotoxic T lymphocytes against synergenic tumor cells by recombinant human tumor necrosis factor. *Cell Immunol* 1989 ; 120 : 154-64.
100. Ostensen ME, Thiele DL, Lipsky PE. Tumor necrosis factor-α enhances activity of human natural killer cells. *J Immunol* 1987 ; 138 : 4185-91.
101. Stashenko P, Dewhirst FE, Peros WJ, Kent RL, Ago JM. Synergistic interactions between interleukin 1, tumor necrosis factor, and lymphotoxin in bone resorption. *J Immunol* 1987 ; 138 : 1464-8.
102. Boyce BF, Aufdemorte TB, Garrett IR, Yates AJP, Mundy GR. Effects of interleukin-1 on bone turnover in normal mice. *Endocrinology* 1989 ; 125 : 1142-50.
103. Johnson RA, Boyce BF, Mundy GR, Roodman GD. Tumors producing human TNF induce hypercalcemia and osteoclastic bone resorption in nude mice. *Endocrinology* 1989 ; 124 : 1424-7.
104. Peetre C, Thysell H, Grubb A, Olsson I. A tumor necrosis factor binding protein is present in human biological fluids. *Eur J Haematol* 1988 ; 41 : 414-9.
105. Engelmann H, Aderka D, Rubinstein M, Rotman D, Wallack D. A tumor necrosis factor-binding protein purified to homogeneity from human urine protects cells from tumor necrosis factor toxicity. *J Biol Chem* 1989 ; 264 : 11974-80.
106. Seckinger P, Isaaz S, Dayer JM. Purification and biologic characterization of a specific tumor necrosis factor inhibitor. *J Biol Chem* 1989 ; 264 : 11966-73.
107. Tsunawaki S, Sporn M, Nathan C. Comparison of transforming growth factor-β and a macrophage-deactivating polypeptide from tumor cells. *J Immunol* 1989 ; 142 : 3462-8.
108. Hart PH, Vitti GF, Burgess DR, Whitty GA, Piccoli DS, Hamilton JA. Potential antiinflammatory effects of interleukin 4 : Suppression of human monocyte tumor necrosis factor α, interleukin 1, and prostaglandin E2. *Proc Natl Acad Sci USA* 1989 ; 86 : 3803-7.
109. Weintraub H. Antisense RNA and DNA. *Sci Am* 1990 ; 40.
110. Heikkila R, Schwab G, Wickstrom E, Loke SL, Pluznik DH, Watt R, Neckers LM. A c-myc antisense oligonucleotide inhibits entry into S phase but not progress from G0 to G1. *Nature* 1987 ; 328 : 445-9.
111. Harel-Bellan A, Durum S, Muegge K, Abbas AK, Farrar WL. Specific inhibition of lymphokine biosynthesis and autocrine growth using antisense oligonucleotides in Th1 and Th2 helper T cell clones. *J Exp Med* 1988 ; 168 : 2309-18.
112. Beutler B, Milsark, IW, Cerami AC. Passive immunization against cachectin/tumor necrosis factor protects mice from lethal effect of endotoxin. *Science* 1985 ; 229 : 869-71.
113. Grau GE, Fajardo LF, Riguet PF, Allet B, Lambert PH, Vassalli P. Tumor necrosis factor (cachectin) as an essential mediator in murine cerebral malaria. *Science* 1987 ; 237 : 1210-2.
114. Kindler V, Sappino AP, Grau GE, Piguet PF, Vassalli P. The inducing role of tumor necrosis factor in the development of bactericidal granulomas during BCG infection. *Cell* 1989 ; 56 : 731-40.
115. Co MS, Deschamps M, Whitley RJ, Queen C. Humanized antibodies for antiviral therapy. *Proc Natl Acad Sci USA* 1991 ; 88 : 2869-73.
116. Brown PS Jr, Parenteau GL, Dirbas FM, Garsia RJ, Goldman CK, Bukowski MA, Junghans RP, Queen C, Hakimi J, Benjamin WR, Clark RE, Waldmann TA. AntiTac-H, a humanized antibody to the interleukin 2 receptor, prolongs primate cardiac allograft survival. *Proc Natl Acad Sci USA* 1991 ; 88 : 2663-7.
117. Saarinen UM, Koskelo EK, Teppo AM, Siimes MA. Tumor necrosis factor in children with malignancies. *Cancer Res* 1990 ; 50 : 592-5.
118. Lindemann A, Ludwig WD, Oster W, Mertelsmann R, Herrmann F. High-level secretion of tumor necrosis factor-alpha contributes to hematopietic failure in hairy cell leukemia. *Blood* 1989 ; 73 : 880-4.
119. Wright SC, Jewett A, Mitsuyasu R, Bonavida B. Spontaneous cytotoxicity and tumor necrosis factor production by peripheral blood monocytes from AIDS patients. *J Immunol* 1988 ; 141 : 99-104.

120. Lichtenstein A, Berenson J, Norman D, Chang MP, Carlile A. Production of cytokines by bone marrow cells obtained form patients with multiple myeloma. *Blood* 1989 ; 74 : 1266-73.
121. Yocum DE, Esparza L, Dubry S, Benjamin JB, Volz R, Scuderi P. Characteristics of tumor necrosis factor production in rheumatoid arthritis. *Cell Immunol* 1989 ; 122 : 131-45.
122. Boswell JM, Yui MA, Burt DW, Kelley VE. Increased tumor necrosis factor and IL-1β gene expression in the kidneys of mice with lupus nephritis. *J Immunol* 1988 ; 141 : 3050-4.
123. Hofman FM, Hinton DR, Johnson K, Merrill JE. Tumor necrosis factor identified in multiple sclerosis brain. *J Exp Med* 1989 ; 170 : 607-12.
124. Larrick JW, Kunkel SL. Hypothesis : Is Reye's syndrome caused by augmented release of tumour necrosis factor ? *Lancet* 1986 ; ii : 132-3.
125. Tracey KJ, Beutler B, Lowry SF, Merryweather J, Wolpe S, Milsark IW, Hariri R, Fahey TJ, Zentella A, Albert JD, Shires GT, Cerami A. Shock and tissue injury induced by recombinant human cachectin. *Science* 1986 ; 234 : 470-4.
126. Tracey KJ, Wei H, Manogue KR, Fong Y, Hesse DG, Nguyen HT, Kuo GC, Beutler B, Cotran RS, Cermani A, Lowry SF. Cachectin-tumor necrosis factor induces cachexia, anemia and inflammation. *J Exp Med* 1988 ; 167 : 1211-27.
127. Mundy GR, Roodman GD, Bonewald LF, Yoneda T, Sabatini M. Effects of TNF and lymphotoxin on bone cells. In : Aggarwal BB, Vilcek J, eds. *Tumor necrosis factors : structure, function and mechanism of action*. New York : Marcel Dekker Press, 1991 : 483-98.
128. Holler E, Kolb HJ, Moller A, Kempeni J, Liesenfeld S, Pechumer H, Lehmacher W, Ruckdeschel G, Gleixner B, Riedner C, Ledderose G, Brehm G, Mittermuller J, Wilmanns W. Increased serum levels of tumor necrosis factor α precede major complications of bone marrow transplantation. *Blood* 1990 ; 75 : 1011-6.
129. Casey ML, Cox SM, Beutler B, Milewich L, MacDonald PC. Cachectin/tumor necrosis factor-α formation in human decidua. Potential role of cytokines in infection-induced preterm labor. *J Clin Invest* 1989 ; 83 : 430-6.

16

Eicosanoids and immunomodulation

Norbert GUALDE, Monique JUZAN

Laboratoire d'Immunologie, URA CNRS 1456, Université de Bordeaux 2, Fondation Bergonié, 33076 Bordeaux Cedex, France.

Some fatty acids, as for example arachidonic acid, modulate the immune response as do other mediators, such as interleukins, many hormones, neuropeptides, etc. Arachidonic acid metabolites, called eicosanoids, include an impressive panel of molecules with numerous biological activities and are the most extensively studied lipid mediators of the immune response. Examination of the immunomodulatory properties of these lipids is an arduous undertaking due to their very special biological characteristics namely, low level synthesis, short half-life, local biological actions and difficult identification and measurement. In spite of these difficulties, it is possible to summarize the major properties of these lipids regarding to their actions on the immune response. Below we briefly outline the most important findings reported in this field.

Eicosanoids and physiology of immune response

Arachidonic acid is an essential fatty acid that man can either synthesize or absorb from food sources as for instance eggs (65 mg of arachidonic acid per egg), calf's liver and meat (95 and 25 mg/100 g, respectively). Arachidonic acid can be synthesized starting with precursors, such as gamma-linolenic acid, which is transformed into dihomo-gamma-linolenic acid and then arachidonic acid. In fact, the young adult can satisfactorily produce arachidonic acid but this is more difficult in aged subjects or those in poor physiological condition. Providing and synthesizing arachidonic acid are not without consequences in the sense that this fatty acid is the most important substrate for the synthesis of a very wide variety of eicosanoids, among which the best known are prostaglandins and leukotrienes. For simplicity's sake, we can say that arachidonic acid has, like other essential fatty acids, a structural function, for example, a component of phospholipid membranes, while its metabolites perform regulatory functions, by playing the role(s) of intercellular mediators. Thromboxane and prostacyclin exert these controls in hemostasis, while prostaglandins and leukotrienes exercise them in inflammation and the immune response.

Cellular release of arachidonic acid (Figure 1)

Arachidonic acid (C20 : 4n-6) is a very important component of the phospholipids forming cell membranes, where it is usually located in position 2 on the glycerol. The fatty acid is released or bound, by deacylation or reacylation. More precisely, arachidonic acid release is associated with the action of two phospholipases : first, phospholipase A2 (PLA2), which releases arachidonic acid from phosphatidyl choline, and then phospholipase C, whose action, in conjunction with that of diglycerine lipase, separates arachidonic acid from phosphatidyl inositol [1-5]

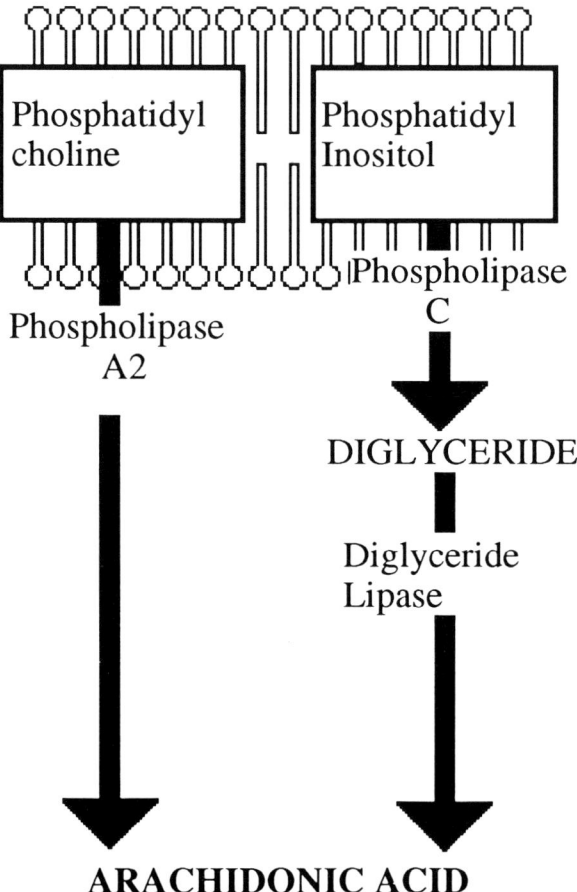

Figure 1. Release of arachidonic acid from the cell membrane.

Phospholipase A2 is inhibited by lipocortin (also called lipomodulin, macrocortin or renocortin), which is formed under the effect of steroids. It is also generally accepted that a lipocortin or endogenous lipocortins exist even in the absence of any pharmacological activation by steroids. In fact, one might keep in mind that the effect of steroids on eicosanoids'metabolite and/or actions is not merely mediated by lipocortin [6, 7]

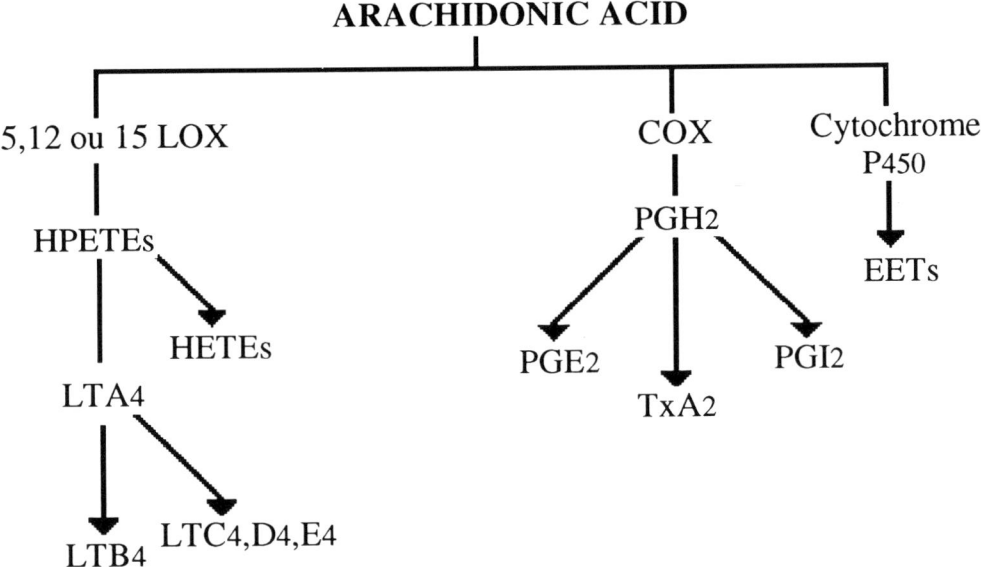

Figure 2. The principle eicosanoids.

Arachidonic acid metabolites (Figure 2)

Released arachidonic acid can be metabolized *via* three pathways : cytochrome P-450, cyclooxygenase (cox) and lipoxygenases (lox). Cytochrome P-450 produces the hydroxyeicosatrienoic acids (eets) ; cyclooxygenase is responsible for the endoperoxides (pgg$_2$ and pgh$_2$) transformed into prostaglandins (pgs) and thromboxanes (txs). That enzymic activity is quite important among macrophages and eosinophils [2-4, 8-10]. The more heterogeneous lipoxygenases transform arachidonic acid into diverse hydroperoxyeicosatetraenoic (HPETEs) and hydroxyeicosatetraenoic acids (HETEs) which even regulate eicosanoid production by macrophages [11]. 5-HPETE is the source material for leukotrienes A4 (LTA$_4$) and B4 (LTB$_4$), and peptidoleukotrienes C4, D4 and E4. These different mediators are responsible of primarily local reactions, occurring in the area surrounding their production site. The terminology, inspired by endocrinological semantics, usually refers to concepts of autocriny and paracriny for eicosanoids, as for interleukins.

The existence of receptors for the various eicosanoids is widely accepted as for instance PGE$_2$, LTB$_4$ and, in such circonstances, the fatty acid can be considered as a mediator acting as an hormone. In other situations, the released metabolite is transferred from the « donor » cell to another cell that, in turn, transforms it into an active derivative. This cell-to-cell transfer differs from classical endocrinological processing and is probably very important. Some of these various possibilities are summarized in Figure 3, where one can see, for example, that prostacyclin (PGI_2) can be produced by vascular endothelium and/or lymphocytes starting with platelet-derived PGH_2. In a similar manner, LTA, produced by neutrophils, can be transformed into either LTC_4 (by vascular endothelium or platelets) or LTB_4 (by red blood cells). Thus, we are very far from a model in which a cell produces a dominant metabolite ; in this case, not only is a cell the source of diverse eicosanoids, but it is the combined efforts of the different elements involved that give rise to a remarkable metabolic richness. In any case the eicosanoids are, above all, local mediators acting in their immediate vicinity, the microbiological environment of the cell producing them [12-14].

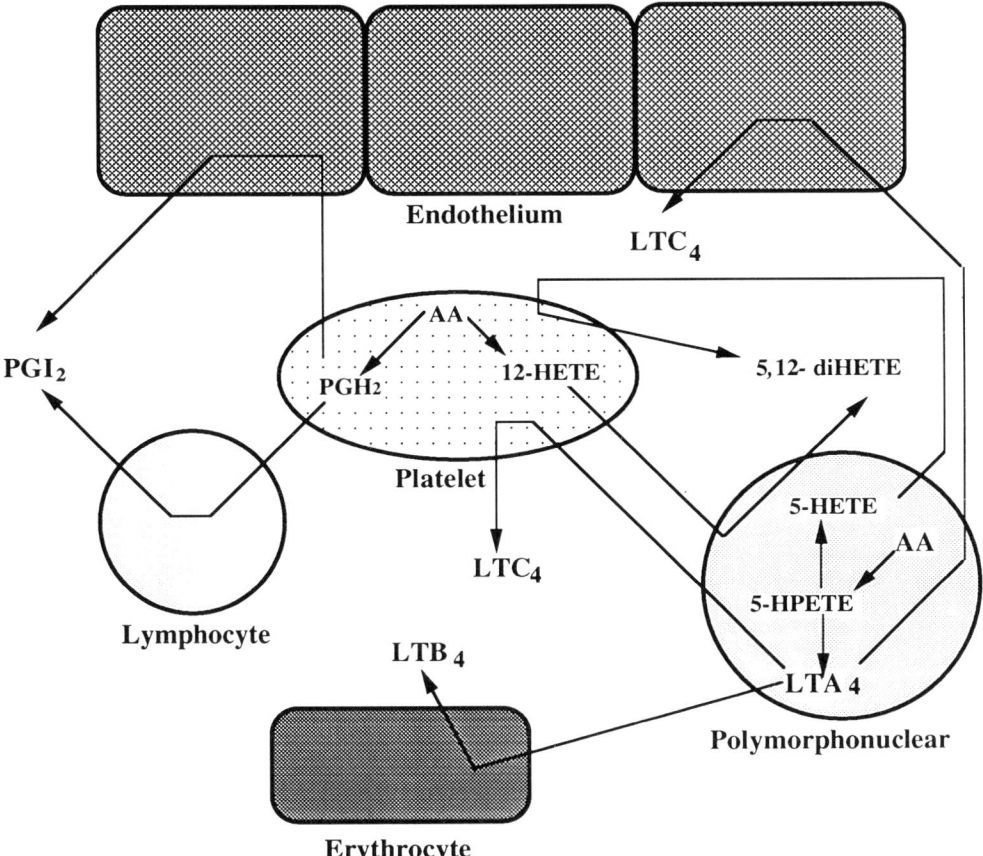

Figure 3. Cell interactions during the synthesis of eicosanoids.

Eicosanoid structure (Figure 4)

Prostaglandins are fatty acids containing 20 carbon atoms and a cyclopentane ring ; they belong to the family of prostanoids [1, 15]. The carbon atoms of prostaglandins are numbered starting at the carboxy terminal. Prostaglandins belong to two series, E and F, each composed of three members, respectively : E_1,

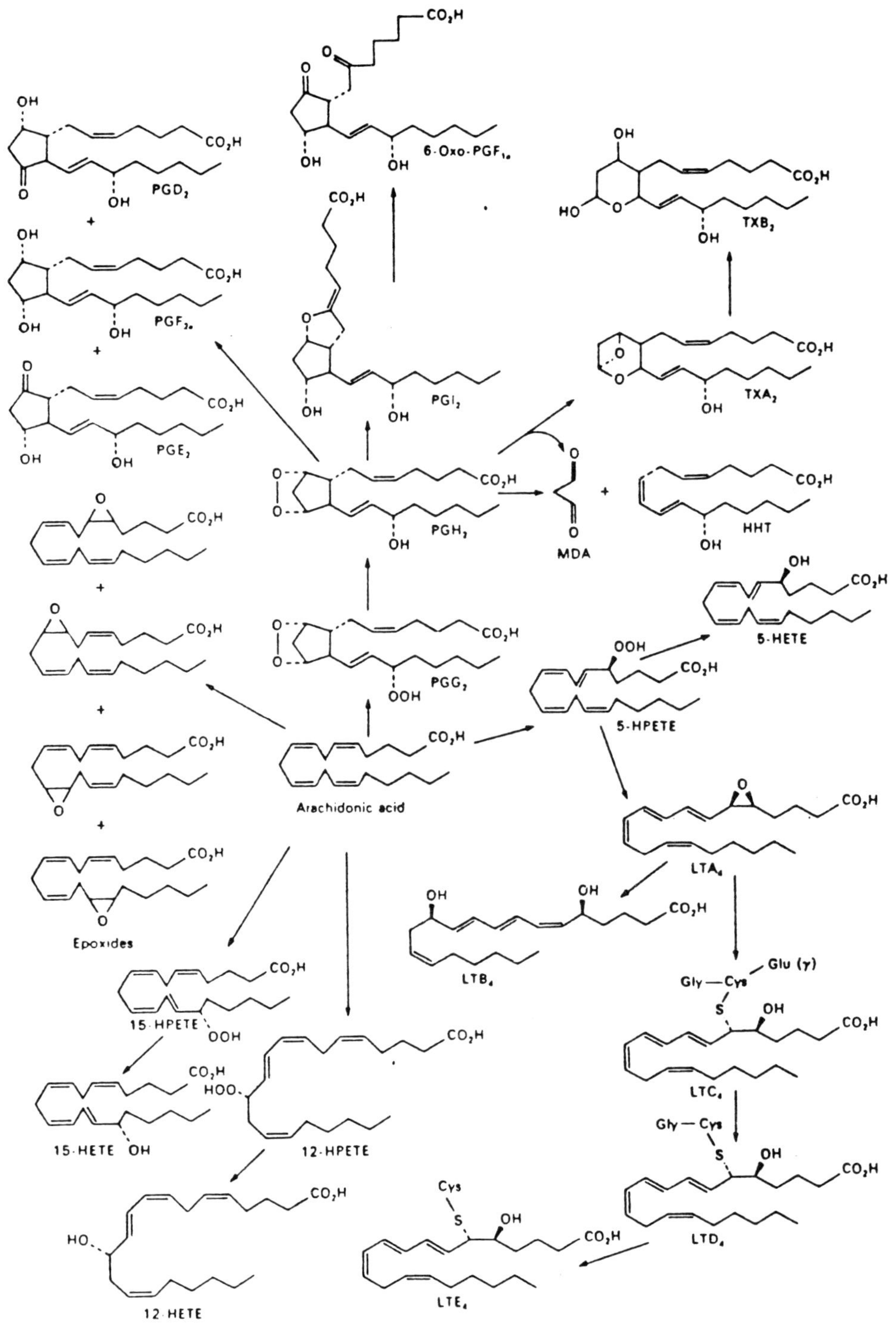

Figure 4. Molecular structure of the principle eicosanoids (from [12]).

E_2 and E_3, and F_1 and F_3. Each cyclopentane ring bears two side chains. These side chains are common to different prostaglandins. Like the prostaglandins, the leukotrienes are 20-carbon fatty acids but they do not have a pentane ring and are characterized by the presence of three conjugated double bonds. The letters assigned to them were given in the order of their discovery. LTC_4 is derived from LTA_4 conjugated to glutathione ; LTD_4 and LTE_4 are derivatives of this peptidoleukotriene. Lipoxins are derivatives of 15-lipoxygenase of which two species are known : lipoxin A and lipoxin B.

Eicosanoid production by cells involved in immunity

It has been clearly proved that among interacting cells involved in the immune response monocytes and macrophages are important producers of eicosanoids. In 1977 Humes *et al.* [16] reported that macrophages were the main source of prostaglandins (PGs) following stimulation by inflammatory products. This former report was confirmed by several authors such as Bankhurst *et al.* who actually demonstrated that prostaglandins produced by peripheral blood mononuclear cells originate from monocytes [17]. Since these reports, prostaglandin E production by phagocytes was demonstrated among various species such as the mouse [8], guinea pig [3], human circulating monocytes [2, 4, 18, 19] or peritoneal macrophages [10]. In fact, it is very well demonstrated that the monocyte-macrophage lineage does not only produce prostaglandins of the E series but also other metabolites from the cyclooxygenase pathway such as thromboxane [10, 20] and prostaglandin D2. There is also evidence that macrophages express a lipoxygenase-activity yielding a large variety of arachidonic acid lipoxygenase-derivatives such as hydroxycicosatetraenoic acids (HETEs) [21], and leukotrienes (LTs) [18, 19, 22]. It has even been reported that in terms of eicosanoid production the population of monocyte-macrophages is heterogeneous since for instance some of these phagocytes produce more PGE2 than others [23, 24] and because the production of eicosanoids depends upon immunostimulation [25], endotoxin treatment [22], drugs [19], presence of interleukins [19], lipoxygenase metabolites themselves [11], lipopolysaccharide [26], calcium-ionophore, lectins, toxins, indomethacin, steroids [20], and various *in vitro* conditions [27]. To summarize the above reports, one can consider as clearly demonstrated that cells from the monocyte-macrophage lineage produce eicosanoids but that in terms of arachidonic acid metabolism these cells are quite heterogeneous. It should be underlined that the *in vivo* production of eicosanoids by macrophages is probably more complex regarding the regulation of synthesis than what has been observed *in vitro* since *in vivo* the cells are kept under the influence of interleukins such as IL-1, IL-6, IL-8, various growth factors and even eicosanoids themselves [12]. Mastocytes are also involved in the immune response and produce eicosanoids but, other than in certain pathological situations, it does not seem that their eicosanoids are physiologically involved in any process regulating the immune response. As regards lymphocytes in terms of eicosanoid production, their role remains highly controversial. Prostaglandin, HETE and leukotriene productions by T and B lymphocytes and leukemic cell lines (for example, Jurkatt cells) have been reported. For other authors, the eicosanoids are the products of « contaminating » cells (macrophages, platelets) or cells having a pathological metabolism (cell lines). The truth in this conflict must be located somewhere in between these two positions and nothing prevents one from reasoning that a lymphocyte is capable of synthesizing a small amount of eicosanoid(s), *via* an autocrine process, like a cellular automessenger. The question concerning the production of eicosanoids by the thymus is quite puzzling. Production of eicosanoids by the thymus was reported, since 1963, by Bergström and Samuelson who demonstrated the presence of PGE_1 in an ethanol extracted material [28]. This former article does not give any information about the lineage of the PGE-producing cells in the thymus. Similarly Tomar et al. reported that thymus cells produced a small quantity of prostaglandins [29]. More information concerning this question was given by the Papiernik group [30] which studied the synthesis of cyclooxygenase metabolites by phagocytic cells of the thymic reticulum in culture. By using both high pressure liquid chromatography and radioimmunoassay, Homo-Delarche et al. [30] demonstrated the synthesis of thromboxane B2, prostaglandin E2, 6-ketoprostaglandin $F_{1\alpha}$, and $PGF_{2\alpha}$ by thymus-phagocytes. Papiernik et al. also demonstrated that phagocytic cells of the thymic epithelium which may be issued from thymic-interdigitating cells cultured in vitro did not only produce PGE2 but also IL-1 and were therefore able to modulate thymocyte proliferation [31] via antagonistic influences, PGE_2 giving the negative signal and IL-1 the positive one. The evidence that prostaglandins could be produced by the so-called « non adherent cells » of the thymus is more controversial and the fact that the prostaglandin-producing cells of the thymus are non-adherent cells in a short-incubation experiment [32] does not mean that these cells belong to the thymocyte lineage. It is likely that production of PGE_2 is an early event during thymus ontogeny and is necessary for the proliferation and differentiation of thymocytes [33]. For example, the production of PGE_2, 6 Keto-$PGF_{1\alpha}$ and $PGF_{2\alpha}$ by fetal thymic cells was reported as well as the expression of thymocyte markers such as Thy-1 and Lyt-1 surface molecules in relation to prostaglandin production [33]. Once again the cell lineage origin of thymus prostaglandins was not clearly demonstrated [33, 34] even if the presence of lipoxygenase metabolites such as HETEs was evidenced during cultures of fetal thymic lobes, and even if cyclooxygenase immunoreactivity appeared to be localized to stromal, i.e. non-lymphoid cells of the fetal thymus [34]. There is a good deal of evidence that thymic epithelial cells produce prostaglandins and that this synthesis is stimulated by cell-to-cell contact between epithelial cells and thymocytes [35]. The data showing that a thymic hormone, thymulin, increases the production of PGE_2 and PGD_2 by human immature T cells support the fact that prostaglandins might be synthesized by thymocytes within the thymus [36]. In fact, the influence of thymic hormone on prostaglandin synthesis by T cells remains controversial and might depend upon the experimental conditions since thymosin fraction 5 induces both a release of PGE2 and an expression of theta antigen by spleen cells from adult thymectomized mice but not by spleen cells from normal mice [37]. These data were not confirmed by Homo-Delarche et al. [21]. There are fewer reports concerning the production of lipoxygenase metabolites by thymus cells [34, 38]. Using both thin layer chromatography and high pressure liquid chromatography of chloroform extracts of culture supernatant, Duval demonstrated the production of 12-HETE by thymic cells [38]. The interesting fact underlined by this report is that the thymic-12-HETE-producing cells release only small amounts of prostaglandins and leukotrienes and are unaffected by steroid treatment [6]. It is likely that leukotrienes as well as HETEs are produced by macrophages of the thymus microenvironment as it was assessed by using thymus-macrophage hybridomas [39]. The question of eicosanoids production by T lymphocytes remains controversial; for example, according to Goldyne, even mature thymocytes are not able to synthetize LTB_4 [40] as was reported by other groups. One cannot exclude a cooperation or more precisely some metabolic interactions between cells of the thymus as it was reported for cells from blood and the vascular system [12]. Hence, that could explain the involvement of thymocytes in eicosanoid production and more precisely the stimulation of the metabolism of arachidonic acid by thymic epithelial cells [35]. The production of eicosanoids by cells of the thymus microenvironment may participate to their modulation of the activation of thymocytes [31, 41-44]. Among the cells of the microenvironment, macrophages which express an intensive metabolism of arachidonic acid [45], are probably the most efficient in terms of binding to thymocytes of the cortex and the medulla [46].

Eicosanoids and cyclic nucleotides

It is generally accepted that the interaction between PGE_2 and the cell *via* a prostaglandin-specific receptor activates adenylate cyclase, thereby transforming adenosine triphosphate (ATP) into 3'5'-cyclic adenosine monophosphate (cAMP). LTB_4, in contrast, activates guanylate cyclase, thereby causing the formation of 3'5'cyclic guanosine monophosphate (cGMP). The cyclic nucleotides participate in the activation of lymphocytes ; although their respective roles remain under discussion [47], it is known that the prolonged increase of intracellular cAMP levels contributes to the inhibition of lymphocyte proliferation, whereas increasing the cGMP concentration has opposite effects [48]. Briefly it was demonstrated that an increase of cAMP intra-lymphocyte concentration diminish the proliferative response of T cells [49, 50] and that cGMP augmentation induce an opposite effect [47].

Effects of eicosanoids on macrophages

The major function of macrophages in the initiation of the immune response is the presentation of epitopes to T lymphocytes. This presentation puts into play the class products of the major histocompatibility complex, called HLA-DR, DP, DQ, etc. in man and Ia in mouse. It has been shown that PGE_2 inhibits the expression of class II products by mouse peritoneal macrophages ; this effect of PGE_2 is blocked by an another eicosanoid, TXB_2 [51]. PGE_2 was reported to inhibit IL-1 production [52]. Dibutyryl-cAMP gives results similar to those obtained with PGE_2, in fact, the majority of eicosanoids produced by macrophages are synthesized *via* the lipoxygenase pathways, in particular that of 5-lipoxygenase. Thus, we can conclude that, under basal conditions, PGE_2 and the other prostaglandins have little effect on macrophage physiology, but this is a hypothesis that remains to be demonstrated. Indeed, a given macrophage, at a precise moment in time, synthesizes prostaglandins or leukotrienes and nothing prevents the supposition that, by means of these metabolites, macrophages « speak » to other macrophages and affect their current activity. In these circumstances, it is completely possible that prostaglandins, like leukotrienes, influence macrophages. For instance, it was reported the modulation of Fcg receptor on monocyte menbrane by HPETE [53], an augmentation of NADPH-dependent superoxyde generation [54] as well as an increase of IL-6 production by LTB_4 [55]

Eicosanoids and thymocyte apoptosis

One cannot discuss the role(s) of eicosanoids on thymocyte proliferative response without arguing about apoptosis or programmed cell death of thymocytes which involves arachidonic acid metabolites. Apoptosis is a mechanism of programmed cell death which is characterized by cleavage of DNA, therefore which looks like a programmed suicide of the cell starting by an intranuclear biochemical phenomenon. Endonuclease activation results in the production of oligonucleosome-length DNA fragments giving an electrophoretic aspect of « DNA ladder » [56]. It is likely that apoptosis is related with education and/or selection of thymocytes in the thymus [57], *i.e.* that autoreactive cells are genetically programmed to die in the organ and hence submitted to a negative selection. The question remains if arachidonic acid metabolites produced in the thymocyte-microenvironment play a critical role in physiological apoptosis. It was reported by McConkey *et al.* that agents that elevate cyclic-AMP stimulate DNA fragmentation in rat thymocytes [58], among these agents PGE_2 is one of the most efficient in terms of programmed cell death. On the contrary PGD_2, $PGF_{2\alpha}$ or analogs of cyclic-GMP are inefficient. PGE_2 induces an endonuclease activation which occurs before cell death. Apoptosis linked to cyclic-AMP-increase is related to an increase of protein kinase A activity (but not protein kinase C activation) and a subsequent protein phosphorylation. Suzuki *et al.* did not observe any effect of PGE_2 on mouse-thymocyte programmed cell death [59], *i.e.* the transient increase of cAMP induced by PGE_2 was not sufficient to induce any DNA fragmentation. However, when PGE_2 and forskolin are added together to thymocytes, there was an effect mediated *via* activation of protein kinase C. It was reported that the DNA cleavage is mostly significant in CD4+ CD8+ (double positive) immature thymocytes suggesting that the stage of differentiation and maturation of thymocytes in an important factor in PGE_2-induced DNA fragmentation. The discrepancy between the Suzuki data on mouse thymocytes [59] and those on rat thymocytes reported by McConkey [58] is still being elucidated. The report of Harford *et al.* [60] is even more confusing since it suggests that murine thymocyte lysis by corticosteroids may be explained by the inhibition of arachidonic acid metabolism. More specifically the lytic effect of the 5 lipoxygenase inhibitors, AA 861 and caffeic acid suggests that part of the thymolytic effect of corticosteroids is linked to inhibition of the production of metabolites of arachidonic acid and among them it is likely that LTB_4 is the more potent anti-apoptosis eicosanoid [60]. One can speculate that arachidonic acid metabolites have dualistic effects on programmed cell death, *i.e.* PGE_2 induces apoptosis while LTB_4 prevents it. The question remains if the depression of thymic weight induced by arachidonic acid [61] may be linked to a cyclooxygenase linked apoptosis since indomethacin prevents this effect of arachidonic acid.

Effects of eicosanoids on T lymphocytes

These actions are polymorphic. Briefly, prostaglandins inhibit the response of T lymphocytes, whereas leukotrienes induce different phenomena, depending upon the cell subpopulation affected by these eicosanoids. First of all, it has been clearly demonstrated that PGE_2 inhibits the proliferative response of thymus-dependent cells [62-66]. This was observed *in vitro*, for instance numerous studies revealed the inhibition by exogenous PGE_2 of tritiated-thymidine incorporation by T lymphocytes independent of the nature of the stimulus (lectin, anti-CD3 antibodies, antigen, calcium ionophore). This phenomenon was confirmed in experimental models and has been the subject of general reviews. The mechanism by which PGE_2 inhibits the T lymphocyte response is linked to the intra-lymphocyte production of cAMP and is accompanied by an inhibition of the activity of these cells. In addition, PGE_2 activation of suppressor T cells, which have been described as short-lived T lymphocytes, CD8+ cells or those expressing the receptor for the Fc fragment of IgG has been reported [67, 68]. PGE_2 can also, directly or indirectly through a T lymphocyte subpopulation, inhibit the production of IL-2. The PGE_2-dependent blockade of IL-2 production has been reported in various species (man, mouse, guinea pig) [62]. In fact, these events are probably not all that simple. The generation of suppressor T cells by PGE_2 recognized and, furthermore it has been reported that even CD4+ cells treated with PGE2 could manifest suppressive activity. It should also be noted that under certain conditions, PGE_2 could increase the proliferative response of T lymphocytes and that the phenomenon would be linked to the absence of short-lived and radiosensitive suppressor T cells [44, 69]. In addition, under the influence of PGE2, T lymphocyte production of suppressive factors has been described. These remarks must not let us lose sight of the primordial effect of PGE2 on T lymphocytes, *i.e.* its suppressive action. Physiologically, the macrophage-synthesized prostaglandins can modulate lymphocyte activity, as shown by *in vitro* experiments in which any stimulation of mononucleated cells (monocytes and lymphocytes), in the presence of inhibitors of prostaglandin synthesis, was accompanied by an increased incorporation of tritiated thymidine. In a similar manner, the *ex vivo* proliferation of T lymphocytes from subjects treated with indomethacin, an inhibitor of prostaglandin synthesis, is enhanced. The actions of the lipoxygenase pathway metabolites of arachidonic acid, HETEs and leukotrienes on T lymphocytes have not yet been studied as extensively.

Briefly, it can be said that the HETEs have an inhibitory action on the proliferative response of mononucleated blood cells [70, 71]; this inhibition is less clear with LTB_4. In fact, LTB_4 blocks the proliferation of CD4+ cells and increases that of CD8+ cells. LTB_4 plays an important role in generating suppressor CD8+ cells that have been discovered by means of models using thymocyte suspensions previously separated into CD4+ and CD8+ subpopulations [72]. 15-HPETE, a metabolite that is probably not strongly implicated in physiological processes, is able to convert CD8- cells into CD8+ cells [73-75]. In fact, leukotrienes play a very important role in thymocyte differentiation. Initially, an elevated production of eicosanoids, especially PGE2 but also leukotrienes, was observed in the thymus. PGE2 was recently shown to be able, under certain conditions, to affect *in vitro* the kinetics of the proliferative response of thymocytes, whereas LTB4 could play a fundamental role by participating in the intrathymic generation of self-specific suppressor T lymphocytes and thus contributing to self tolerance. Finally, the lipoxygenase pathway metabolites of arachidonic acid are the protagonists involved in the production of interferon-γ and IL-1.

The effect of eicosanoids on T cell function might explain the regulatory role of macrophages in antigenic stimulation [51]. One may also underline that the sensitivity to eicosanoids might be linked to both HLA type [65, 76] and age [77].

Interactions between eicosanoids and thymic hormones

The thymus is an endocrine gland which produces hormones involved in the differentiation and the maturation of thymocytes [78]. Bach's group was the first to report the role of prostaglandins in the expression of membrane molecules and their interaction with the thymic factor, thymulin (previously called FTS, *facteur thymique sérique*) [79, 80]. Garaci *et al.* reported similar data since they demonstrated that after adult thymectomy the *in vivo* expression by splenocytes of the theta marker was induced when animals were treated by an analog of PGE_2 [81]. This phenomenon was later reported to be linked to the induction of a serum thymic-like activity [82]. It is likely that the role of thymic hormones such as thymosin fraction 5 depends upon the immunological status of the animal since the hormone reinduces the expression of membrane theta molecules *via* the production of PGE_2 in thymectomized mice (this phenomenon is inhibited by indomethacin) [37]. In contrast, PGE$_2$ production by splenocytes from normal mice is inhibited by the hormone [37]. Thymic hormones act *via* the production of cyclic AMP and/or PGE$_2$ [83], and it is probable that thymic hormones induce an increase of the intra-thymocyte cyclic-AMP either directly or *via* the production of PGE$_2$ [80, 84]. The effect of thymic hormones depends upon the level of maturation of thymocytes, for example, thymulin increases the intracellular cyclic-AMP/cyclic-GMP ratio of immature but not mature thymocytes, and under some experimental conditions has reverse effects in terms of PGE$_2$ production [83]. This is in agreement with the fact that peripheral blood human T cells respond to thymulin by an increase of prostaglandin production [36]. As regards to the effects of thymic hormones on prostaglandins production, more controversial data were reported by Homo-Delarche *et al.* [21, 85].

Role of eicosanoids in thymocyte differentiation and maturation

The thymus plays a critical role in the education of thymocytes by controlling the positive and negative selection of thymocytes, the education of immature thymocytes, and the selection of the repertoire of T cells [27, 57, 86-88]. There is a good deal of evidence that eicosanoids participate in the differentiation and the maturation of thymocytes as they do for bone marrow stem cells during hematopoiesis. Broadly speaking, it was reported that prostaglandins and metabolites of 15-lipoxygenase had an inhibitory effect on myelopoiesis but that 5-lipoxygenase metabolites usually stimulated hematopoiesis [89-94]. Therefore, cyclooxygenase and lipoxygenase metabolites of arachidonic acid can modulate the differentiation of commited and uncommited stem cells. Concerning the thymus, it was reported that prostaglandin production is very low in this organ in the lupus prone NZB/NZW mouse which is characterised by a defect in suppressor cells [95]. This may be related to abnormalities of early T-cell development. Recently, by using Northern blots and *in situ* hybridization to thymus macrophage RNA, we demonstrated the presence of 5 lipoxygenase transcripts within the thymus. The activity of the 5 lipoxygenase enzyme was demonstrated by assessment of leukotrienes produced by thymic-macrophage hybridomas [39]. It was reported that LTB$_4$ plus IL-2 treatment of immature CD4- CD8- double negative thymocytes induces them to express the CD8 antigen [96] which is the marker of both the suppressor and the cytotoxic T lymphocytes. Later, we demonstrated that the LTB4-induced CD8+ thymocytes are suppressor cells [97] which are mainly involved in tolerance to self [98]. This is in agreement with the already reported role of lipoxygenase metabolites in the generation of suppressor cells [99-103]. Hence, we speculated that immature double negative thymocytes in the context of self environment and leukotrienes are induced to differentiate into CD8+ self-specific suppressor T cells involved in tolerance to self [98]. Considering the fact that thymic prostaglandin production is modulated by thymic hormones and that PGE$_2$ plays a role in apoptosis which is probably related to the negative selection of immature thymocytes, it is likely that eicosanoids are quite important mediators during the early steps of their maturation and selection of thymocytes. Therefore, we speculate that prostaglandins and leukotrienes play a fundamental role in thymus physiology, more precisely that they participate in the thymus-driven tolerance to self either by inducing apoptosis and/or generating suppressor cells which shut-off autoreactive lymphocytes [99, 100]. On the one hand, anti-self immature double positive (CD4+, CD8+) thymocytes which are both in the context of self antigens (expressed by cells of the thymus microenvironment) and in the presence of PGE$_2$ initiate their program of cell death and then are negatively selected. On the other hand immature double negative thymocytes (CD4-,CD8-) which are also in the context of self-antigens are, in the presence of LTB4, induced to give rise to CD8+ suppressor cells involved in tolerance to autologous antigens. Hence, in both cases, eicosanoids play a critical role in tolerance to self; in the first case, tolerance to self results from a PGE_2-induced apoptosis which is in agreement with the model of the « forbidden-clone » [104-106]. A forbidden clone is a clone of lymphocytes capable of reaction with self-components of the body but which is regularly eliminated by the normal homeostatic mechanism [106]. In the second case, auto-tolerance is produced *via* the generation of suppressor cells which is in agreement with the theory of clonal anergy involved in tolerance to self [104, 107, 108]. Clonal anergy means that the forbidden clone is still present but that some homeostatic mechanism (for example suppressor cells) induces its (clonal) unresponsiveness to self-components.

Effects of eicosanoids on B lymphocytes

The influence of eicosanoids on B lymphocytes has been studied less thoroughly. When PGE_2 is added to purified B cells stimulated, for example, by *Staphylococcus aureus*, the presence of the prostaglandin diminishes the synthesis of immunoglobulins. This PGE_2-induced inhibition seems to be linked to the intralymphocyte B increase of cAMP; in addition, forskolin gives analogous results. In fact, it is probable that, under physiological conditions, the effect of PGE_2 on the production of antibodies acts *via* T lymphocytes. In the case of autoimmune disorders, PGE_2 could favor the production of autoantibodies by inhibiting the activity of suppressor T cells. This was demonstrated in rheumatoid arthritis patients treated with an inhibitor of prostaglandin synthesis. In these subjects, the abnormally elevated production of PGE_2 inhibited the activity of CD8+ suppressor T cells more than that of B cells synthesizing the rheumatoid factor.

Eicosanoids and cytotoxic cells not restricted by the major histocompatibility complex

Such cells include natural killer (NK) cells, which have a spontaneous cytolytic activity against certain tumoral cell lines, *e.g.* K562 in man, and other cells called lymphokine-activated killers (LAK), which are induced *in vitro* by treating normal mononucleated cells with IL-2. LAK cells can be distinguished from NK cells by their ability to lyse tumor cells that are normally NK-resistant, for example, Daudi cells in man. NK and LAK cells have repertoires that are not restricted by the major histocompatibility complex. PGE_2 is a potent inhibitor of the natural cytolytic activities [109, 110]; this inhibitory capacity is associated with the higher level of intracellular cAMP. Thus molecules such as forskolin, by increasing the intracellular cAMP level, block the tumoricidal activities described above exactly like the cAMP analogues, *e.g.*, dibutyryl cAMP. Under physiological conditions, macrophage-produced PGE_2 is probably responsible for modulation of the natural cytotoxic activity; indeed, it has been shown that the macrophage-dependent inhibition can be lifted either by macrophage depletion or by treating the cells with a cyclooxygenase inhibitor. Lipoxygenase pathway metabolites antagonize the activities of PGE_2; for example, LTB_4 and 5-HETE increase NK activity whereas lipoxygenase inhibitors, like nordihydroguaretic acid (NDGA), or decrease it [111-114]. In addition, the amplifying effect of lipoxygenase pathway metabolites could be linked to their effect favoring the synthesis of interferon, which is also an activator of natural cytotoxic cells.

Eicosanoids and immunopathology

Autoimmune diseases

Among autoimmune disorders or those suggestive of an autoimmune phenomenon, rheumatoid diseases are perhaps the best studied in terms of their relationships with eicosanoids. This is probably linked to the fact that prostaglandins are important protagonists of inflammation, since abundant amounts of them are found in the joints of subjects suffering from chronic and acute arthritides [115].

Rheumatoid arthritis is the model for these diseases. In this case, PGE_2 is synthesized in the pathological joint by synoviocytes and macrophages. In fact, patients' monocytes produce a mononuclear cell factor that acts on synoviocytes, inducing collagenase synthesis simultaneously with that of PGE_2 [116]. *A priori*, this elevated production of prostaglandin can be considered as a potential source of immunosuppression. Indeed, Goodwin showed that inhibitors of prostaglandin synthesis, *e.g.* piroxicam, could induce a reduction in the serum level of rheumatoid factor. This observation was explained by an excess PGE_2-induced inhibition of suppressor cells and thus an inability to control the production of autoantibodies. In these circumstances, cyclooxygenase inhibitors can reestablish physiological regulation. The overproduction of PGE_2 in rheumatoid arthritis explains the low-level synthesis of IL-2 by the patients' lymphocytes which are affected by prostaglandins either directly or *via* the activation of CD8+ suppressor cells. Metabolites issued from the lipoxygenase pathway might be involved in autoimmune disease as well [117] but it is not clear if lipoxygenase induced suppressor cells are involved in autoimmune disease regulation [118]

Allergies

It is well known that the eicosanoids are important mediators of allergies, responsible for numerous clinical manifestations in cases of hypersensitivity [119-121]. The standard model of such states linked to the production of eicosanoids is represented by atopy or hypersensitivity type I reactions. In these instances, lipid mediators are released primarily by mastocytes and basophils bearing allergen-specific IgE. Thus, we are not dealing directly with eicosanoids participating in an immunomodulation but with soluble agents synthesised and released during a hypersensitivity crisis, playing a role absolutely essential to the appearance of the observed symptoms (coryza, bronchial spasm, transit disorders, blood pressure changes, etc.).

The eicosanoids involved (PGD_2, $PGF_{2\alpha}$, leukotrienes) are not stored in the cells. They are released during a crisis when the binding of the allergen to IgE triggers the activation of phospholipase A_2 and the release of arachidonic acid, which in turn is susceptible to being transformed by cyclooxygenase and/or lipoxygenases. Among the 5-lipoxygenase metabolites, leukotrienes C_4, D_4 and E_4 are the fundamental elements in the disorders observed ; they were identified as such when discovered as the slow reacting substance of anaphylaxis (SRS-A).

Asthma is typically a disease of allergic origin [120], whose clinical manifestations are in large part associated with the release of arachidonic acid metabolites and, among these, the components of SRS-A. This explains the presence in atopic patients of allergen-specific IgE and mastocytes in the pulmonary tissue (which is not specific to asthmatics). We point out that the proposed explanation of aspirin-induced asthma, according to which the non-steroidal anti-inflammatory drug blocks the cylooxygenase pathway and provides more substrate for the 5-lipoxygenase, seems rather irrelevant in light of the fact that, in all cases, mastocytes produce 9 times more leukotrienes than prostaglandins. In other terms, if aspirin induced asthma is really linked to cyclooxygenase inhibition, it is unlikely that the manifestations observed result from an excess supply of arachidonic acid shunted from the cyclooxygenase pathway to the lipoxygenase pathway [122].

Grafts and transplants

Taking into consideration what is known about the immunomodulatory effects of eicosanoids, the presence of prostaglandins at a possible rejection site can potentially inhibit the reaction, whereas the presence of leukotrienes can amplify it. It has been shown in murine secondary mixed-lymphocyte cultures that the recipient's responding cells produce prostaglandins, probably under the effect of the interleukins released [25]. It is now generally accepted that the rejection of an allograft is accompanied by PGE_2 synthesis ; this was demonstrated for skin grafts and kidney transplants. Practical experience with grafts and transplants has shown that the production of PGE_2 does not prevent rejection crises [123, 124], although experiments in mice bearing skin allografts showed that administration of PGE_2 or dimethyl-PGE_2 to the recipient prolonged graft survival, whereas indomethacin reduced it [125-127]. In clinical practice, it has been reported that urinary excretion of PGE2 could precede renal insufficiency and the increase in the level of serum creatinine. As regards to the role of lipoxygenase metabolites during rejection episodes, at the present time, the supposed effects are purely speculative and it is difficult to determine if the eicosanoids produced are the protagonists of the rejection or simply witnesses of the phenomenon.

Cancer

Without too much exaggeration, this section on eicosanoids and cancers shares certain similarities with the preceding one. As in the case of grafts, entire volumes have been devoted to the production of arachidonic acid metabolites during cancer. And, as above, nothing definitive has been decided for time being, which in no way means that nothing important exists in terms of the biological reality. The short discussion that follows summarizes the principle concepts reported concerning this domain. Eicosanoids can affect cancerous diseases by interfering in three different processes : (1) tumor initiation and promotion [128, 129] ; (2) metastatic spread ; and (3) immunomonitoring [130-133].

It has been shown that many tumor cell lines and spontaneous tumors (cancers of the breast, kidney and bronchus, and malignant lymphomas) produce large amounts of prostaglandins [134-140]. The prostaglandins synthesized have a potential effect on the initiation and promotion of the tumor by participating, *via* their free radicals, in the oxidation of carcinogens. Tumor promotion due to phorbol esters is partially linked to the production of prostaglandins.

As far as metastases are concerned, eicosanoids have antagonistic effects seen in light of thromboxane's ability to aggregate platelets, which can favor the grafting at a distance of the tumor cells, whereas prostacyclin has opposing effects, as demonstrated experimentally *in vivo* by using nafazatrom, a promoter of PGE_2 synthesis. PGE_2 produced during malignant proliferation has immunosuppressive effects, as shown by Goodwin in Hodgkin's disease [141].

Monocytes from patients with Hodgkin's disease inhibit *ex vivo* the proliferation of circulating lymphocytes stimulated by phytohemagglutinin (PHA); this inhibition is lifted by indomethacin, an inhibitor of prostaglandin synthesis. The clearest experimental proof of the effect of eicosanoids on cells potentially implicated in immunomonitoring concerns cytotoxic cells not restricted by the major histocompatibility complex *(see above)*. The role(s) that can be played by arachidonic acid metabolites in cancer provide more or less plausible explanations for an association between dietary fatty acid content and the occurrence of cancers *(see below)*. In fact, many epidemiological reports attempt to demonstrate a relationship, for example, between high lipid content in the diet and breast cancer.

Diet

Observations made on Eskimos, Japanese fishermen and Icelanders have demonstrated that populations consuming a diet rich in fish from cold oceans (mackerel, menhaden) had lower frequencies of cardiovascular diseases and prolonged bleeding times. These modifications of biological parameters are attributed to the high levels of w-3 fatty acids (at the expense of series w-6) in the diet [142-144]. Eicosapentaenoic acid (EPA) and docosahexaenoic acid (DHA) are among the omega-3 fatty acids present in the oils of these fishes. These fatty acids, constituents of phospholipids, are metabolised like arachidonic acid but give rise to series 3 prostaglandins and series 5 leukotrienes which have low biological activities [145-148]. These findings justify the use of EPA in experimental inflammatory diseases and its attempted application to human pathology [149-155].

In a similar manner, because on the one hand Eskimos seem to have fewer cancers of the colon and breast and, on the other, that lipid-rich diets seem to favor cancer development, it was proposed that w-6 fatty acids could favor the appearance of malignant tumors. To recommend dietary changes to prevent the appearance of neoplasms based on these observations is a small step but a rapidly made one; however, it is still too early to know if such lifestyle alterations will provide relevant contributions to the prevention of cancers.

Conclusion

The biological effects of eicosanoids are truly fascinating. Their fact that a given eicosanoid can act on different natural processes and that the eicosanoids include a remarkable panoply of molecules. During a « regular » immune response, it is difficult to determine if arachidonic acid derivatives play a notable role and, if so, the production sequences of these metabolites and the possible result(s) of their action(s). In pathological circumstances and in cases of known oversynthesis of one or several eicosanoids, it is possible, within certain limits, to explain the clinical and/or biological manifestations by the presence of these excess eicosanoids.

Nonetheless, it must be recognized that this is, for the most part, speculative. Finally, as far as therapeutic applications are concerned, it must be admitted that, to date, the pharmaceutical industry was unable to produce selective inhibitors of the synthesis of the different eicosanoids.

References

1. Samuelsson B. An elucidation of the arachidonic acid cascade discovery of prostaglandins, thromboxane and leukotrienes. *Drugs* 1987 ; 33 : suppl.1 : 2-9.
2. Goldyne ME, Stobo JD. Synthesis of prostaglandins by subpopulations of human peripheral blood monocytes. *Prostaglandins* 1979 ; 18 : 687-95.
3. Morley J, Bray MA, Jones RW, Nugteren DH, VanDorp DA. Prostaglandin and thromboxanes production by human and guinea pig macrophages and leucocytes. *Prostaglandins* 1979 ; 17 : 729-36.
4. Kennedy MS, Stobo JD, Goldyne ME. *In vitro* synthesis of prostaglandins and related lipids by populations of human peripheral blood mononuclear cells. *Prostaglandins* 1980 ; 20 : 135-45.
5. Johnson M, Carey F, McMillan M. Alternative pathways of arachidonate metabolism : prostaglandins thromboxane and leukotrienes. In : Campbell PN, Marshall rd. *Essays in Biochemistry*. New York : Academic Press, 1983 ; 19 : 41-141.
6. Duval D, Huneau JF, Homo-Delarche F. Effects of serum on the metabolism of exogenous arachidonic acid by phagocytic cells of the mouse thymic reticulum. *Prostaglandins Leukotrienes Med* 1989 ; 23 : 67-71.
7. Errasfa M, Rothhut B, Russo-Marie F. Phospholipase A2 inhibitory activity in thymocytes of dexamethasone-treated mice-possible implication of lipocortins. *Biochem Biophys Res Commun* 1989 ; 159 : 53-60.
8. Kurland JI, Bockman R. Prostaglandin E production by human blood monocytes and mouse peritoneal macrophages. *J Exp Med* 1978 ; 147 : 952-5.
9. Bockman RS. Prostaglandin production by human blood monocytes and mouse peritoneal macrophages : synthesis dependent on *in vitro* culture conditions *Prostaglandins* 1991 ; 21 : 9-31.
10. Foegh ML, Maddox YT, Ramwell PW. Human peritoneal eosinophils and formation of arachidonate cyclooxygenase products. *Scand J Immunol* 1986 ; 23 : 599-603.
11. Humes JL, Opas EE, Galavage M, Soderman D, Bonney RJ. Regulation of macrophage eicosanoid production by hydroperoxy and hydroxy-eicosatetraenoic acids. *Biochem J* 1986 ; 233 : 199-206.
12. Lagarde M, Gualde N, Rigaud M. Metabolic interactions between eicosanoids in blood and vascular cells. *Biochem J* 1989 ; 257 : 921-34.
13. Fitzpatrick F, Liggett W, McGee J, Bunting G, Morton S, Samuelsson B. Metabolism of leukotriene A4 by human erythrocytes. A novel cellular source of leukotriene B_4. *J Biol Chem* 1984 ; 259 : 11403-7.
14. Maclouf J, Fruteau de Laclos B, Borgeat P. Effects of 12-hydroxy-and 12-hydroperoxy-5, 8, 10, 14-eicosatetraenoic acids on the synthesis of 5-hydroxy-6, 8, 11, 14-eicosatetraenoic acid and leukotriene B_4 in human blood leukocytes. *Adv Prostaglandin Thromboxane Leukotriene Res* 1983 ; 11 : 159-62.
15. Parker CW. Lipid mediators produced through the lipoxygenase pathway. *Annu Rev Immunol* 1987 ; 5 : 65-84.
16. Humes JL, Bonney RW, Pelus L, Dahlgren ME, Sadowski SS, Kuehl FA, Davies P. Macrophages synthetize and release prostaglandins in response to inflammatory stimuli. *Nature* 1977 ; 269 : 149-51.
17. Bankhurst AD, Hastain E, Goodwin JS, Peake GT. The nature of the prostaglandin-producing mononuclear cell in human peripheral blood. *J Lab Clin Med* 1981 ; 97 : 179-86.
18. Goldyne ME, Burrish GF, Poubelle P, Borgeat P. Arachidonic acid metabolism among human mononuclear leucocytes. *J Biol Chem* 1984 ; 259 : 8815-9.

19. Bonney RJ, Humes JL. Physiological and pharmacological regulation of prostaglandin and leukotriene production by macrophages. *J Leukocyte Biol* 1984 ; 35 : 1-10.
20. Lewis RA, Austen FK. The biologically active leukotrienes. Biosynthesis, metabolism, receptors, functions, and pharmacology. *J Clin Invest* 1984 ; 73 : 889-97.
21. Homo-Delarche F, Bach JF, Dardenne M. Thymic hormones and prostaglandins. I. Lack of stimulation of prostaglandin production by thymic hormones. *Prostaglandins* 1989 ; 38 : 183-96.
22. Lüderitz Th, Rietschele Th, Schade H. Leukotriene C4-release from endotoxin-stimulated macrophages. *Ann Immunol Hung* 1983 ; 23 : 81-91.
23. Khansari N, Chou YK, Fudenberg HH. Human monocyte heterogeneity : interleukin 1 and prostaglandin E_2 production by separate subsets. *Eur J Immunol* 1985 ; 15 : 48-51.
24. Ujihara M, Urade Y, Eguchi N, Hayashi H, Ikai K, Hayaishi O. Prostaglandin D_2 formation and chatacterization of its synthetases in various tissues of adult rats. *Arch Biochem Biophys* 1988 ; 260 : 521-31.
25. Dy M, Astoin M, Rigaud M, Hamburger J. Prostaglandin (PG) release in the mixed lymphocyte culture ; effect of presensitization by a skin allograft ; nature of the PG-producing cell. *Eur J Immunol* 1980 ; 10 : 121-6.
26. Nichols FC, Schenkein HA, Rutherford RB. Prostaglandin E2,prostaglandin E1 and thromboxane B2 release from human monocytes treated with C3b or bacterial lipopolysaccharide. *Biochim Biophys Acta* 1987 ; 927 : 149-57.
27. Bevan MJ. Thymic education. *Immunol Today* 1981 ; 2 : 216-9.
28. Bergström S, Samuelsson B. Isolation of prostaglandin E1 from calf thymus. Prostaglandins and related factors 20. *Acta Chem Scand* 1963 ; 17 : S282-7.
29. Tomar RH, Darrow TL, John PA. Response to and production of prostaglandin by murine thymus, spleen, bone marrow, and lymph node cells. *Cell Immunol* 1981 ; 60 : 335-46.
30. Homo-Delarche F, Duval D, Papiernik M. Prostaglandin production by phagocytic cells of the mouse thymic reticulum in culture and its modulation by indomethacin and corticosteroids. *Immunology* 1985 ; 135 : 506-12.
31. Papiernik M, Homo-Delarche F. Thymic reticulum in mice.III. Phagocytic cells of the thymic reticulum in culture secrete both prostaglandin E2 and interkeukin 1 which regulate thymocyte proliferation. *Eur J Immunol* 1983 ; 13 : 689-92.
32. Borda E, Genaro AM, Perez Leiros C, Cremaschi G, Peredo H, Sterin-Borda L. Prostaglandins, cyclic AMP production and biological activity of alloimmune thymocytes. *Prostaglandins Leukotrienes Med* 1985 ; 19 : 197-208.
33. Shipman PM, Schmidt RR, Chepenik KP. Relation between arachidonic acid metabolism and development of thymocytes in fetal thymic organ cultures. *J Immunol* 1988 ; 140 : 2714-20.
34. Appasamy PM, Pendino K, Schmidt RR, Chepenik KP, Prystowsky MB, Goldowitz D. Expression of prostaglandin G/H synthase (cyclooxygenase) during murine fetal thymic development. *Cell Immunol* 1991 ; 330 : 341-57.
35. Sun L, Piltch AS, Liu P-S, Johnson LA, Hayashi J. Thymocytes stimulate metabolism of arachidonic acid in rat thymic epithelial cells. *Cell Immunol* 1990 ; 131 : 86-97.
36. Gualde N, Rigaud M, Bach JF. Stimulation of prostaglandin synthesis by the serum factor (FTS). *Cell Immunol* 1982 ; 70 : 362-6.
37. Garaci RL, Favalli C, Del Gobbo V, Garaci E, Jaffe BM. Is thymosin action mediated by prostaglandin release ? *Science* 1983 ; 220 : 1163-5.
38. Duval D. Effect of dexamethasone on arachidonate metabolism in isolated mouse thymocytes. *Prostaglandins Leukotrienes Essential Fatty Acids* 1986 ; 37 : 149-56.
39. Delebassée S, Cogny Van Weydevelt F, Gualde N. Effect of arachidonic acid metabolites on thymus tolerance. *Ann NY Acad Sci* 1988 ; 524 : 227-9.
40. Goldyne ME, Laidler R. Stimulated T cell and natural killer (NK) cell lines fail to synthesize leukotriene B_4. *Prostaglandins* 1987 ; 34 : 783-95.
41. Papiernik M, Nabbara B, Savino W, Pontoux C., Barbey S. Thymic reticulum in mice.II.Culture and characterization of nonepithelial phagocytic cells of the thymic retic-

ulum : their role in the syngeneic stimulation of thymic medullary lymphocytes. *Eur J Immunol* 1983 ; 13 : 147-55.
42. Papiernik M, Penit C, El Rouby S. Control of prothymocyte proliferation by thymic accessory cells. *Eur J Immunol* 1987 ; 17 : 1303-10.
43. Denning SM, Kurtzberg J, Le PT, Tuck D, Singer KH, Haynes BF. Human thymic epithelial cells directly induce activation of autologous immature thymocytes. *Proc Natl Aca Sci USA* 1988 ; 85 : 3125-9.
44. Hayari Y, Kukulansky T, Globerson A. Regulation of thymocyte proliferative response by macrophage-derived prostaglandin E2 and interleukin 1. *Eur J Immunol* 1985 ; 15 : 43-7.
45. Milicevic NM, Milicevic Z, Colic M, Mujovic S. Ultrastructural study of macrophages in the rat thymus, with special reference to the cortico-medullary zone. *J Anat Physiol Norm Pathol Homme Animaux* 1987 ; 150 : 89-98.
46. Wood GW. Macrophages in the thymus. *Survey Immunol Res* 1985 ; 4 : 179-91.
47. Mexmain S, Cook J, Aldiger JC, Gualde N, Rigaud M. Thymocyte cyclic AMP and cyclic GMP responses to treatment with metabolites issued from the lipoxygenase pathway. *J Immunol* 1985 ; 135 : 1361-5.
48. Segal J. Opposite regulatory effects of cAMP and cGMP on sugar uptake in rat thymocytes. *Am J Physiol* 1987 ; 252 : E588-94.
49. Goodwin JS, Kaszubowski PA, Williams RC Jr. Cyclic adenosine monophosphate response to prostaglandin E_2 on subpopulations of human lymphocytes. *J Exp Med* 1979 ; 150 : 1260-4
50. Goodwin JS, Bromberg S, Messner RP. Studies on the cyclic AMP response to prostaglandin in human lymphocytes. *Cell Immunol* 1981 ; 60 : 298-307
51. Unanue ER. The regulatory role of macrophages in antigenic stimulation. II. Symbiotic relationship between lymphocytes and macrophages. *Adv Immunol* 1981 ; 31 : 1-136.
52. Brandwein SR. Regulation of interleukin 1 production by mouse peritoneal macrophages. Effects of arachidonic acid metabolites, cyclic nucleotides, and interferons. *J Biol Chem* 1986 ; 261 : 8624-32.
53. Goodwin JS, Gualde N, Aldigier JC, Rigaud M, Vanderhoeck JY. Modulation of Fc IgG receptors on T cells and monocytes by 15 hydroperoxyeicosatetranoic acid. *Prostaglandins Leukotrienes Med* 1984 ; 13 : 109-12
54. Bromberg Y, Pick E. Unsaturated fatty acids stimulate NADPH-dependent superoxide production by cell-free system derived from macrophages. *Cell Immunol* 1984 ; 88 : 213-21.
55. Rola-Pleszczynski M, Stankova J. Leukotriene B4 enhances interleukin-6 (IL-6) production and IL-6 messenger RNA accumulation in human monocytes *in vitro* : transcriptional and posttranscriptional mechanisms. *Blood* 1992 ; 80 : 1004-11
56. Wyllie AH. Glucocorticoid-induced thymocyte apoptosis is associated with endogenous endonuclease activation. *Nature* 1980 ; 284 : 555-8.
57. MacDonald HR, Lees RK. Programmed death of autoreactive thymocytes. *Nature* 1990 ; 343 : 642-4.
58. McConkey DJ, Orrenius S, Jondal M. Agents that elevate cAMP stimulate DNA fragmentation in thymocytes. *J Immunol* 1990 ; 145 : 1227-30.
59. Suzuki K, Tadakuma T, Harutoshi K. Modulation of thymocyte apoptosis by isoproterenol and prostaglandin E_2. *Cell Immunol* 1991 ; 134 : 235-40.
60. Harford AM, Shopp GM, Goodwin JS, Ebbesen MA, Gibel L, Smith AY, Sterling WA. Murine thymocyte lysis by inhibitors of arachidonic acid metabolism. *Ad Prostaglandins Thromboxane Leukotriene Res* 1991 ; 21B : 489-92.
61. Meade CJ. How arachidonic acid depresses thymus weight. *Int Arch Allergy Applied Immunol* 1979 ; 59 : 432-6.
62. Chouaib S, Chatenoud L, Klatzmann D, Fradelizi D. The mechanism of inhibition of human IL-2 production. II. PGE_2 induction of suppressor T lymphocytes. *J Immunol* 1984 ; 132 : 1-7.
63. Rigaud M, Breton JC, Gualde N, Malinvaud G. *In vitro* inhibition of human lymphocyte transformation by natural or synthetic prostaglandins. *Prostaglandins Med* 1979 ; 3 : 167-9.

64. Gualde N, Rigaud M, Rabinovitch H, Durand J, Beneytout JL, BretonJC. Inhibition de la réponse lymphocytaire par les métabolites libérés par la lipoxygenase des macrophages chez la souris. *CR Acad Sci (Série D) Paris* 1981 ; 293 : 359-62.
65. Gualde N, Rabinovitch H, Fredon M, Rigaud M. Effects of 15-hydroperoxyeicosatetraenoic acid on human lymphocyte sheep erythrocyte rosette formation and response to concanavalin A associated with HLA system. *Eur J Immunol* 1982 ; 12 : 773-7.
66. Gualde N, Chable-Rabinovitch H, Motta C, Durand J, Beneytout JL, Rigaud M. Hydroperoxyeicosatetraenoic acids potent inhibitors of lymphocyte responses. *Biochem Biophys Acta* 1983 ; 750 : 429-33.
67. Fischer A, Durandy A, Griscelli C. Role of prostaglandin E_2 in the induction of non-specific T lymphocyte suppressor activity. *J Immunol* 1981 ; 126 : 1452-5.
68. Aldigier JC, Gualde N, Mexmain S, Chable-Rabinovitch H, RatinaudMH, Rigaud M. Immunosuppression induced *in vivo* by 15 hydroeicosatetraenoic acid (15-HETE). *Prostaglandins Leukotrienes Med* 1984 ; 13 : 99-107.
69. Stobo JD, Kennedy MS, Goldyne ME. Prostaglandin E modulation of the mitogenic response of human T cells. *J Clin Invest* 1979 ; 64 : 1188-92.
70. Gualde N, Goodwin JS. Induction of suppressor T cells *in vitro* by arachidonic acid metabolites issued from the lipoxygenase pathway. In : Bailey JM, ed. *Prostaglandins, leukotrienes and lipoxins*. New York : Plenum Press, 1983 : 565-75.
71. Goodman MG. Inhibition of lymphocyte mitogenesis by an arachidonic acid hydroperoxide. *J Supramolecular* 1980 ; 13 : 373-83.
72. Gualde N, Atluru D, Goodwin JS. Effect of lipoxygenase metabolites of arachidonic acid on proliferation of human T cells and T cell subsets. *J Immunol* 1985 ; 134 : 1125-9
73. Gualde N, Rigaud M, Goodwin JS. Induction of suppressor cells from peripheral blood T cells by 15-hydroperoxyeicosatetraenoic acid (15-HPETE). *J Immunol* 1985 ; 135 : 3424-9
74. Rola-Pleszczynski M. Differential effects of leukotriene B4 on T4+ and T8+ lymphocyte phenotype and immunoregulatory functions. *J Immunol* 1985 ; 135 : 1357-60
75. Goodwin JS. Regulation of T cell activation by leukotriene B4. *Immunol Res* 1986 ; 5 : 233-48
76. Staszak C, Goodwin JS, Troup GM, Pathak DR, Williams RC Jr. Decreased sensitivity to prostaglandin and histamine in lymphocytes from normal HLA-B12 individuals : a possible role in autoimmunity. *J Immunol* 1980 ; 125 : 181-5
77. Goodwin JS, Messner RP. Sensitivity of lymphocytes to prostaglandin E2 increases in subjects over age 70. *J Clin Invest* 1979 ; 64 : 434-9.
78. Sprent J. T lymphocytes and the thymus. In : Paul WE, ed. *Fundamental immunology*. New York : Raven Press, 1984 : 69.
79. Bach MA, Bach JF. Effets de l'AMP cyclique sur les cellules formant les rosettes spontanées. *CR Acad Sci (Série D) Paris* 1972 ; 275 : 2783-6.
80. Bach MA, Bach JF. Studies on thymus products.VI.The effects of cyclic nucleotides and prostaglandins on rosette-forming cells. Interactions with thymic factor. *Eur J Immunol* 1973 ; 3 : 778-83.
81. Garaci E, Rinaldi-Garaci C, Del Gobbo V, Favalli C, Santoro G, *et al*. A synthetic analog of prostaglandin E_2 is able to induce *in vivo* theta antigen on spleen cells of adult thymectomized mice. *Cell Immunol* 1981 ; 62 : 8-14.
82. Rinaldi-Garaci C, Del Gobbo V, Favalli C, Garaci E, Bistoni F, *et al*. Induction of serum thymic-like activity in adult thymectomized mice by a synthetic analog of PGE_2. *Cell Immunol* 1982 ; 72 : 97-101.
83. Rinaldi-Garaci C, Jezzi T, Baldassare AM, Dardenne M, Bach JF, Garaci E. Effect of thymulin on intracellular cyclic nucleotides and prostaglandins E_2 in peanut agglutinin- fractionated thymocytes. *Eur J Immunol* 1985 ; 15 : 548-52.
84. Kook AI, Trainin N. The control exerted by thymic hormone (THF) on cellular cAMP levels and immune reactivity of spleen cells in the MLC assay. *J Immunol* 1975 ; 115 : 8-14.

85. Homo-Delarche F, Gagnerault MC, Bach JF, Dardenne M. Thymic hormones and prostaglandins. II. Synergistic effect on mouse spontaneous rosette forming cells. *Prostaglandins* 1990 ; 39 : 299-318.
86. Nikolic-Zubic J, Bevan MJ. Role of self peptides in positively selecting the T cell repertoire. *Nature* 1990 ; 344 : 65-7.
87. Von Boehmer H, Teh HS, Kisielow P. The thymus selects the useful, neglects the useless and destroys the harmful. *Immunol Today* 1989 ; 10 : 57-61.
88. Saito T, Germain RN. The generation and selection of the T cell repertoire : insights from the studies of the molecular basis of T cell recognition. *Immunol Rev* 1988 ; 101 : 81-113.
89. Simantov R, Sachs L. Role of phospholipase A_2 and prostaglandin E in growth and differentiation of myeloïd leukemic cells. *Biochim Biophys* Acta 1982 ; 720 : 111-9.
90. Malinvaud G, Gaillard S, Chable H, Allegros A, Rigaud M. Effet inhibiteur du 15HPETE sur les cellules souches granulocytaires (CFU-GM). *Nouv Rev Fr Hematol (Paris)* 1983 ; 25 : 319-22.
91. Patchen ML. Immunomodulators and hemopoiesis. *Survey Immunol Res* 1983 ; 2 : 237-42.
92. Claesson HE, Dahlberg N, Gahrton G. Stimulation of human myelopoiesis by leukotriene B_4. *Biochim Biophys Acta* 1985 ; 131 : 579-85.
93. Snyder DS, Desforges JF. Lipoxygenase metabolites of arachidonic acid modulate hematopoiesis. *Blood* 1986 ; 67 : 1675-9.
94. Pelus LM, Gentile PS. In vivo modulation of myelopoiesis by prostaglandin E2.III. Induction of suppressor cells in marrow and spleen capable of mediating inhibition of CFU-GM proliferation. *Blood* 1988 ; 6 : 1633-40.
95. Nieburgs AC, Korn JH, Picciano PT, Cohen S. Thymic epithelium *in vitro*. IV. Regulation of growth and mediator production by epidermal growth factor. *Cell Immunol* 1987 ; 108 : 396-404.
96. Gualde N, Cook JM. Role of double negative thymocytes (CD4[-]CD8[-]) in the induction of tolerance to self. *FASEB J* 2 : A478 (abstract).
97. Delebassée S, Cogny Van Weydevelt F, Gualde N. Effects of eicosanoids on thymocyte physiology. *Immunobiol* 1988 ; Suppl 3 : 227-8.
98. Gualde N, Cogny Van Weydevelt F, Buffière F, Jauberteau MO, Daculsi R, Vaillier D. Influence of LTB_4 on CD4[-], CD8[-] thymocytes. Evidence that LTB_4 plus IL-2 generate CD8[+] suppressor thymocytes involved in tolerance to self. *Thymus* 1991 ; 18 : 111-28.
99. Gualde N, Rigaud M, Goodwin JS. Induction of suppressor cells from peripheral blood T cells by 15-HPETE. *Clin Res* 1983 ; 31 : 490-2.
100. Gualde N, Goodwin JS. Induction of suppressor T cells *in vitro* by arachidonic acid metabolites issued from the lipoxygenase pathway. In : Bailey M, ed. *Prostaglandins, leukotrienes and lipoxins*. New York : Plenum Press, 1985 : 565.
101. Atluru D, Goodwin JS. Control of polyclonal immunoglobulin production from human lymphocytes by leukotrienes ; leukotriene B_4 induces an OKT8(+), radiosensitive suppressor cell from resting human OKT8(-)T cells. *J Clin Invest* 1984 ; 74 : 1444-50.
102. Rola-Pleszczynski M. Leukotriene B4 induces human suppressor lymphocytes. *Biochim Biophys Acta* 1985 ; 4 : 1531-7.
103. Swat W, Ignatowicz L, Von Boehmer H, Kisielow P. Clonal deletion of immature CD4+8+ thymocytes in suspension culture by extrathymic antigen-presenting cells. *Nature* 1991 ; 351 : 150-3.
104. Ohashi P, Pircher H, Burki Z, Zinkernagel AM, Hengartner H. Distinct sequence of negative or positive selection implied by thymocyte T-cell receptor densities. *Nature* 1990 ; 346 : 861-3.
105. Fry AM, Jones LA, Kruisbeek AM, Matis LA. Thymic requirement for clonal deletion during T cell development. *Science* 1989 ; 246 : 1044-6.
106. Burnet FM. *The clonal selection theory of acquired immunity*. London : Cambridge University Press, 1959.

107. Blackman MA, Gerhard-Burgert H, Woodland DL, Palmer E, Kappler JW, Marrack P. A role for clonal inactivation in T cell tolerance to MIS-1. *Nature* 1990 ; 345 : 540-2.
108. Cohen IR, Wekerle H. Regulation of autosensitization.The immune activation and specific inhibition of self-recognizing thymus-derived lymphocytes. *J Exp Med* 1973 ; 330 : 224-38.
109. Vaillier D, Daculsi R, Gualde N, Bezian JH. Effect of LTB4 on the inhibition of natural cytotoxic activity by PGE2. *Cell Immunol* 1992 ; 139 : 248-58.
110. Vaillier D, Daculsi R, Gualde N. Effects of LPS on IL-2-induced cytotoxic activity of murine splenocytes cultures. Role of PGE2 and Interferons. *Cancer Immunol Immunother* 1992 ; 35 : 395-400.
111. Vaillier D, Daculsi R, Gualde N. PGE2 and LTB4 modulate both cytokines production and natural cytotoxic activity. *Biochem Pharmacol (Life Science Advances)* 1990 ; 9 : 347-55.
112. Rola-Pleszczynski M, Gagnon L, Sirois P. Leukotriene B4 augments human natural cytotoxic cell activity. *Biochem Biophys Acta* 1983 ; 113 : 531-7.
113. Rola-Pleszczynski M, Gagnon L, Rudzinska M, Borgeat P, Sirois S. Human natural cytotoxic cell activity :enhancement by leukotrienes (LT) A4,B4 and D4,but not by stereoisomers of LTB4 or HETES. *Prostaglandins Leukotrienes Med* 1984 ; 13 : 113-7.
114. Gagnon L, Girard M, Sullivan AK, Rola-Pleszczynski M. Augmentation of human natural cytotoxic cell activity by leukotriene B4 mediated by enhanced effector- target cell binding and increased lytic efficiency. *Cell Immunol* 1987 ; 110 : 243-52.
115. Whittum-Hudson J, Ballow M, Zurier RB. Effect of PGE1 treatment on *in vitro* thymocyte function of normal and autoimmune mice. *Immunopharmacology* 1988 ; 16 : 71-8.
116. Wolinski SI, Goodwin JS, Messner RP, Williams RJ Jr. Role of prostaglandin in the depressed cell-mediated immune response in rheumatoid arthritis. *Clin Immunol Immunopathol* 1980 ; 17 : 31-7.
117. Kato K, Koshihara Y, Fujiwara M, Murota S. Augmentation of 12-lipoxygenase activity of lymph node and spleen T cells in autoimmune mice MRL/1. *Prostaglandins Leukotrienes Med* 1983 ; 12 : 273-280.
118. Aldigier JC, Cook J, Delebassée S, Guibert F, Touchard G, Juzan M, Gualde N. NZB/NZW mouse nephritis and immune response are not changed by treatment with a 15-lipoxygenase derivative. *Prostaglandins Leukotrienes Essential Fatty Acids* 1992 ; 47 : 159-64.
119. Talbot SF, Atkins PC, Goetzl EJ, Zweiman B. Accumulation of leukotriene C4 and histamine in human allergic skin reaction. *J Clin Invest* 1985 ; 76 : 650-6.
120. Murray JJ, Tonnel A-B, Brash AR, Roberts JL, Gosset P, Workman R, Capron A, Oates J. Prostaglandin D2 is released during acute allergic bronchospasm in man. *Trans Assoc Am Phys* 1985 ; 98 : 275-80.
121. Bisgaard H, Ford-Hutchinson AW, Charleson S, Taudorf E. Production of leukotrienes in human skin and conjunctival mucosa after specific allergen challenge. *Allergy* 1985 ; 40 : 417-23.
122. Guez S, Gualde N, Bezian JH, Cabanieu G. *In vitro* study of platelets and circulating mononuclear cells of subjects presenting an intolerance to aspirin. *Int Arch Allergy Immunol* 1992 ; 97 : 233-6.
123. Lapp WS, Mendes M, Kirchner H. Prostaglandin synthesis by lymphoid tissue of mice experiencing a graft-versus-host reaction : relationship to immunosuppression. *Cell Immunol* 1980 ; 50 : 271-281.
124. Saffe BM, Moore TC, Vigran TS. Tissue levels of prostaglandin E following heterotopic rat heart allograft. *Surgery* 1975 ; 78 : 481-4.
125. Anderson CB, Jaffe BM, Graff RJ. Prolongation of murine skin allografts by prostaglandin E. *Transplantation* 1978 ; 23 : 444-7.
126. Strom TB, Carpenter CB. Prostaglandin as an effective antirejection therapy in rat renal allograft recipients. *Transplantation* 1983 ; 35 : 279-81.
127. Mangino MJ, Anderson CB, Deschryver K, Turk J. Arachidonate lipoxygenase products and renal allograft rejection in dogs. *Transplantation* 1987 ; 44 : 805-8.
128. Werner EJ, Nalenga RW, Dubowy RL, Boone S, Stuart MJ. Inhibition of human malig-

nant neuroblastoma cell DNA synthesis by lipoxygenase metabolites of arachidonic acid. *Cancer Res* 1985 ; 45 : 561-3.
129. Rozengurt E. A role for arachidonic acid and its metabolites in the regulation of p21ras activity. *Cancer Cells* 1991 ; 3 : 397-8.
130. Goodwin JS, Husby G, Williams RC Jr. Prostaglandin E and cancer growth. *Cancer Immunol Immunother* 1980 ; 8 : 3-7.
131. Goodwin JS. Prostaglandin synthetase inhibitors as immunoadjuvants in the treatment of cancer. *J Immunopharmacol* 1980 ; 2 : 397-424.
132. Ceuppens J, Goodwin JS. Prostaglandins and the immune response to cancer (review). *Anticancer Res* 1981 ; 1 : 71-8.
133. Rose DP, Connolly JM. Effects of fatty acids and inhibitors of eicosanoid synthesis on the growth of a human breast cancer cell line in culture. *Cancer Res* 1990 ; 50 : 7139-44.
134. Shimakura S, Boland CR. Eicosanoid production by the human gastric cancer cell line AGS and its relation to cell growth. *Cancer Res* 1992 ; 52 : 1744-9.
135. Hokama Y, Cripps C, Sumida K, Mookini RK, Oishi N. Significant increase of plasma prostaglandins in cancer patients. *Res Commun Chem Pathol Pharmacol* 1981 ; 31 : 379-82.
136. Ikemoto S, Kishimoto T, Nishio S, Wada S, Maekawa M. Correlation of tumor necrosis factor and prostaglandin E2 production of monocytes in bladder cancer patients. *Cancer* 1989 ; 64 : 2076-80.
137. Bockman R, Bellin A, Hickok N. Disorded prostaglandin production and cell differentiation/Proliferation in cancer. In : Thaler-Dao H, Crastes de Paulet A, Paoletti R, eds. *Eicosanoids and cancer*. New York : Raven Press, 1984 : 169-82.
138. Porteder H, Matjejka M, Ulrich W, Sinzinger H. The cyclo-oxygenase and lipoxygenase pathways in human oral cancer. *J Maxillofac Surg* 1984 ; 12 : 145-7.
139. Ikemoto S, Kishimoto T, Nishio S, Wada S, Maekawa M. Correlation of tumor necrosis factor and prostaglandin E2 production of monocytes in bladder cancer patients. *Cancer* 1989 ; 64 : 2076-80.
140. Lehnert T, Deschner EE, Karmali RA, DeCosse JJ. Effect of flurbiprofen and 16,16-dimethyl prostaglandin E2 on gastrointestinal tumorigenesis induced by N-methyl-N'-nitro-N-nitrosoguanidine in rats : glandular epithelium of stomach and duodenum. *Cancer Res* 1990 ; 50 : 381-4.
141. Goodwin JS, Messner RP, Bankhurst AD, Peake GT, Saiki JH, Williams RC Jr. Prostaglandin-producing suppressor cells in Hodgkin's disease. *N Engl J Med* 1977 ; 297 : 963-8.
142. Lee TH, Hoover RL, Williams JD, Sperling RI, Ravalese J, Spur BW, Robinson DR, Corey EJ, Lewis RA, Austen FK. Effect of dietary enrichment with eicosapentaenoic and docosahexaenoic acids on *in vitro* neutrophil and monocyte leukotriene generation and neutrophil function. *N Engl J Med* 1985 ; 312 : 1217-24.
143. Terano T, Salmon JA, Moncada S. Effect of orally administered eicosapentaenoic acid (EPA) on the formation of leukotriene B4 and leukotriene B5 by rat leukocyte. *Biochem Pharmacol* 1984 ; 33 : 3071-6.
144. Tou JS. Incorporation of arachidonic acid and eicosapentaenoic acid into phospholipids by polymorphonuclear leukocytes *in vitro*. *Lipids* 1984 ; 19 : 573-7.
145. Weiner TW, Sprecher H. Arachidonic acid, 5, 8, 11-eicosatrienoic acid and 5, 8, 11, 14, 17-eicosapentaenoic acid. Dietary manipulation of the levels of these acids in rat liver and platelet phospholipids and their incorporation into human lipids. *Biochim Biophys Acta* 1984 ; 792 : 293-303.
146. Ishinaga M, Takamura H, Rarita H, Kito M. Changes of linoleic, arachidonic and eicosapentaenoic acids in rat platelet, aorta and plasma lipids after changing from a sardine oil diet to a corn oil diet. *Agric Biol Chem* 1985 ; 49 : 2741-6.
147. Chapkin RS, Carmichael SL. Effects of dietary N-3 and N-6 polyunsaturated fatty acids on macrophage phospholipid classes and subclasses. *Lipids* 1990 ; 25 : 827-34.
148. Prickett JD, Robinson DR, Steinberg AD. Effects of dietary enrichment with eicosapen-

taenoic acid upon autoimmune nephritis in female NZBxNZW/F1 mice. *Arthritis Rheum* 1983 ; 26 : 133-9.
149. Prickett JD, Robinson DR, Steinberg AD. Dietary enrichment with the polyunsaturated fatty acid eicosapentaenoic acid prevents proteinuria. *J Clin Invest* 1981 ; 68 : 556-9.
150. Lee TH, Mencia-Huerta JM, Shih C, Corey EJ, Lewis RA, Austen FK. Characterization and biologic properties of 5,12-dihydroxy derivatives of eicosapentaenoic acid, including leukotriene B5 and the double lipoxygenase product. *J Biol Chem* 1984 ; 259 : 2383-9.
151. Lokesh BR, Kinsella JE. Modulation of prostaglandin synthesis in mouse peritoneal macrophages by enrichment of lipids with either eicosapentaenoic or docosahexaenoic acids *in vitro*. *Immunobiol* 1987 ; 175 : 406-19.
152. Lokesh BR, German B, Kinsella JE. Differential effects of docosahexaenoic acid and eicosapentaenoic acid on suppression of lipoxygenase pathway in peritoneal macrophages. *Biochim Biophys Acta* 1988 ; 958 : 99-107.
153. Weaver BJ, Holub BJ. The inhibition of arachidonic acid incorporation into human platelet phospholipids by eicosapentaenoic acid. *Nutr Res* 1985 ; 5 : 31-7.
154. Kobatake Y, Kuroda K, Jinnouchi H, Nishide E, Innami S. Differential effects of dietary eicosapentaenoic and docosahexaenoic fatty acids on lowering of triglyceride and cholesterol levels in the serum of rats on hypercholesterolemic diet. *J Nutr Sci Vitamin* 1984 ; 30 : 357-72.
155. Magrum LJ, Johnston PV. Effect of culture *in vitro* with eicosatetraenoic (20 :4(n-6)) and eicosapentaenoic (20 :5(n-3)) acids on fatty acid composition, prostaglandin synthesis and chemiluminescence of rat peritoneal macrophages. *Biochim Biophys Acta* 1985 ; 836 : 354-60.

17

Anti-inflammatory drugs and immunomodulation

L.F. PERRIN[1], *P.E. LAURENT*[2]

[1] Faculté des Sciences, Université Catholique, Lyon, France.
Faculté de Médecine, Lyon, France.
[2] Institut Pasteur, Lyon, France.

Anti-inflammatory agents include two large classes of drugs:
a) the glucocorticosteroids, a.k.a. glucocorticoids or corticosteroids, derived from the adrenal cortex, such as corticone and hydrocortisone, or synthetic analogues,
b) the non-steroidal anti-inflammatory drugs (NSAID).

Both groups are used in inflammatory processes and both have effects on the immune response, but there, at times their effects appear to be antagonistic.

Glucocorticosteroids

Since their introduction in 1950, corticosteroids have assumed a major role in the treatment of inflammatory and immunologically mediated diseases. Along with their anti-inflammatory properties, they have indeed potent immunosuppressive effects, which is the main reason of their use when the immune system has to be slowed down, as in auto-immune diseases for instance.

Cortisone (coupound E) was first isolated by Kendall *et al.* in 1935. Sufficient quantities were obtained in 1948 for its administration to patients by Hench and associates.

Cortisol (or hydrocortisone) is the major glucocorticoid in man. A number of synthetic analogues of cortisol are available for clinical usage. All glucocorticoids consist of a basic steroid nucleus with varying side groups. They have different potencies and duration of action, as shown in Table I.

Table I. Comparison of commonly used corticosteroids (data from [1]).

Name	Equivalent dose (mg)	Relative anti-inflammatory potency
Hydrocortisone	20.00	1.00
Cortisone	25.00	0.8
Prednisone	5.0	4.0
Prednisolone	5.0	4.0
Methylprednisolone	4.0	5.0
Triamcinolone	4.0	5.0
Betamethasone	0.6	20-30
Dexamethasone	0.75	30-30

Absorption of glucocorticoids occur in the upper jejunum and peak plasma levels are attained in 30 to 100 min. In the blood, these agents are largely bound to plasma proteins (transcortin, and to a far lesser extent, albumin). The bound steroid is inactive in this form, and serves as a store in equilibrium with the free hormone. Only the unbound fraction is active therapeutically. Approximately 95 % of the cortisol present is bound to plasma proteins. Synthetic glucocorticoids bind less tightly to both transcortin and albumin than natural cortisol and therefore diffuse more completely into tissue.

Regarding the evaluation of the literature of the effects of glucocorticoids on immune response, an important point has to be mentionned : the difference between the effects of glucocorticoids in different species.

The mouse, rat and rabbit are corticoid-sensitive species. On the other hand, man, as well as the monkey and guinea pig, is much less susceptible to the effects of glucocorticoids and is termed corticosteroid-resistant. Thus, many studies showing profound effects on immunological parameters in a corticosteroid-sensitive animal do not apply to man. Nevertheless, some of them have been shown to be operative in humans. Another pitfall is that many studies using *in vitro* systems have shown effects only at concentrations of corticosteroids unattainable *in vivo* for any significant period of time.

Nevertheless, steroids have a depressive effect on the immune response. This effect is achieved through several ways :
— by inhibiting leukocyte movements and migration of cells to areas of inflammation,
— by inhibiting mediator release and cytokines release,
— by suppressing cell-mediated hypersensitivity,
— perhaps, but to a far lesser extent, by influencing humoral antibody titers.

The mechanisms of action of steroids have to be considered at different levels.

Corticosteroid-mediated immunoregulation mechanisms have been reviewed in detail [2, 3].

Subcellular mechanisms

One of the main findings has been the discovery of glucocorticoid receptors.

- *Glucocorticoid receptors*

Steroids interact with specific receptors in order to modify the behaviour of target cells.

Glucocorticoids can freely penetrate cellular membranes and bind to a specific cytoplasmic receptor in the target cell. The steroid-receptor complex undergoes modification and is translocated to the nucleus of the cell. There the complex binds to nuclear chromatin causing formation of a protein lipomodulin with a molecular weight of 40,000. This lipomodulin was shown to be a potent inhibitor of phospholipase A2 and of neutrophil chemotaxis.

This cellular model of glucocorticoid action has been shown to be applicable to the immune response in steroid-sensitive species.

In humans, specific receptors have been identified in normal lymphocytes [4], monocytes [5], neutrophils and eosinophils [6], but corticosteroid responsiveness does not appear to directly correlate with receptor-related parameters. For instance, circulating peripheral blood leukocytes, with demonstrable different responses to *in vivo* administered corticosteroids, have similar intracytoplasmic corticosteroid receptors profiles.

Nevertheless, macrophages and bone marrow cells have much more glucocorticoid receptors (about 13,920 for each cell) than peripheral blood B and T lymphocytes that have a mean of 4,000 receptors/cell.

Other subcellular mechanisms may be important in the immunoregulatory effects of glucosteroids : level of intracellular ATP, accumulation of cyclic-AMP, perturbation in cell membranes.

Cellular mechanisms

- *Leukocyte movement :* shifts in traffic of circulating cells.

A portion of the normal pool of peripheral blood lymphocytes recirculates between intravascular and extravascular compartments [7]. In corticosteroid-sensitive species, glucocorticoid administration produces a profound circulating lymphopenia due to cell death. In man, glucocorticoid administration results in a circulation lymphopenia too, not due to cell death but due to the redistribution of lymphocytes out of the circulation into other body compartments.

Another feature of the corticosteroid-induced lymphopenia in man is its relative selectivity for T lymphocytes and particularly for $CD4^+$. Studies in man have demonstrated that T cells from the normal circulating lymphocytes pool enter bone marrow parenchyma in the same way as in guinea pigs. Fauci *et al.* [8], as well as Moretta *et al.* [9], have shown that the lymphopenia involves a greater depletion of those T cells with a Fc receptor for IgM, compared to those cells with an Fc receptor for IgG. This may be one mechanism by which corticosteroids can exert a selective effect on immunologic regulation.

A profound monocytopenia is observed following corticosteroid administration, probably due to a redistribution phenomenon similar to that of the lymphocytes.

Monocytes are even more sensitive than lymphocytes to the redistribution effect of lower doses of glucocorticoid. Monocyte chemotaxis is inhibited by *in vitro* glucocorticoids in the pharmacological concentration range while neutrophil chemotaxis is unaffected by as high as 30 times as much corticosteroid [10]. On the other hand, administration of glucosteroid produces a neutrophilic leukocytosis. The neutrophil count rise is due to the accelerated release of mature neutrophils from the bone marrow and their decreased egress from the blood. The most important effect of corticosteroids on inflammation is to suppress leukocyte accumulation at an inflammatory site.

At the same time, a profound decrease in circulating eosinophils is observed (basis of the Thorn test) probably due to redistribution of cells to other body compartments.

• *Leukocyte function*. Investigation of glucocorticoid effects on leukocyte function are difficult to interpret. Many of the *in vitro* studies are done at concentrations of drug that are seldom if ever achieved *in vivo*.

Moreover, studies on isolated cells have yielded results somewhat different from those obtained with specific *in vitro* immunological models of cellular immunity. The latter have shown that the corticosteroid-induced changes of the function of individual lymphoid cells may not be directly extended to situations where these cells are only part of a more complex *in vivo* immunologic system.

Lymphocyte proliferation responses to antigens and mitogens have been extensively studied. *In vitro*, the lymphocyte blastogenic response to mitogens is blocked by high concentrations of glucocorticoids.

The proliferative response of the allogenic mixed leukocytic reaction (MLR) is inhibited by pharmacologic concentrations of glucocorticoids. The autologuous MLR is inhibited by both *in vitro* and *in vivo* glucocorticoids. Conflicting results have produced some confusion about the effect of corticosteroids on lymphocyte proliferation, presumably deriving mainly from differences in culture methods and assay systems [11]. Studies in humans treated with corticosteroids have shown that lymphocyte responses to antigen are more easily suppressed than responses to several non specific mitogens. This suggests either a differential sensitivity to corticosteroids of the various subpopulations of lymphocytes or a selective depletion from the circulation of certain of these subpopulations.

At physiological concentrations, glucocorticoids produce a lymphopenia which is more important for T-helper lymphocytes ($CD4^+$) than for T-suppressor cells ($CD8^+$).

• *Degranulation and mediator release*. Degranulation of mast cells and basophils, and subsequent inflammatory mediator release are recognized as a classic mechanism in an allergen-induced immune response.

Inhibition of this mediator release is known to be an important anti-inflammatory mechanism of steroids. *In vitro*, it has been shown that degranulation of rodent mast cells and basophils is inhibited by low concentrations of steroids, but that human mast cells are not sensitive. Conversely, steroids inhibit degranulation of human basophils stimulated by IgE-directed stimuli.

Steroids also inhibit the release of eicosanoids, products of arachidonic acid metabolism, from a variety of cell types.

Actually, it is now known that the ability of steroids to inhibit eicosanoid release is due to the inhibition of the enzyme responsible for release of arachidonic acid, phospholipase A2. The name of « lipocortin » was assigned for the proteins (initially named « macrocortin » and « lipomodulin ») which mediate the action of steroids on eicosanoid release. Lipocortins were shown to have immunomodulatory actions, and to inhibit neutrophil chemotaxis [12]. (A major step in the study of lipocortins was the production of recombinant material. The gene for the protein now known as « lipocortin I » has been cloned, and the recombinant human protein expressed in *E. coli.*).

Finally, steroids are good inhibitors of arachidonic acid metabolites release, as well as PAF formation, in many cell types.

• *Leukocyte priming.* Primed inflammatory cells release many more mediators than unprimed cells. For instance, primed eosinophils or basophils release 3 to 10 times as much leucotriene as unprimed leukocytes. Priming is induced by different cytokines. Glucocorticoids prevent the priming response of neutrophils to gamma-interferon, and of eosinophils to GM-CSF, but not the priming of basophils by IL3.

So it appears that steroids can selectively inhibit the response of granulocytes to the priming cytokines. Moreover, they can also block the release of these priming cytokines.

• *Cytokine release.* Inhibition of cytokine release is probably one of the most important anti-inflammatory effects of steroids, since it can be regarded as a main link in the chain of immunosuppressive mechanisms.

« Cytokines and cytokine networks are part of a complex, multifaceted regulatory apparatus that involves the nervous system, endocrine system and other modulators of cell function such as histamine, serotonine, kinins, prostaglandins, leukotrienes, neuropeptides and neuro-transmitters » [13]. Glucocorticosteroids block production of a variety of cytokines, and so, cut communications between the cells of the immune system, and also between the immune and nervous systems.

Several peptides mediators, like IL-1, are secreted in response to various forms of stress and are suppressed by corticosteroids.

Thus corticosteroids can be regarded as serving the physiological function in stress of protecting the organism from its own activated defence mechanisms, preventing these mechanisms from overshooting and themselves causing damage.

Corticosteroids and infection

From a clinical viewpoint, steroids can alter the course of most infectious diseases ; many types of infection occur more frequently in patients receiving long-term treatment with steroids.

However, the risk is variable. Gram-negative bacterial and staphylococcal infections, tuberculosis, as well as certain types of fungal and viral infections, are most frequently encountered.

Most of our current knowledge indicates that it is chiefly the leukocytes rather than the humoral components of the defence mechanisms that are altered. The bactericidal activity of monocytes from patients receiving steroids is reduced. Steroids seem to suppress phagocytosis by peripheral monocytes and macrophages *in vitro* [10], and it has been shown *in vivo* that corticosteroids block reticuloendothelial system clearance of opsonized and non-opsonized material.

Corticosteroids and hypersensitivity reactions

After antigen challenge in a sensitive patient, there is a release of direct acting mediators resulting in immediate bronchoconstriction : this is the early phase pulmonary response. There is also cell recruitment that results in additional mediator release and sustained bronchoconstriction, occurring several hours after the challenge : this is the late phase pulmonary response. Even administered by aerosol before the challenge, corticosteroids have no definite effects on the early phase but block the late phase pulmonary response, cell recruitement being inhibited.

In skin testing, immediate response is not altered by corticosteroids, but cutaneous delayed hypersensitivity is suppressed, as a result of a decrease in the recruitment of macrophages necessary to the expression of cellular immunity.

In contrast with the action in cell-mediated immunity, glucocorticoid effects on humoral factors involved in the immune response appear to be clinically insignificant. Suppression of antibody production following glucocorticoid administration can be demonstrated in corticosteroid-sensitive species, but in man specific antibody synthesis is not suppressed. Serum IgG and IgA levels have been reported to be decreased after glucocorticoid treatment, but in some allergic patients both total IgE and specific IgE increased. IgE production appears to be sensitive to the regulatory suppressive effects of T lymphocytes. The decrease in T cell mediated suppressor activity, after glucocorticoid treatment, may explain this increase in serum IgE levels [14]. Complement metabolism is not affected by glucocorticoids in man.

Conclusion

Corticosteroids have a potent anti-inflammatory action. They suppress acute and chronic inflammation by inhibiting virtually every step in the inflammatory process. They cause redistribution of leukocytes, suppress the recruitment of monocytes/macrophages, and they inhibit a wide variety of leukocyte functions that are involved in immunologic and inflammatory processes.

Along with their anti-inflammatory action, corticosteroids have potent immunosuppressive effects, that are widely used in the treatment of auto-immune diseases. But these effects are also responsible for a diminished resistance to infections.

Non-steroidal anti-inflammatory drugs

Non-steroidal anti-inflammatory drugs (NSAID) are extensively used in a wide range of diseases, not only in the field of rheumatology but in many clinical disorders such as ENT diseases, vascular process or after trauma and plastic surgery.

These drugs are highly effective in many stages of the inflammatory process and have also other effects, particularly on the immune response.

It must be emphasized that these effects are quite different from those of the corticosteroids. Nevertheless, in France NSAID are often assimilated to corticosteroids regarding their effect on the immune function, because of their action on leukocytes movements. Table II shows the most commonly used NSAID.

Table II. Principal chemical types of NSAID.

Salicylates	Aspirin
Pyrazole derivatives	Phenylbutazone
	Oxyphenbutazone
Indoleacetic acids	Indomethacin
	Sulindac
Propionic acid derivatives	Ibuprofen
	Indoprofen
	Fenoprofen
	Ketoprofen
	Naproxen
	Fenbufen
	Pirprofen
Fenamates	Mefenamic acid
	Flufenamic acid
Anthranilic acid derivatives	Tolfenamic acid
Oxicams	Piroxicam
Phenylacetic acid derivative	Sulindac
Nicotinic acid derivatives	Niflumic acid

Actions of NSAID on the migration of leucocytes

Several NSAID have been reported to decrease the migration of total leukocytes into inflammatory exudates.

Di Rosa et al. [15] showed that indomethacin, phenylbutazone, flufenamic acid and even aspirin, suppressed the migration of mononuclear cells into inflamed tissues. Perper et al. [16] demonstrated effective inhibition of mononuclear cells after oral administration of indomethacin, phenylbutazone and mefenamic acid.

Indomethacin, naproxen and ketoprofen, when administered prophylactically, have been shown able to suppress mononuclear cell migration into the pleural cavity of rats 24 h after injections of carrageenin.

Conversely, the inhibitory effects of indomethacin on mononuclear cells were not demonstrated in other studies at the same dose levels, but only at higher dose levels [17].

No corresponding effects were observed on polymorphonuclear (PMN) migration in these studies.

However, many studies have shown that, at least some but not all, NSAID at therapeutic drug concentrations inhibit the migration of polymorphonuclear leukocytes or monocytes, or both, *in vitro* as well as *in vivo* [18].

The mechanisms whereby the NSAID exert their effects, when they exist, against leukocyte migration are not well defined. It was suggested by Vane (1971) that the effects of aspirin-like drugs were attributable to their ability to inhibit the cyclo-oxygenase enzyme, and hence the production of inflammatory prostaglandins. But the profile activity of indomethacin, one of the most potent inhibitors of prostaglandin-synthetase *in vitro*, did not totally fall in line with this theory, as this agent failed to reduce the accumulation of leukocytes *in vivo* in implanted polyester sponges. It appears therefore that whereas the role of prostaglandins in inflammation is well documented, their role in the control of leukocyte movements is not established.

Moreover, the effects of NSAID on mononuclear cells and PMN differ widely. Analysis of the effects of NSAID on cell movement revealed that the random movements and the chemotactic migration are dissociated events. Rivkin *et al.* [18] demonstrated that naproxen, ibuprofen and aspirin inhibited the chemotaxis of human peripheral blood PMN, but that these same drugs, at the same concentration, had no effect on random or spontaneous movements of these cells.

On the contrary, it must be reminded that glucocorticosteroids inhibit both chemotaxis and spontaneous movements, and hence differ from the NSAID, and do not share the same effects on the immune response.

On the other hand, Dawson (1980) reported that ibuprofen inhibited monocyte chemotaxis *in vitro*, whereas indomethacin, naproxen and salicylate did not. He also found differences in the effects of various NSAID on polymorphonuclear leukocytes chemotaxis. Several NSAID caused significant inhibition, but indomethacin did not.

Other authors had different results when the assay was carried out under other methods.

Reports on the effects of NSAID tend to vary considerably and this may be due to differences in cell sources and in techniques used for the assessment of chemotaxis.

Because all NSAID inhibit cyclo-oxygenase, these results show that their interference with leukocytic migration is not related to their effects on prostaglandins.

Furthermore, whether or not these effects *in vitro* can be extrapolated to effects *in vivo* remains to be established [19].

NSAID, prostaglandins and the immune response

Inflammatory mediators that alter the tissue microenvironment may be either released from secretory granules of mast cells and basophils, or they may be derived from the membrane phospholipids and generated during cell activation, as is the case for metabolites of arachidonic acid.

Arachidonic acid may be metabolized *via* the lipo-oxygenase enzyme pathway with the formation of leukotrienes, or *via* the cyclo-oxygenase pathway with the formation of endoperoxides, thromboxane A2 and prostaglandins. Prostaglandins exert an important influence on the immune response at different levels, particularly as agents which modulate the response of sensitized cells to antigens and alter the release of mediators of immediate and delayed hypersensitivity, and also as agents which alter the response of migrating leukocytes to chemotactic stimuli and thereby influence immunologically mediated inflammation.

Now, we know that NSAID inhibit cyclo-oxygenase, and thus the production of prostaglandins. As prostaglandins have important immunoregulatory properties, NSAID by inhibiting prostaglandin production should be able to modulate immune responses *in vitro* and *in vivo*.

• *Effects of NSAID on cellular immunity* in vitro. The effects of prostaglandins have been studied on *in vitro* lymphocyte proliferation. Physiologic concentrations of PGE2 suppress many *in vitro* manifestations of T lymphocytic function : antigenic stimulation, mitogen responsiveness, lymphokine production, among other effects. Natural killer activity and antibody-dependant cytotoxic activity are also inhibited by PGE2.

In human blood, the cell responsible for PGE2 production is a monocyte. An increased activity of these monocytes has been shown to be at least partly responsible for depressed immune responses. The role of the prostaglandin producing monocyte in the hyporesponsiveness to PHA of monocytes from patients with untreated Hodgkin's disease is well documented [20]. The addition of indomethacin to the cell culture almost totally reverses the depressed PHA response.

Thus indomethacin, and probably other NSAID, can be considered as stimulating the immune response *in vitro*.

• *Effects of NSAID on cellular immunity* in vivo. Several studies showed that NSAID *in vivo* act as general immunostimulants, increasing cellular immune responses in humans and experimental animals. Inhibition of endogenous prostaglandins biosynthesis by indomethacin shortened allograft survival, and this effect was completely abrogated by concurrent injections of PGE2 [21].

In guinea pigs previously sensitized to *Mycobacterium bovis*, the intradermal injection of *M. bovis* antigen resulted in a more than two-fold increase in delayed skin test reaction when guinea pigs were given indomethacin.

Natural killer cell activity is also enhanced *in vivo* by NSAID. It has been shown that the BCG-induced augmentation of natural killer cell activity is potentiated by NSAID as a result of inhibition of prostaglandins synthesis [22].

In normal man, indomethacin did not influence the delayed hypersensitivity skin testing ; but when indomethacin was administered to subjects with depressed cellular immunity, there was an enhancement of delayed hypersensitivity [23]. These studies, among others, confirm that cellular immune responses can be enhanced *in vivo* as well as *in vitro* by administration of NSAID.

Immunodeficient anergic patients can become reactive to skin tests during indomethacin treatment, and are anergic again when the medication is stopped.

Thus it appears that PGE acts as a feedback inhibitor of delayed hypersensitivity and that the administration of NSAID, by suppressing PGE production, can restore cellular immune response. These studies among others confirm that cellular immune responses can be enhanced *in vivo* as well as *in vitro* by administration of NSAID.

In one approach to this problem, we studied the influence of niflumic acid, a potent NSAID, on the consequences of the immunodeficiency induced by major thermal injury. The immunodeficiency results, in part, to enhanced susceptibility to infection, related mainly to activation of T lymphocytes with suppressive effects. It has been shown that peripheral blood contains toxic factors which alter the lymphocyte functions. Among these substances, prostaglandins, mostly PGE2, are known to produce T suppressor activation. Furthermore, prostaglandin biosynthesis is dramatically increased at the site of injury. Thus, NSAID would be expected to reduce this T suppressor effect.

Thirty-two patients were studied, 16 controls and 16 niflumic acid treated burned patients (burn surface area range : 30 % to 90 %). Although no statistically significant difference was observed between the two groups, the number of patients with non suppressive effects of serum was greater in the treated groupe (using the mixed lymphocyte culture test or the PHA lymphoblastogenic test) but the difference was not significative. These results suggest that production of prostaglandin in damaged tissues is not the main factor of altered immunity, and also that the physiological role of PGE2 is more complex than previously stated [24, 25].

• *Effects of NSAID on the humoral response.* The influence of NSAID on the humoral response seems to be mediated through effects on prostaglandins. Pharmacological doses of PGE2 inhibit immunoglobulin production by human B cells *in vitro* [26]. Thus, it can be expected that NSAID, by blocking prostaglandin synthesis, increase immunoglobulin production by B cells. This is precisely what can be seen in several experimental models.

Most effects of PGE seem to be mediated through the T cell regulation of antibody production. Suppressor T cells have a much higher density of PGE2 receptors on their membrane than helper T cells. By blocking prostaglandin synthesis, NSAIDs interfere with suppressor T cells more than with helper T cells, and so enhance *in vitro* B cell function. *In vivo* studies have also shown an enhancement of humoral immune responses with an NSAID (indomethacin) [23].

• *Effects of NSAID on autoantibody production.* A culture of human mononuclear cells stimulated with pokeweed mitogen was used to evaluate the *in vitro* effect of PG and PG-synthetase inhibitors on autoantibody production [20].

Lymphocytes from patients with rheumatoid arthritis produce IgM rheumatoid factor ; PGE is normally produced in these cultures. When an NSAID (indomethacin) is added to the culture, the IgM rheumatoid factor production is inhibited. Thus, it seems that endogenous PGE stimulates IgM rheumatoid factor production ; when PGE synthesis is inhibited rheumatoid factor falls, and when PGE is added rheumatoid factor rises.

Conclusion

A number of NSAIDs are available and are highly efficient on inflammatory processes. The effects of these drugs on the immune response are not so well defined as those of the corticosteroids. On the whole, they inhibit the migration of leukocytes, a fact which can suggest a depression of the immune response. But the results differ widely according to techniques, and the relevance of this action remains to be established in clinical practice. On the contrary, by inhibiting prostaglandin synthesis, NSAID appear to stimulate cellular and humoral immune response. Experimental data, *in vitro* and *in vivo*, as well as a some clinical observations, tend to prove that, far from being immunodepressant, NSAID possess some immunostimulant properties.

References

1. Townley RG, Suliaman F. *Ann Allergy* 1987 ; 58 : 1-6.
2. Parillo JE, Fauci AS. Mechanisms of glucocorticoid action on immune processes. *Annu Rev Pharmacol Toxicol* 1979 ; 19 : 179-201.
3. Cupps TR, Fauci AS. Corticosteroid-mediated immunoregulation in man. *Immunol Rev* 1982 ; 65 : 133-55.
4. Lippman ME, Barr R. Glucocorticoid receptors in purified subpopulations of human peripheral blood lymphocytes. *J Immunol* 1977 ; 118 : 1977-81.
5. Werb Z, Foley R, Munck A. Interaction of glucocorticoid with macrophages. Identification of glucocorticoids receptors in monocytes and macrophages. *J Exp Med* 1978 ; 147 : 1684.
6. Peterson AP, Altman LC, Hill JS, *et al*. Glucocorticoid receptors in normal human eosinophils. Comparison with neutrophils. *J Allergy Clin Immunol* 1981 ; 62 : 212.
7. Scott JL, Davidson JG, Marino JV, *et al*. Leukocyte labelling with ^{51}chromium. The kinetics of normal lymphocytes. *Blood* 1972 ; 40 : 276.
8. Fauci AS, Dale DC, Balow JE. Glucocorticosteroid therapy : mechanisms of action and clinical considerations. *Ann Intern Med* 1976 ; 84 : 304-15.
9. Moretta L, Webb SR, Grossi CE, *et al*. Functionnal analysis of two human T cell subpopulations : help and suppression of B cell responses by T cells bearing receptors for IgM or IgG. *J Exp Med* 1977 ; 146 : 184-200.
10. Rinehart JJ, Balcerzak SP, Sagone AI, *et al*. Effects of corticosteroids on human monocyte function. *J Clin Invest* 1974 ; 54 : 1337.
11. Heilman DH, Gambrill M, Leichner JP. The effect of hydrocortisone on the incorporation of tritiated thymidine by human blood lymphocytes cultured with phytohaemaglutinin and pokeweed mitogen. *Clin Exp Immunol* 1973 ; 15 : 203.
12. Sertl K, Clark T, Kaliner M. Corticosteroids : their biologic mechanisms and applications to the treatment of asthma. *Am Rev Respir Dis* 1990 ; 141 : S1-S96.
13. Elias JA, Zitnik RJ. Cytokine-cytokine interactions in the context of cytokine networking. *Am J Respir Cell Mol Biol* 1992 ; 7 : 365-7.
14. Saxon A, Stevens RH, Ramer SJ, *et al*. Glucocorticoids administered *in vivo* inhibit human suppressor T lymphocyte function and diminish B lymphocyte responsiveness *in vitro* immunoglubilin synthesis. *J Clin Invest* 1977 ; 61 : 922.
15. Di Rosa M, Sorrentino L, Parente L. Non-steroidal anti-inflammatory drugs and leukocyte emigration. *J Pharm Pharmacol* 1972 ; 24 : 575.

16. Perper RJ, Sanda M, Chinea G, et al. Leukocytes chemotaxis *in vivo* : II. Analysis of the selective inhibition of neutrophils or mononuclear cell accumulation. *J Lab Clin Med* 1974 ; 84 : 394.
17. Warne PJ, West GB. Inhibition of leukocyte migration by salicylates and indomethacin. *J Pharm Pharmacol* 1978 ; 30 : 783.
18. Rivkin L, Foschi GV, Rosen CH. Inhibition of *in vitro* neutrophil chemotaxis and spontaneous motility by anti-inflammatory agents. *Proc Soc Exp Biol Med* 1976 ; 153 : 236.
19. Perrin LF, Laurent PE. Aspirine et immunité. *Med Hyg* 1989 ; 47 : 1887.
20. Ceuppens IL, Goodwin JS. Immunological responses in treatment with non-steroidal anti-inflammatory drugs, with particular reference to the role of prostaglandins. In : Rainsford KD, ed. *Anti-inflammatory and anti-rheumatic drugs.* Vol. I. Boca Raton : CRC Press, 1985.
21. Anderson CB, Jaffee BM, Graff RJ. Prolongation of murine skin allograft by prostaglandin E. *Transplantation* 1977 ; 23 : 444.
22. Tracey DE, Adkinson NF. Prostaglandin synthesis inhibitors potentiate the BCG-induced augmentation of natural killer cell activity. *J Immunol* 1980 ; 125 : 136.
23. Goodwin JS, Selinger DS, Messner RP, et al. Effect of indomethacin *in vivo* on humoral and cellular immunity in humans. *Infect Immun* 1978 ; 19 : 430.
24. Gros P, Laurent PE, Marichy J, Freidel AC, Perrin LF, Bienvenu J, Betuel H. The effect of a non-steroidal anti-inflammatory agent (NSAID) on lymphocyte activity after burn. *Int Arch Allerg Appl Immunol* 1987 ; suppl. avril : 16.
25. Perrin LF, Laurent PE, Gros P. Anti-inflammatoires non stéroidiens et immunodépression, risques réels ou innocuité ? *Med Hyg* 1987 ; 45 : 1816.
26. Morito T, Bankhurst, Willimas RC. Studies on the modulation of immunoglobulin production by prostaglandins. *Prostaglandins* 1980 ; 20 : 383.

18

Immunological effects of neuropsychotropic substances

B. Deleplanque, P.J. Neveu

*INSERM U 259, Université de Bordeaux II,
Domaine de Carreire, rue Camille Saint-Saens
33077 Bordeaux, France.*

The central nervous system (CNS) has recently been shown to regulate activity of the immune system. CNS modulates the neuroendocrine system and especially the hypothalamo-pituitary axis which is known to have immunoregulatory functions [1]. Furthermore, lymphoid tissues including the thymus, spleen, lymph nodes, mesenteric patches, are innervated by sympathetic and parasympathetic components of the autonomic nervous system (ANS). Morphological features of both parts of the ANS have been described extensively [2-4].

Neurotransmitters and neuropeptides, apart from neuroendocrine hormones, may be the major mediators of the neuroimmune interactions. Clinical studies have shown that most neuropsychiatric diseases accompanied by immunological changes have central neurochemical correlates. Examples include the degeneration of cholinergic neurons and receptors in Alzheimer's dementia, dysfunction of the central dopaminergic pathways in schizophrenia and Parkinson's disease, alteration of various monoaminergic and opiate peptide neuronal networks associated with depression and stress.

The modes of action of neurotransmitters and neuropeptides are quite diversified. They can modulate the ANS outflow [5, 6] and the neuroendocrine secretion, for example, dopaminergic neurons of the tuberoinfundibular region inhibit prolactine release and its immunoregulatory consequence [7]. Opiate peptides stimulate pituitary secretion of growth hormone, prolactine and corticotropin [8-10]. Circulating opiates and monoamines are themselves released by pituitary and/or adrenal glands under physiological conditions or during stress [11]. Finally, the release of neurotransmitters and neuropeptides by nerve endings not only regulates blood outflow but also participates in the biochemical microenvironment of immune cells [3].

There is also a growing body of evidences for a specific binding of neurotransmitters and neuropeptides with lymphocytes and macrophages.

Most drugs with neuropsychotropic effects interact with neurotransmitter systems, either directly as receptor agonists or antagonists, or indirectly by inhibiting their reuptake or degradation. Similarly, most of these drugs have immunoregulatory properties that may only be side effects. Still conversely, these drugs may be potential candidates for immunotherapy.

The immunological effects of neurotransmitters, neuropeptides or drugs may be mediated by central and/or peripheral mechanisms. On a methodological point of view, the role of central pathways may be demonstrated *in vivo* either by chemical or surgical lesions of specific CNS regions or by the intracisternal injections of agonists or antagonists. The peripheral role of neurotransmitters can be shown by denervation experiments or by *in vitro* assays. Likewise, the peripheral effects of neuropeptides and drugs have been studied *in vitro*. Usually, *in vitro* concentrations of these substances should be similar to physiological plasma levels. However, higher concentrations may be justified for their relevance to physiology as they could be compatible to that found to occur in the vicinity of nerve endings or in inflammatory sites.

The involvement of specific receptors on immune cells, in contrast to non-specific membrane effects, must be demonstrated by the examination of dose-dependent effects and by their suppression by specific receptor blockage.

A neuroimmune network not only involves connections between the brain and the lymphoid tissues in the periphery but also implies cell communications at the level of the immune microenvironment which may be considered as an immune neuroendocrine complex.

Immunoregulatory roles of neurotransmitters

Noradrenaline

The lymphoid tissues are mainly innervated by the sympathetic nervous system [2-4]. The suggestion is that catecholamines may have some immunomodulatory roles. The immunomodulatory role of peripheral noradrenaline (NA) has been first assessed either by chemical (using 6-hydroxydopamine : 6-OHDA) or surgical spleen sympathectomy experiments in animals. In neonates sympathectomy normally enhances the number of plaque forming cells (PFC) in response to thymus dependent [12, 13] and thymus independent antigens [14]. Chemical sympathectomy also stimulates natural killer cell (NK) activity even though the effect is transient [15]. In adult animals, NK cell activity is enhanced also after chemical sympathectomy [16]. Similar to neonates, the PFC response to T independent antigens is enhanced with sympathectomy [14], while the PFC response to T dependent antigens is suppressed [17]. Blockade of catecholamine synthesis by α-methyl-p-tyrosine (AMPT) has been shown to depress NK cell activity, however AMPT is active on both central and peripheral catecholamines [18]. The differences in the immunological effects of neonatal or adult sympathectomy may be explained, at least partly, by differences in the development of the noradrenergic innervation of lymphoid tissues. Indeed in the newborn, NA innervation is not fully developed [19] and 6-OHDA treatment produces a definitive neuronal destruction, while in adults, the drug only induces a reversible axotomy. Furthermore, 6-OHDA crosses the blood-brain barrier in neonates but not in adults. Therefore, in neonates, 6-OHDA may impair the central noradrenergic transmission which is possibly involved in neuroimmunomodulation.

The role of catecholamines in immunomodulation may also be demonstrated by modifications of the NA-turnover in lymphoid tissues during immune responses. The first experiment [20] showed that after immunization against sheep erythrocytes, the content of noradrenaline in the spleen dropped just before the peak of the PFC response. A recent study [21] using the same antigen does not confirm the decrease of spleen adrenaline content but shows an enhanced neuronal activity as assessed by the increase of the catecholamine metabolite (DOPAC) levels.

Systemic administration of catecholamines modifies the immune response when using doses found in stressfull situations. In humans and animals, adrenergic agonists depress mitogen-induced T lymphocyte proliferation, increase NK cell activity and modulate the primary antibody response to sheep erythrocytes [22, 23]. Catecholamines modify the immune responses by acting on lymphocytes and also by changing the lymphocyte traffic in the spleen and lymph nodes.

The modulatory effects of adrenergic agonists at the lymphocyte level is evidenced by *in vitro* studies. Adrenaline, noradrenaline and isoproterenol depress PHA induced T cell proliferation [3] but enhance B cell mitogenesis, immunoglobulin production [24] and the primary PFC response [25]. However, only high concentrations (10^{-4}, 10^{-6}M) which may be found in the *in vivo* microenvironment of lymphocytes are effective. Adrenaline also modulates human NK cell activity at concentrations (10^{-7}, 10^{-9}M) which are more compatible with a specific binding [26]. Preincubation of lymphocytes with adrenaline enhances NK cell activity whereas adrenaline depresses this activity when added to the lymphocyte-target cell culture.

The immunomodulating effects of catecholamines appear to be mediated by specific receptors. Specific antagonism by propanolol [24] and coupled stimulation of adenylate cyclase activity [27] show that the immune effects of NA are mediated by β-receptor located on lymphocytes. Binding studies have also demonstrated the presence of β-adrenergic receptors on lymphocytes [28, 29] even though the characteristics of these receptors remain controversial. Recent studies using stereospecific β antagonists with high affinity confirm the presence of β-adrenoreceptors on B and T lymphocytes but not on thymocytes [30]. The order of agonist potencies suggests that these receptors are of the β_2 subtype. Moreover, the density of β adrenoreceptors on lymphocytes appears to be down regulated by adrenaline [31] as well as by antigenic stimulation [30].

That *in vivo* immunomodulatory effects of dopaminergic agonists and antagonists are centrally mediated or involved receptors on immune cells remains unclear. A dopamine receptor of a D1 type located on mammalian lymphocytes has been first described by Le Fur *et al.* using a specific D1 antagonist [32]. The lymphocyte dopamine receptor differs from the central nervous dopaminergic binding sites by its stereospecificity. No binding may be observed with D1 agonists and reverse stereospecificity may be observed with D2 antagonists [33]. Recent evidence suggests saturable stereospecific dopaminergic binding sites of high affinity on mouse thymocytes [34]. This receptor appears to be unlike the known D1 and D2 subtypes. *In vitro*, dopamine depresses mitogen-induced B cell mitogenesis and immunoglobulin synthesis [35], but the effective doses of 10^{-4}-10^{-5} M are not compatible with a specific binding to dopamine receptors. Dopamine usually increases cAMP in lymphocytes and thymocytes [35, 36] but this metabolic coupling appears to result from a non-specific binding of dopaminergic agonists to lysosomes [36]. Although having some immmunomodulatory effects *in vivo*, no binding sites for haloperidol and apomorphine have been found on immune cells [33]. Possibly these substances regulate immune responses through the central dopaminergic pathways ; the latter clearly are related to other neurotransmitter systems such as opiate peptides, the autonomic nervous system [5] and prolactin secretion [7].

Serotonin

Serotonin plays an important role in immunomodulation mainly at the peripheral level. Peripheral administration of serotonin (5-HT) or of its precursor 5-hydroxytryptophane (5-HTP) depresses IgM and IgG PFC responses in mice. Yet, inhibition of serotonin synthesis by para-chlorophenylalanine (PCPA) enhances PFC responses [37]. PCPA and 5-HTP cross the blood brain barrier and may act, at least partly, on central serotoninergic pathways. Serotonin does not cross the blood brain barrier and, therefore, can be active only in the periphery when injected systemically. Furthermore, the involvement of central serotonin in neuroimmunomodulation is not well established. The destruction of the raphe nucleus (a central serotoninergic structure) stimulates antibody production [38] whereas central depletion of serotonin by intracisternal injection of 5-7 dihydroxytryptamine does not modify PFC responses [37]. The peripheral effects of serotonin are confirmed by *in vitro* experiments. High concentrations of serotonin (10^{-3} M) depress mitogen-induced proliferation of human or murine lymphocytes [39, 40] and the *in vivo* primary antibody response [40]. At lower doses (10^{-5} to 10^{-7} M) serotonin depresses the macrophage Ia expression induced by γ interferon [41]. Several experiments have shown that immune cells may have receptors which bind serotonin [42]. The decrease of Ia expression induced by serotonin is antagonized by a receptor antagonist of the 5-HT2 type [41]. On the other hand, saturable, stereospecific bindings sites of the 5-HT1 subtype have been found on T and B murine lymphocytes but not on thymocytes [43].

Peripheral serotonin is mainly released by thrombocytes in inflammatory sites at concentrations (10^{-6} to 10^{-8} M) compatible with the *in vitro* effects of serotonin on macrophage Ia expression and in accordance with the affinity constant of 5-HT receptors. The role of serotonin released by nerve endings is uncertain.

Acetylcholine

Evidence for parasympathetic innervation of lymphoid tissues [4] suggests the hypothesis that acetylcholine has immunomodulatory functions. This has been demonstrated by *in vitro* studies. Cholinergic agonists enhance the cytotoxic lymphocyte responses [44, 45] as well as the proliferation of both unstimulated lymphocytes [46], lymphocytes stimulated by mitogens [44], or by mixed lymphocyte culture [47]. This cholinergic stimulation of lymphocytes is associated with an increase of cGMP and a decrease of cAMP and may be reversed by atropin. The mechanism appears to be related to stimulation of M2 muscarinic receptors. On the contrary, a selective M1 muscarinic agonist, pilocarpine, has inhibitory effects on PHA-induced mitogenesis [48] suggesting that M1 and M2 receptors may have opposite effects on lymphocyte reactivity. Nicotinic receptors could also be involved in the cholinergic modulation of the immune system. Carbamylcholine, a mixed muscarinic-nicotinic agonist, suppresses or augments lymphocyte proliferation, depending on the dosage. Suppression of lymphoproliferation by low doses of carbamylcholine appears to be related to nicotinic receptors because it is blocked by a nicotinic antagonist [49]. Muscarinic [(50, 51] and nicotinic [52, 53] binding sites with high affinity have been demonstrated on peripheral blood cells. Their relative density on T and B lymphocytes is not known. Density and binding capacity of cholinergic receptors may vary under different physiological or pharmacological situations. The muscarinic receptors on lymphocytes, as well as those in the brain, appear not to be regulated by systemic atropin. Moreover, binding capacity increases with old age [54].

The physiological impact of central cholinergic pathways on immune regulation remains to be established. Some immunological impairment has been described during Alzheimer's disease [55], but the bilateral lesions of the basal nucleus of Meynert rich in cholinergic neurons, paradoxically enhances NK cell activity and T-cell mitogenesis in rats [56]. Central and peripheral anticholinergic properties could account for some of the immunoregulatory effects of some psychotropic drugs such as tricyclic antidepressants and neuroleptics.

Immunoregulatory roles of neuropeptides

Neuropeptides are distributed largely in neuronal, but are also found in non neuronal endocrine cells. They are involved in cell communications by means of neurotransmission and by paracrine or endocrine secretion. Their involvement in the control of numerous peripheral functions suggests influence on the immune system as well. Although their synthesis involves identical mechanisms, peptides usually are classified in three functional categories for comprehensive purposes : (i) neuropeptides of the hypothalamo-pituitary axis, (ii) cerebrointestinal peptides, (iii) opiate peptides.

Non-opiate neuropeptides

The first category includes thyreotropic, gonadotropic, corticotropic and somatotropic factors. Each are a primary source of neuroimmunomodulation, mainly *via* stimulatory effects on hormone production. The immunomodulatory roles of hormones have been described in details elsewhere [1] and will not be discussed further here.

Gastrointestinal peptides, including somatostatine (SOM), vasoactive intestinal peptide (VIP), substance P (SP), substance K (SK), neuropeptide Y (NPY), and neurotensine are produced by the diffuse endocrine system. Yet the peptides also are components of the CNS with specific functions, for example as mediators of pain. Calcitonin gene-related peptide (CGRP) is another peptide, also found in the brain.

The immunomodulatory properties of non-opiate peptides [57, 58] is suggested by the rich peptidergic innervation of lymphoid organs. In lymph nodes and thymus, neuropeptides such as NPY are colocated with noradrenaline [59, 60] and neuropeptides SP, SK, CGRP and VIP are present in sensory nerve endings which are in close contact with immune cells.

Non-opiate peptides are mediators of inflammation. For instance, intestinal concentrations of VIP are increased during Crohn's disease [61] and SP plays a role in experimental arthritis [62-64]. Neuropeptides not only regulate blood flow and vascular permeability, but they also directly modulate chemotactism, phagocytosis and mast cell degranulation [65]. SP and neurotensine enhance lymphocyte traffic in lymph nodes [66] chimiotactism [67, 68] and phagocytosis [69]. SP may also reverse VIP induced inhibition of lymphocyte traffic and monocyte production of superoxide and peroxide ions [70].

In vitro data favor a direct influence of neuropeptides on immune cells. Efficient concentrations (10^{-9} to 10^{-10} M) are similar to those presumed to occur locally in lymphoid tissues. Furthermore, dose-effect curves are consistent with the characteristics of the specific binding sites on monocytes and lymphocytes. SP stimulates *in vitro* Con A-induced T cell proliferation [71, 72] and T-cell mediated antibody synthesis [73]. Specific binding sites for SP have been demonstrated in murine T-lymphocytes but not on monocytes [74]. VIP, SOM and CGRP suppress T-lymphocyte blastogenesis induced by ConA or PHA [75-78] *via* the enhancement of cellular cAMP levels [77, 79, 80] but do not affect B cell mitogenesis. VIP and SOM also depress NK cell activity [81]. These results are consonant with the presence of specific and saturable receptors for VIP and CGRP which have been found on T-cells and human monocytes [75, 76, 82-84] but not on other immune cells [75]. Two types of binding sites for VIP with high [10^{-9} M] and low [10^{-7} M] affinity, have been described on T-cells [76, 85]. The inhibitory effects of these peptides are maximal when added at the beginning of the culture, and less effective when added 24 hours later. As demonstrated for VIP, decreased efficiency correlates with a lower binding capacity of lymphocytes [86]. Furthermore, pretreatment of lymphocytes with VIP, a few hours before the introduction of mitogens or target cells, has stimulatory effects [81] suggesting a bimodal immunomodulating activity of VIP. The immunomodulatory activities of non-opiate neuropeptides have been demonstrated in inflammatory sites where they are released with other neurotransmitters. However, neuropeptides in the general circulation also may play an immunoregulatory role in spite of their low serum concentrations. Monocytes and blood lymphocytes are highly sensitive even to very slight variation of neuropeptide levels.

Neuropeptides in the CNS could have immunoregulatory properties but possibly through other transmitter pathways. These complex networks in the brain will require considerable further investigations.

Opiate peptides

Opiate peptides are active in a variety of brain functions. β-endorphins are implicated in nociception and enkephalins likely modulate moods such as depression and anxiety, and serve as anticonvulsivants, at least in animals. Interest in the immunoregulatory role of endogenous opiates comes from their connections to some stressfull situations known to be immunosuppressive. Additional support is found in the immunological impairment of many opium related drug addicts. Immunological consequences of the endogenous opiates may be mediated by their activity on the pituitary and adrenal glands and on the sympathetic outflow. However, *in vitro* studies reveal that circulating endogenous opiates, in stress situations and in basal conditions, directly can act on immune cells. The existence of specific opiate receptors on immune cells is suggested by dose dependent effects in 10^{-9}-10^{-12} M range and its reversal by the opiate antagonist naloxone. Numerous studies have identified binding sites with high affinity for enkephalins and morphine on lymphocytes and phagocytes [87, 88] although the binding experiments were not completely convincing [89]. More recently [90], δ and κ receptors similar to those of the neuroendocrine tissue have been described on B and T lymphocytes and on macrophages. They are coupled to intracellular metabolism (adenyl-cyclase) and affect conductance of ion channels. Indeed, the four known receptor subtypes (φ, δ, κ and ϵ) are possibly involved in immunomodulation. Agonists and antogonists are required to test this hypothesis. Moreover, endogenous opiates modulate immune functions *via* non-opiate receptors [91].

The immunoregulatory function of endogenous opiates have been widely studied. In humans, NK cell activity is enhanced by β-endorphin, Leu- and Met-enkephalins *in vitro* [92-94]. Enhancement is observed in about 50 % of both healthy humans [101] and those with cancer [95] but is more pronounced when the baseline of NK cell activity is relatively low [96, 97]. Opiate peptides particularly may be benefical to cancer patients who normally exhibit defective NK cell activity. β-endorphins and Met-enkephalin also enhance superoxide production by human and rat macrophages [98, 99]. Reversal of this enhancing effect by naloxone demonstrates the involvement of a specific opioid receptor interacting with the N-terminal region of the peptide. Modulation of lymphoproliferation by opiate peptides is more complex and involves two different receptors. Opiates have been shown to enhance mitogen-induced lymphoproliferation *via* the stimulation specific δ opiate receptor [100] or of a nonopiate receptor [101, 102]. In contrast, some authors have reported that β-endorphin may suppress mitogenesis [103]. These contradictory findings may result from the opposite effects of small *versus* large doses of β-endorphin. Moreover there is a great variability in individual susceptibility of lymphocytes to the peptide [104]. Finally, β-endorphin has been reported to induce the suppressive activity of T-lymphocytes in synergy with ConA [105]. This could be related to the reported immunosuppressive effects of β-endorphin. Antibody production *in vitro* is more or less inhibited by the different opioid peptides. The greatest inhibition is induced by α-endorphin, the weakest by α- and γ-endorphin, while intermediate inhibition is induced by Met- and Leu-enkephalin. The inhibitory activity of α-endorphin is reversed by naloxone [106].

Physiological relevance of the *in vitro* data has been assessed *in vivo* by systemic administration of endogenous opiates using doses compatible with plasma levels found in basal or stress conditions. β-endorphin, as well as Met- and Leu-enkephalin prolong the survival of leukemic mice, enhance PHA- and ConA-induced mitogenesis and modulate PFC response [107, 108]. The *in vivo* effects of opiates on NK cell activity remain unclear. In rats, NK cell activity is depressed in stress conditions which are assumed to involve opiate peptides [109]. In contrast, physical exercise in human enhances NK cell activity even though it also increases the plasma levels of enkephalins and β-endorphin [110, 111]. These *in vivo* data are difficult to interpret because endogenous opiates also may act on central receptors implicated in neuromodulation. Furthermore, the central opiate receptors may be differently involved depending on the various types of stress. Finally, precursors and transduction products of opiate peptides are found in lymphocytes and macrophages from both humans and animals [112-114]. The suggestion is that opiate and non-opiate receptors could be involved in autocrine or paracrine regulation of lymphocyte functions independently of their modulating activity of the neuroendocrine system.

Immunological effects of neuropsychotropic drugs

Neuro-psychotropic drugs are prescribed widely and, with a few exceptions, interact with central and peripheral neurotransmitters and peptides which have been noted earlier to have immunoregulatory functions. Therefore, these drugs have the potential to influence the immune system. For example, one of the possible side effects of the drugs may be to compromise the functioning of the immune system. Unfortunately, few experiments have been performed to test this possibility. Psychotropic-immune relations could provide new insights in neuroimmunomodulation, but also may be responsible for immune side effects that are not yet well definite. Unfortunately, the litterature on this subject is very sparse.

Tricyclic anti-depressants have been shown to depress NK cell activity, mitogen-induced lymphoproliferation and delayed hypersensitivity following systemic administration to mice or to humans [115-117]. These effects could be related to the monoaminergic modulation of the immune response cited earlier. Tricyclic anti-depressants inhibit central and peripheral noradrenaline and block scrotonin uptake by nervous endings. Dimethylimipramine specifically inhibits the reuptake of NA but has no effect on NK cell activity [115]. Tricyclic anti-depressants also may have immunosuppressive effects *via* their binding to muscarinic or histamine receptors. *In vitro*, experiments have reported that these drugs depressed T and B cell proliferation and NK cell activity [115, 118, 119]. The high doses used are far above therapeutic ranges and leave those data open to question.

Benzodiazepines are widely prescribed as anxiolytic, anticonvulsant, sedative and myorelaxant. Benzodiazepine receptors are distributed in the central nervous system and in peripheral tissues where they have been found on monocytes, polymorphonuclear neutrophils and thymocytes [13, 120, 121]. However, the presence of an endogenous ligand is still debated [122]. Systemic administration of diazepam that binds to central and peripheral receptors has been shown to depress delayed hypersensitivity in mice [117] but to enhance *in vivo* mitogenic activity [123]. These *in vivo* immunomodulations involve both central nervous receptors and peripheral binding sites on immune cells with opposite effects. Peripheral ligands depress phagocyte oxidative metabolism, production of monokines and mitogenesis [123]. These inhibitory effects of peripheral ligands are confirmed by *in vivo* experiments where diazepam depresses lymphoproliferation [124]. By contrast, there is evidence that central ligands enhance mitogenesis and NK cell activity [123, 125]. Central benzodiazepine receptors influence sympathetic activity and hypothalamic-pituitary secretion. In particular, the drug stimulates the production of growth hormone which is known to be immunostimulant [126].

Neuroleptics also may influence the immune response. Some clinical studies have investigated the immune consequences of long term administration of neuroleptics. Treatment of schizophrenic patients with chlorpromazine enhance IgM and IgG plasma levels and lower T cell number in the blood stream [127, 128]. But, this psychotic disease directly induces immunological changes [127-129] that are difficult to dissociate from those of the drugs. Experimental studies with mice have yielded conflicting results, dependent upon the class of drugs used, phenothiazine or butyrophenones, and on the immune parameters investigated. Post-vaccination, daily administration of chlorpromazine, a phenothiazine, impairs the development of humoral and/or cellular immunity against viral or mycobacterial antigens [130]. Treatment also inhibits delayed hypersensitivity reactions to DNCB [131] and to sheep erythrocytes [117]. As the immune response is depressed both at the afferent and the efferent levels, it has been proposed this drug has a non-specific effect on lymphocytes [117]. That also may be true for haloperidol which is a butyrophenone. However, immune effects of haloperidol are probably more complex; daily injections enhance delayed hypersensitivity to DNCB when given prior to antigenic challenge but does the opposite when administered from the day of immunization and has no effect on the elicitation phase of the reaction. These results suggest that the effects of haloperidol may be mediated by central dopaminergic receptors [131].

Morphine is used extensively as a narcotic analgesic and is known to be immunosuppressive. Morphine addiction is associated with a higher incidence of infections and has been reported to depress several lymphocyte functions such as mitogenesis or T cell rosetting [132], macrophage respiratory burst [133] and phagocytosis [132]. In animals, systemic injection of high doses of morphine (30-50mg/kg) depresses NK cell activity [134], mitogenesis [135], phagocytosis [136] and antibody response to sheep erythrocytes [137]. These morphine-induced effects appear to be mediated by central opiate receptors. Indeed, the intracerebroventricular injection of morphine reduces NK cell activity whereas the peripheral injection of dihydromorphine does not cross the blood brain barrier and is ineffective. Similarly, morphine has little or even no effect on lymphocytes or mast cells *in vitro* [138, 139].

Conclusion

This short overview of the neuroimmune relations suggests that:

— the immune system is not isolated from other factors influencing the individual. At the minimum, the immune system is regulated by the nervous system at either the level of the brain or the periphery;
— molecules involved in neuronal networks also have immunological activities;
— immune cells appear to possess functional receptors for neurotransmitters and neuropeptides.

This review is intended as a mechanism to introduce new concepts in immunomodulation rather than to compile a set of conclusive findings. This approach is necessitated by the relative youth of the neuroimmunomodulation field and by the enormous complexity of both neuronal and immune networks.

Acknowledgements

We would like to thank Pr George Taylor for his critical review of the manuscript.

References

1. Weigent D, Blalock JE. Structural and functional relationship between the immune and neuroendocrine systems. *Bull Institut Pasteur* Paris, 1989 ; 87 : 61-92.
2. Felten DL, Livnat S, Felten S, Carlson SL, Bellinger DL, Yeh P. Sympathetic innervation of lymph nodes in mice. *Brain Res Bull* 1984 ; 13 : 693-9.
3. Livnat S, Felten S, Carlson S, Lorton, Bellinger D, Felten DL. Involvement of peripheral and central catecholamine systems in neural immune interactions. *J Neuroimmunol* 1985 ; 10 : 5-30.
4. Bullock K. The innervation of immune system tissues and organs. In : Cotman CW, Brinton RE, Galaburda A, McEwen B, Schneider DM, eds. *The neuro-immune-endocrine connections*. New York : Raven Press, 1987 : 33-47.
5. Lindvall O, Björklund A, Skagergerg G. Dopamine-containing neurons in the spinal cord : anatomy and some functional aspects. *Ann Neurol* 1983 ; 14 : 255-60.
6. Van Loon GR, Appel NM. β-Endorphin-induced hyperglycemia is mediated by increased central sympathetic out-flow to adrenal medulla. *Brain Res* 1981 ; 204 : 236-41.
7. Bernton EW. Prolactin and immune host defense. *PNEI Perspective* 1989 ; 1 : 21-9.
8. Dupont A, Cusan L, Caron M, Labrie F, Li CH. β-Endorphin : stimulation of growth hormone release *in vivo*. *Proc Natl, Acad Sci USA* 1977 ; 74 : 358-9.
9. Van Loon GR, De Souza EB, Shin SH. β-Endorphin-induced prolactin secretion is mediated by suppression of release of newly synthetized hypothalamic dopamine. *Can J Physiol Pharmacol* 1980 ; 58 : 436-9.
10. Van Loon GR, de Souza EB. Development of tolerance to the ACTH-releasing effects of β-endorphin. *Res Commun Chem Pathol Pharmacol* 1978 ; 22 : 203-4.
11. Akil H, Watson SJ, Young E, Lewis ME, Khachaturian H, Walker JM. Endogenous opioids : biology and function. *Ann Rev Neurosci* 1984 ; 7 : 223-55.
12. Besedovsky HO, Del Rey EA, Sorkin M, DA Prada M, Keller HH. Immunoregulation mediated by the sympathetic nervous system. *Cell Immunol* 1979 ; 48 : 346-55.
13. Williams JM, Peterson RG, Shea PA, Schmedtje JF, Bauer DC, Felten DL. Sympathetic innervation of murine thymus and spleen. Evidence for a functional link between the nervous and immune systems. *Brain Res Bull* 1981 ; 6 : 83-94.
14. Miles KE, Quintans E, Chilmicka-Schorr E, Arnason BGW. The symphathetic nervous system modulates antibody response to thymus-independent antigens. *J Neuroimmunol* 1981 ; 1 : 101-5.
15. Reder A, Checinski M, Chelmicka-Schorr E. The effect of chemical sympathetomy on natural killer cells in mice. *Brain Behav Immun* 1989 ; 3 : 110-8.
16. Felten DL, Felten SY, Bellinger DL, Carlson SL, Ackerman KD, Madden KS, Olschowka JA, Livnas S. Noradrenergic sympathetic neural interactions with the immune system : structure and function. *Immunol Rev* 1987 ; 100 : 225-67.
17. Hall NR, McClure JE, Hu SK, Tare NS, Seals CM, Goldstein AL. Effects of 6-hydroxydopamine upon primary and secondary thymus dependent immune responses. *Immunopharmacology* 1982 ; 5 : 39-48.
18. Won SJ, Lin MT. Depletion of catecholamines with α-methyl-p-thyrosine suppresses splenic NK cell activity. *Int J Immunopharmacol* 1989 ; 11 : 451-7.
19. Ackerman KD, Felten SY, Dijkstra DD, Livnat S, Felten DL. Parallel development of noradrenergic innervation and cellular compartmentation in the rat spleen. *Exp Neurol* 1989 ; 103 : 239-55.
20. Besedovsky HO, Del Rey A, Sorkin EA, Da Prada M, Keller HH. Immunoregulation mediated by the sympathetic nervous system. *Cell Immunol* 1979 ; 48 : 346.
21. Fuchs BA, Campbell KS, Manson AE. Norepinephrine and serotonin content of the murine spleen : its relationship to lymphocyte β-adrenergic receptor density and the humoral immune response *in vivo* and *in vitro*. *Cell Immunol* 1988 ; 117 : 339-51.
22. Feldman RD, Hunninghake GW, McArdle WL. β-Adrenergic receptor-mediated suppression of interleukin-2 receptors in human lymphocytes. *J Immunol* 1987 ; 139 : 3355-9.

23. Ekladios EM, Higashi GI, El Ghorab NM, Ayeeb M. *In vivo* modulation of T lymphocytes and dermal sensitivity by propanonol. *J Egypt Med Assoc* 1977 ; 60 : 60 : 241-9.
24. Kouassi E, Li YS, Boukhris W, Millet I, Revillard JP. Opposite effects of the catecholamines dopamine and norepinephrine on murine polyclonal B-cell activation. *Immunopharmacology* 1988 ; 16 : 125-37.
25. Sanders VM, Manson AE. Norepinephrine and the antibody response. *Pharmacol Rev* 1985 ; 37 : 229-48.
26. Hellstrand K, Hermodsson S, Strannegard Ö. Evidence for a β-adrenoreceptor-mediated regulation of human natural killer cells. *J Immunol* 1985 ; 134 : 4095-9.
27. Carlson SL, Brooks WH, Roszman TL. Neurotransmitter-lymphocyte interactions : dual receptor modulation of lymphocyte proliferation and cAMP production. *J Neuroimmunol* 1989 ; 24 : 155-62.
28. Williams LT, Snyderman R, Lefkowitz RJ. Identification of β-adrenergic receptors in human lymphocytes by (-)^{3}H-alprenolol binding. *J Clin Invest* 1976 ; 57 : 149-55.
29. Loveland BE, Jarrot B, McKenzie IFC. The detection of β-adrenoreceptors on murine lymphocytes. *Int J Immunopharmacol* 1981 ; 3 : 45-55.
30. Fuchs BA, Albright JW, Albright JF. β-adrenergic receptors on murine lymphocytes : density varies with cell maturity and lymphocyte subtype and is decreased after antigen administration. *Cell Immunol* 1988 ; 114 : 231-35.
31. Krall JF, Connelly M, Tuck ML. Acute regulation of beta-adrenergic catecholamine sensitivity in human lymphocytes. *J Pharmacol Exp Ther* 1980 ; 214 : 554-60.
32. Le Fur G, Phan T, Uzan A. Identification of stereospecific [3H] spiroperidol binding sites in mammalian lymphocytes. *Life Sci* 1980 ; 26 : 1139-48.
33. Shaskan EG, Ballow M, Lederman M, Margoles SM, Melchreit T. Spiroperidol binding sites on mouse lymphoid cells. Effects of ascorbic acid and psychotropic drugs. *J Neuroimmunol* 1984 ; 6 : 59-66.
34. Stefano GB, Zhao J, Bailey D, Metlay M, Leung MK. High affinity dopamine binding to mouse thymocytes and mytilus edulis (Bivalvia) hemocytes *J Neuroimmunol* 1989 ; 21 : 67-74.
35. Kouassi E, Li YS, Boukhris W, Millet I, Revillard JP. Opposite effects of the catecholamines, dopamine and norepinephrine on murine polyclonal B-cell activation. *Immunopharmacology* 1988 ; 16 : 125-37.
36. Kouassi E, Li YS, Flacher M, Revillard JP. Cyclic adenosine 3'-5-monophosphate response to dopamine in mouse lymphoid cells and cell lines. *Life Sci* 1987 ; 40 : 2385-92.
37. Jackson JC, Cross RJ, Walker RF, Markesbery WR, Brooks MH, Roszman TL. Influence of serotonin on the immune response. *Immunology* 1985 ; 54 : 505-12.
38. Eremina OF, Devoino LV. Production of humoral antibodies in rabbits following destruction of the nucleus of the midbrain raphé. *Biull Eksp Biol Med* 1973 ; 74 : 58.
39. Slauson DO, Walker C, Kristensen F, Wang Y, De Week AL. Mechanism of serotonin-induced lymphocyte proliferation inhibition. *Cell Immunol* 1984 ; 84 : 240-52.
40. Roszman TL, Jackson JC, Cross RJ, Titus MJ, Markesbery WR, Brooks Wh. Neuroanatomic and neurotransmitter influence on immune function. *J Immunol* 1985 ; 135 : 769-72.
41. Sternberg EM, Trial J, Parker CW. Effect of serotonin on murine macrophage : suppression of Ia expression by serotonin and its reversal by 6-HT2 serotoninergie receptor antagonists. *J Immunol* 1986 ; 137 : 276-82.
42. Roszman TL, Sparks DL, Slevin JT, Markesbery WR, Jackson JC, Cross RJ. The presence of serotonin receptors on murine lymphocytes and macrophages. *Soc Neurosci* (Abst.) 1984 ; 10 : 726.
43. Bonnet M, Lespinats G, Burtin C. Evidence for serotonin (5-HT) binding sites on murine lymphocytes. *Int J Immunopharmacol* 1987 ; 9 : 551-8.
44. Hadden JW, Hadden EM, Haddox MK, Goldberg ND. Guanosine 3'5'-cycli monophosphate : a possible intracellular mediator of mitogenic influences in lymphocytes. *Proc Natl Acad Sci USA* 1972 ; 69 : 3024-7.

45. Strom TB, Sytkowski AJ, Carpenter CB, Merrill JP. Cholinergie augmentation of lymphocyte-mediated cytotixicity. *Proc Natl Acad Sci USA* 1974 ; 71 : 1330-3.
46. McManus JP, Boynton AL, Whitfield JP, Gillan DJ, Isaacs RJ. Acetylcholine-induced initiation of thymic lymphoblast DNA synthesis and proliferation. *J Cell Physiol* 1975 ; 85 : 321-9.
47. Hant T. Enhancement of « one way » human mixed lymphocyte reaction by cholliner-gic agents. *Exp Immunol* 1976 ; 25 : 338-41.
48. Arzt ES, Fernandez-Castelo S, Diaz A, Fuikielman S, Nahmod VC. The muscarinic agonist pilocarpine inhibits DNA and interferon synthesis in peripheral bllod mononuclear cells. *Int J Immunopharmacol* 1989 ; 11 : 275-81.
49. Richman DP, Arnason BGW. Nicotinic acetylcholyne receptors : evidence for a functionally distinct receptor on human lymphocytes. *Proc Natl Acad Sci USA* 1979 ; 76 : 4632-5.
50. Gordon MA, Cohen JJ, Wilson IB. Muscarinic cholinergic receptors in murine lymphocytes. Demonstration by direct binding. *Proc Natl Acad Sci USA* 1978 ; 75 : 2902-4.
51. Strom TB, Lane MA, George K. The parallel time-dependent, bimodal changes in lymphocyte cholinergic-binding activity and cholinergic influence upon lymphocyte-mediated cytotoxicity after lymphocyte activation. *J Immunol* 1981 ; 71 : 1330-3.
52 Maslinksi W, Grabczewska E, Ryzewski J. Acetylcholine receptors of rat lymphocytes. *Biochim Biophys Acta* 1980 ; 633 : 269-73.
53 Atweh SF, Grayback JJ, Richman DP. A cholinergic receptor site on murine lymphocytes with novel binding characteristics. *Life Sci* 1984 ; 35 : 2459-69.
54. Shenkman L, Rabey JM, Gilad GM. Cholinergic muscarinic binding by rat lymphocytes : effects of antagonist treatment, strian and aging. *Brain Res* 1986 ; 380 : 303-8.
55. Mcdonald SM, Goldstone AH, Morris JE, Exton-Smith AN, Callard RE. Immunological parameters in the aged and in Alzheimer's disease. *Clin Exp Immunol* 1982 ; 49 : 123-8.
56. Cherkaoui J, Mayo W, Neveu PJ, Kelley KW, Dantzer R, Le Moal M, Simon H. The nucleus basalis is involved in brain modulation of the immune system in rats. *Brain Res* 1990 ; 516 : 345-8.
57. Morley JE, Kay N. Neuropeptides and pyschoneuroimmunology. *Psychopharm Bull* 1986 ; 22 : 1089-91.
58. Covelli V, Jirillo E. Neuropeptides with immunoregulatory functions : current status of investigations. *Funct Neurol* 1988 ; 3 : 253-61.
59. Fink T, Weihe E. Multiple neuropeptides in nerves supplying mammalian lymphnodes : messenger candidates for sensory and autonomic neuroimmunomodulation ? *Neurosci Lett* 1988 ; 90 : 39-44.
60. Weihe E, Muller S, Fink T, Zentel HJ. Tachykinins, calcitonin gene-related peptide and neuropeptide Y in nerves of the mammalian thymus ; interactions with the mast cells in autonomic and sensory neuroimmunomodulation ? *Neurosci Lett* 1989 ; 100 : 77-82.
61. Bishop AE, Polak JM, Bryant MG, Bloom Hamilton SR. Abnormalities of vasoactive intestinal polypeptide containing nerves in Crohn's disease. *Gastroenterology* 1980 ; 79.
62. Lembeck F, Holzer P. Substance P as a neurogenic mediator of antidromic vasodilatation and neurogenic plasma extravasation. *Nauryn Schiedesbergs Arch Pharmakol* 1979 ; 310 : 175-83.
63. Johnson HM, Smith EM, Torres BA, Blalock JE. Regulation of the *in vivo* antibody response by neuroendocrine hormones. *Proc Natl Acad Sci USA* 1982 ; 79 : 4171-4.
64. Levine TD, Clark R, Devor M, Helms C, Moskowitz MA. Intraneuronal substance P contributes to the severity of experimental arthritis. *Science* 1984 ; 226 : 547-9.
65. Hokfelt TR, Elde R, Johanson D, Ljungdahl A, Schultzberg M, Fuxe K. Distribution of peptide containing neurons. In : Lipton MA, DiMascio A, Killam KF, eds. *Psychopharmacology : a generation of progresses*. New York : Raven Press.
66. Moore TC. Modification of lymphocyte traffic by vasoactive neurotransmitter substances. *Immunology* 1984 ; 52 : 511-7.

67. Ruff MR, Wahl SM, Pert CB. Substance P receptor-mediated chemotaxis of human monocytes. *Peptides* 1985 ; 6 : 507-11.
68. Mc Gillis JP, Organist ML, Payan DG. Substance P and immunoregulation. Federation Proceedings 1987 ; 46 : 196-9.
69. Bar-Shavit Z, Goldman R, Stabinsky Y, Gottlieb P, Fridkin M, Teichberg M, Blumberg S. Enhancement of phagocytoxis. A newly found activity of substance P residing in its N-terminal tetrapeptide sequence. *Biochem Biophys Res Commun* 1980 ; 94 : 1445-50.
70. Wilk P. Vasoactive intestinal peptide inhibits the respiratory hurst in human monocytes by a cyclic AMP-mediated mechanism. *Regul Pept* 1989 ; 25 : 187-97.
71. Payan DG, Levine JD, Goetzl EJ. Modulation of immunity and hypersensitivity by sensory neuropeptides. *J Immunol* 1984 ; 132 : 1601-3.
72. Payan DG, Mc Gillis JP, Renold FK, Mitsuhashi M, Goetzl EJ. Neuropeptide modulation of leukocyte function. In : Jankovic BD, Markovic BM, Spector N, eds. *Neuroimmune interactions. Ann NY Acad Sci* 1987 ; 496 : 182-91.
73. Stanisz AM, Befus D, Bienenstock J. Differential effects of vasoactive intestinal peptide, substance P, and somatostatin on immunoglobulin synthesis and proliferations by lymphocytes from Peyer's patches, mesenteric lymphnodes and spleen. *J Immunol* 1986 ; 136 : 152-6.
74. Stanisz AM, Schicchitano R, Dazin P, Bienenstock J, Payan DG. Distribution of substance P receptors on murine spleen and Peyer's patch T and B cells. *J Immunol* 1987 ; 139 : 749-54.
75 Ottaway CA, Greenberg GR. Interaction of vasoactive intestinal peptide with mouse lymphocytes : specific binding and the modulation of mitogen responses. *J Immunol* 1984 ; 132 : 417-23.
76. Peurière S, Susini C, Estève JP, Vaysse N, Escoula L. Dual effect of vasointestinal peptide on the mitogenic response of rabbit spleen lymphocytes. *Regul Pept* 1990 ; 27 : 117-26.
77 Umeda Y, Takamiya M, Yoshizaki H, Arisawa M. Inhibition of mitogen-stimulated T lymphocyte proliferation by calcitonin gene-related peptide. *Biochem Biophys Res Comm* 1988 ; 154 : 227-235.
78. Ottaway CA, Bernaerts C, Chan B, Greenberg G. Specific binding of a vasoactive intestinal peptide to human circulating mononuclear cells. *Can J Physiol Pharmacol* 1983 ; 61 : 664.
79 O'Dorisio MS, Hermina NS, O'Dorisio TM, Balcerzak SP. Vasoactive intestinal polypeptide modulation of lymphocyte adenylcyclase. *J Immunol* 1981 ; 127 : 2551-4.
80. Guerrero JM, Prieto JC, Calvao JR, Goberna R. Activation of cyclic AMP-dependent protein kinase by VIP in blood mononuclear cells. *Peptides* 1984 ; 5 : 371.
81. Rola-Pleszczynki M, Bolduc D, St-Pierre S. The effects of vasoactive intestinal peptide on human killer cell function. *J Immunol* 1985 ; 135 : 2569-73.
82. Umeda Y, Arisawa M. Characterization of the calcitonin gene-related peptide receptor in mouse T-lymphocytes. *Neuropeptides* 1989 ; 14 : 237-42.
83. Wiik P, Opstad PK, Boyum A. Binding of vasoactive intestinal polypeptide (VIP) by human blood monocytes : demonstration of specific binding sites. *Regul Pept* 1985 ; 12 : 145-63.
84. Danek A, O'Dorisio MS, O'Dorisio TM, George JM. Specific binding sites for vasoactive intestinal polypeptide on nonadherent peripheral blood lymphocytes. *J Immunol* 1983 ; 131 : 1173-7.
85. O'Dorisio MS. Biochemical characteristics of receptors for vasoactive intestinal polypeptide in nervous, endocrine, and immune systems. *Fed Proc* 1987 ; 46 : 192-5.
86. Ottaway CA. Selective effects of vasoactive intestinal peptide on the mitogenic response of murine T cells. *Immunology* 1987 ; 62 : 291-7.
87. Ausiello CM, Roda LG. Leu-enkephalin binding to cultured human T lymphocytes. *Cell Biol Int Rep* 1984 ; 8 : 97-106.

88. Lopker A, Abood LG, Hoss W, Lionetti FJ. Stereoselective muscarinine acetylcholin and opiate receptors in human phagocytic leukocytes. *Biochem Pharmacol* 1980 ; 29 : 1361-5.
89. Sibinga NES, Goldstein A. Opioid peptides and opioid receptors in cells of the immune system. *Annu Rev Immunol* 1988 ; 6 : 219-49.
90. Carr JJ, De Costa BR, Kim CH, Jacobson AE, Guarcello V, Rice KC, Blalock JE. Opioid receptors on cells of the immune system : evidence for and classes. *J Endocrinol* 1989 ; 122 : 161-8.
91. Mathews PM, Froelich CJ, Sibbitt WL, Bankhurst AD. Enhancement of natural cytotoxicity by B-endorphin. *J Immunol* 1983 ; 130 : 1658-62.
92. Faith RE, Liang HJ, Murgo AJ, Plotnikoff NP. Neuroimmunomodulation with enkephalins : enhancement of human natural killer (NK) cell activity *in vitro*. *Clin Immunol Pathol* 1984 ; 31 : 412-8.
93. Kay N, Allen J, Morley JE. Endorphins stimulate normal human peripheral blood lymphocyte natural killer activity. *Life Sci* 1984 ; 35 : 53-9.
94. Wybran J. Enkephalins and endorphins as modifiers of the immune system : present and future. *Fed Proc* 1985 ; 44 : 92-4.
95. Plotnikoff NP, Murgo AJ, Miller GC, Corder CN, Faith RE. Enkephalins : immunomodulators. *Fed Proc* 1985 ; 44 : 118-22.
96. Faith RE, Liang HJ, Plotnikoff NP, Murgo AJ, Mimeh NF. Neuroimmunomodulation with enkephalins : *in vitro* enhancement of natural killer cell activity in peripheral blood lymphocystes from cancer patients. *Nat Immunol Cell Growth Regul* 1987 ; 6 : 88-98.
97. De Sanetis G, De Carolis C, Moretti C, Perricone R, Fabbri A, Gnessi L, Fraioli F, Fontana L. Endogenous opioids and the immune system : demonstration of inhibiting as well as enhancing effects of -endorphin on natural killer activity EDS. *Riv Immunol Immunofarmacol* 1986 ; 6 : 13.
98. Foris G, Medgyesi GA, Gyimesi E, Hauck M. Met-enkephalin induced alterations of macrophage functions. *Mol Immunol* 1984 ; 21 : 747-50.
99. Sharp BM, Keane WF, Suh HJ, Gekker G, Tsukayama D, Peterson PK. Opioid peptides rapidly stimulate superoxide production by human polymorphonuclear leukocytes and macrophages. *Endocrinology* 1985 ; 117 : 793.
100. Huckledbridge FH, Hudspith BN, Lydyard PM, Brostoff J. Stimulation of human peripheral lymphocytes by methionine enkephalin and -selective opioid analogues. *Immunopharmacology* 1990 ; 19 : 87-91.
101. Gilman SC, Schwartz JM, Milner RJ, Bloom FE, Feldman JO. γ-endorphin enhances lymphocyte proliferative responses. *Proc Natl Acad Sci USA* 1982 ; 79 : 4226-30.
102 Gilmore W, Weiner LP. The opioid specificity of beta-endorphin enhancement of murine lymphocyte proliferation. *Immunopharmacology* 1989 ; 17 : 19-30.
103. Puppo F, Corsini G, Mangini P, Bottaro L, Barreca T. Influence of γ-endorphin on phytohemagglutinin induced lymphocyte proliferation and on the expression of mononuclear cell surface antigens *in vitro*. *Immunopharmacology* 1985 : 10 : 119-25.
104. Roscetti G, Ausiello CM, Palma C, Gulla P, Roda LG. Enkephalin activity on antigen-induced proliferation of human peripheral blood mononucleate cells. *Int J Immunopharmacol* 1988 ; 10 : 819-23.
105. Mc Cain HW, Lamster IB, Billota J. Modulation of human T-cell suppressor activity by γ-endorphin and glycyl-L-glutamine. *Int J Immunopharmacol* 1986 ; 8 : 443-6.
106. Johnson HW, Smith EM, Torres BA, Blalock JE. Regulation of the *in vitro* antibody response by neuroendocrine hormones. *Proc Natl Acad Sci USA* 1982 ; 79 : 4171-4.
107. Plotnikoff NP, Kastin AJ, Coy DH, Christensen CW, Schally SV, Spirtes MA. Neuropharmacological actions of enkephalin after systemic administration. *Life Sci* 1976 ; 19 : 1283-8.
108. Kusnecov AW, Husband AJ, King MG, Smith R. Modulation of mitogen induced spleen cell proliferation and the antibody cell response by γ-endorphin *in vivo*. *Peptides* 1989 ; 10 : 473-9.

109. Shavit Y, Lewis JW, Terman GW, Gale RP, Liebeskind JC. Opioid peptides mediate the suppressive effect of stress on natural killer cell cytotoxicity. *Science* 1984 ; 223 : 188-90.
110. Farrel PA, Gates WK, Maksud MG, Morgan WP. Increases in plasma γ-lipotropin immunoreactivity after treadmill running in humans. *J Appl Physiol* 1982 ; 52 : 1245-9.
111. Targan S, Britvan L, Dorey F. Activation of human NKCC by moderate exercise : increased frequency of NK cells with enhanced capability of effector-target lytic interactions. *Clin Exp Immunol* 1981 ; 45 : 352-60.
112. Zurawski G, Benedik M, Kanp BJ, Abrams JS, Zurawski SM, Lee FD. Activation of mouse T-helper cell induced abundant preproenkephalin mRNA synthesis. *Science* 1986 ; 232 : 772-5.
113. Lolait SJ, Clements JA, Markwick AJ, Cheng C, Mc Nally M, Smith AJ, Funder JW. Pro-opiomelanocortin messenger ribonucleic acid and post-translational processing of γendorphin in spleen macrophages. *J Clin Invest* 1986 ; 77 : 1776-9.
114. Martin J, Prystowsky MB, Angeletti RK. Preproenkephalin mRNA in T-cells, macrophages and mast cells. *Neurosci Res* 1987 ; 18 : 82-7.
115. Eisen JN, Irwin J, Quay J, Liunat S. The effect of antidepressants on immune function in mice. *Biol Psychiatry* 1989 ; 26 : 805-17.
116. Albrecht J, Helderman JH, Schlesser MA, Rush AJ. A controlled study of cellular immune function in affective disorders before and during somatic therapy. *Psychiatry Res* 1985 ; 15 : 185-93.
117. Descotes R, Tedone R, Evreux JC. Different effects of psychotropic drugs on delayed hypersensitivity response in mice. *J Neuroimmunol* 1985 ; 9 : 81-5.
118. Audus KL, Gordon MA. Tricyclic antidepressant effects on the murine lymphocyte mitogen response. *J Immunopharmacol* 1982 ; 4 : 13-28.
119. Miller AH, Asnis GM, Van Praag HM, Norin AJ. Influence of desmethylimipramine on natural killer cell activity. *Psychiatry Res* 1986 ; 19 : 9-15.
120. Ruff MR, Pert CB, Weber RJ, Wahl LM, Wahl SM, Paul SM. Benzodiazepine receptor mediated chemotaxis of human monocytes. *Science* 1985 ; 229 : 1281-3.
121. Bond PA, Cundall RL, Rolfe B. (^{3}H) diazepam binding to human granulocytes. *Life Sci* 1985 ; 37 : 11.
122. Stephenson FA. Benzodiazepines innthe brain. *TINS* 1987 ; 10 : 185-6.
123. Slepien H, Pawlikowska A, Pawlikowska M. Effects of benzodiazepines on thymus cell proliferation. *Thymus* 1988 ; 12 : 117-21.
124. Pawlikowski M, Slepien H, Kunert-Radek J. Diazepam inhibits proliferation of the mouse spleen lymphocytes *in vitro*. *Pol J Pharmacol Pharm* 1986 ; 38 : 167-70.
125. Arora PK, Hanna EE, Paul SM, Skolnick P. Suppression of the immune response by benzodiapezine receptor inverse agonists. *J Neuroimmunol* 1987 ; 15 : 1-9.
126. Monroe WG, Roth JA, Grier RL, Arp LH, Naylor PH. Effects of growth hormone on the adult canine thymus. *Thymus* 1987 ; 9 : 173-87.
127. Solomon GF. Immunologic abnormalities in mental illness. In : Ader R, ed. *Behavioral Medicine Series*. Academic Press, 1981 ; 259-78.
128. Truma I, Zapletalek M, Krejsek J, Pidrman V. Some parameters of the immune system at schizophrenia therapy with chlorpromazin and zetidoline. *Act Nerv Super* 1989 ; 31 : 272-3.
129. De Lisi LE, Ortaldo JR, Malwish AE, Wyatt RJ. Deficient natural killer activity and macrophage functioning in schizophrenic patients. *J Neurol Transm* 1983 ; 58 : 99-106.
130. Mitrova E, Mayer V. Phenothiazine-induced alterations of immune response in experimental tick-borne encephalist morphological model analysis of events. *Acta Virol* 1976 ; 20 : 479-85.
131. Descotes J, Eurens JC. Effect of chlorpromazine on contact hypersensitivity to DNBC in the guinea pig. *J Neuroimmunol* 1982 ; 2 : 21-5.
132. Yahda MD, Watson RR. Minireview : immunomodulation by morphine and marijuana. *Life Sci* 1987 ; 41 : 2503-10.

133. Peterson P, Gekker G, Brummitt C, Pentel, Bullock M, Simpson M, Hitt J, Sharp B. Suppression of human peripheral blood monunuclear cell function by methadone and morphine. *J Infect Dis* 1989 ; 159 : 480-7.
134. Shavit Y, Depaulis A, Martin FC, Terman GN, Pechnick RN, Zane CJ, Gale RP, Liebeskind JC. Involvement of brain opiate receptors in the immune suppressive effect of morphine. *Proc Natl Acad Sci USA* 1986 ; 83 : 71114-7.
135. Ho WKK, Leung A. The effect of morphine addition on concanavalin A mediated blastogenesis. *Pharmacol Res Commun* 1979 ; 11 : 413-9.
136. Tubaro E, Santiangeli C, Belogi L, Borelli G, Cavallo G, Avico V. Methadone vs morphine : comparison of their effect on phagocytic functions. *Int J Immunopharmacol* 1987 ; 9 : 79-88.
137. Güntor M, Gene E, Sagduyu H, Eroglu L, Koyun Cuoglu H. Effect of chronic administration of morphine on primary immune response in mice. *Experienta* 1980 ; 36 : 1309-10.
138. Liu JS, Garrett KM, Lui SCC, Way EL. The effects of opiates on calcium accumulation on rat peritoneal mast cells. *Eur J Pharmacol* 1983 ; 91 : 335.
139. Yamasaki Y, Shimamura O, Kizu A, Nakagawa N, Ijichi H. Interaction of morphine with PGE_1 isoproterenol, dopamine and aminophylline in rat mast cells : their effects of IgE mediated ^{14}C serotonine release. *Agent Actions* 1983 ; 13 : 21.

19

An alternative concept of immunomodulation

Madeleine BASTIDE, Frédéric BOUDARD

Laboratoire d'Immunologie, Faculté de Pharmacie, Université de Montepellier-I,
34060 Montpellier Cedex 1, France.

The novel concept of immunomodulation proposed herein does not involve a new molecule or extract but rather a new approach to the use of conventional substances to modulate the immune response.

Presentation of the concept

Over the past few decades, immunopharmacologists have been searching for agents or molecules able to modulate the immune system. These substances are intended to improve the anti-infectious and anti-tumoral defence mechanisms or to prevent or treat autoimmune diseases. Various compounds of chemical or biological origin, termed immunomodulators, have been studied by classical pharmacological methods which are based on the toxicological and pharmacokinetic data of the test compounds. Since the effect of these drugs is a function of their half-life and serum level, they have to be used at particularly high doses to attain high blood levels and tissue concentrations. The case of the cytokine interferon α exemplifies this point. This substance is used in human therapy at doses equivalent to several million units. As expected, such a treatment is associated with severe side effects. Administration of such high doses is also in contradiction with the fact that interferon α is secreted in a microenvironment and acts according to a paracrine mechanism.

The classical immunopharmacological approach often leads to a marked modification of the subtle multifactorial balance of the immune system, whereas in fact the aim of the therapy is to improve the functionning of the system. To this end, we propose a new model of immunomodulation. Given the fact that the immune system is subjected to a multiplicity of interwoven regulatory mechanisms characteristic of systemic organization, we suggest that the regulation of biological systems involves the notion of « information » rather than the quantity of molecules it receives. Indeed, the immune response is under the control of the idiotypic network, which is a reservoir of information on antigenic structures. Therefore, it is possible that besides the regulatory mechanisms in living organisms reacting in response to hormones or cytokines and obeying the laws of classical pharmacokinetics, other mechanisms reacting in response to « information » might exist. These regulatory effects could be expressed at another level than those of the classical effector mechanisms of the cells. To transmit this information, we studied the effect of a series of highly diluted test substances. Our results indicate that high dilutions of several test molecules have immunomodulatory activity.

Test molecules and their preparation

We studied thymic hormones, bursin which participates to B lymphocyte maturation and cytokines. Although most of our investigations were carried out with thymulin [1] and natural mouse interferon $\alpha\beta$, we sometimes tested other thymic hormones, interleukin 2 (IL-2) and tuftsin.

The immunomodulating agents were prepared as follows : the mother solutions (1 mg/ml) were prepared in distilled water. Next, successive 100-fold dilutions vortexed 30 s were carried out using an alcohol-water-glycerine solvent that had been filtered through a 0.45-μm Sartorius membrane ; the dilutions used for injections or in *in vitro* tests were prepared in 0.15 M NaCl. The following solutions were prepared : thymulin (Serva, Le Perray en Yvelines, France) at 10^{-x} mg/ml (where x = 5, 6, 7, 8, 9, 11, 13, 15, 17, 19, 23) ; thymopoietin II (Serva) at 10^{-x} mg/ml (where x = 9, 15, 19, 23) ; thymosin 5 (kindly supplied by Hoffman-LaRoche) at 10^{-x} mg/ml (where x = 9, 15, 19, 23) ; tuftsin (Serva) at 10^{-x} mg/ml (where x = 9, 19) ; natural murine interferon $\alpha\beta$, 2×10^7 IU/mg of protein (kindly provided by Dr. Michael G. Tovey (Paris) or Interchim, Montluçon France) at 10 IU/ml in 0.15 M NaCl and 10^{-9} IU/ml ; natural semi-purified human IL2, 330 IU/mg of protein (kindly provided by D. Fradelizi, Paris) at 10 IU/ml and 10^{-9} IU/ml. Aliquots of all test solutions were stored at $-20\,°C$ until use and vortexed again before experimentation. The controls (mice or cultured macrophages) received the solvent diluted in the same manner as the test substances.

Experimental results in mice

Classical immunopharmacological *ex vivo* models were used to evaluate the effect of the diluted immunomodulators. The specific humoral immune response was studied by the Jerne plaque forming cell technique (PFC) on Swiss (OF1) or New Zealand Black (NZB) mice challenged with SRBC. The specific cellular immune response of C57BL/6 or NZB mice against P 815 mastocytoma cells or EL4 cells, respectively, was evaluated using the 51Cr-release technique after *in vivo* immunization. The non-specific natural killer response of C57BL/6 mice against YAC-1 cells was also evaluated using the 51Cr-release technique. The *in vitro* techniques used were the lymphocyte transformation test (LTT) and chemiluminescence evaluation of adherent peritoneal cells from BALB/c mice.

Ex vivo pharmacological studies in healthy mice

• *Effect of thymulin :* Swiss mice pretreated with 10^{-9}, 10^{-15}, 10^{-19}, or 10^{-23} mg/ml of thymulin showed a significantly depressed specific humoral immune response to sheep red blood cells (SRBC) [2-5]. All control mice received solvent intraperitoneally under the same conditions as the test mice (four injections 0.2 ml i.p.). We studied the effect of pretreatment of different groups of C57BL/6 mice treated at days -15, -13, -11 and -8 before sacrifice with 0.2 ml of thymulin solutions ranging from 10^{-5} mg/ml to 10^{-19} mg /ml ; we observed a significantly depressed specific cellular immune response with the highest dilutions as shown in Figure 1 [3, 6, 7]. The concentration of 10^{-19} mg/ml showed a reproducible effect (Table I). In other experiments, thymulin significantly stimulated the NK response (P < 0.001) [7, 8].

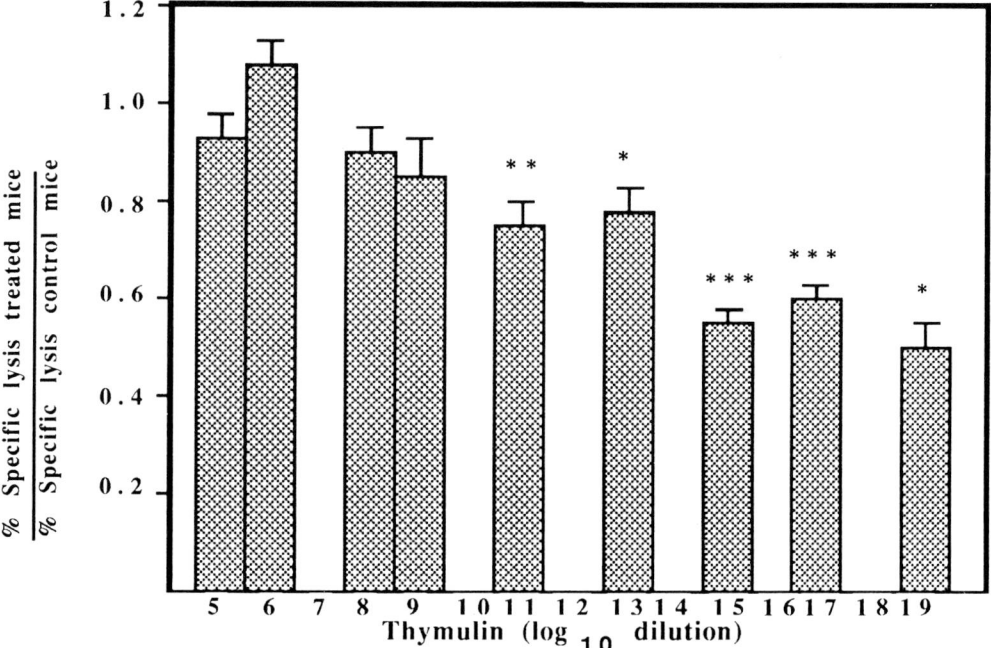

Figure 1. Allospecific cellular immune response of mice treated with different concentrations of thymulin.
Effector cells/target cell = 200. Newman-Keuls multiple comparison test.
* P<0.05 ** P<0.025 *** P<0.001

• *Effect of leucocytary interferon :* We also studied the effect of pretreatment with natural murine interferon $\alpha\beta$ on the specific humoral response of Swiss (OF1) mice. The mice received four injections of either 2 IU or 2×10^{-10} IU before challenge with SRBC. The lowest concentration significantly increased the specific humoral immune response in the four experiments as shown in Table II [3, 7].

Table I. Allospecific cellular immune response of C57BL/6 mice treated with very low concentrations of thymulin.

	Effector cells/ Target cells	Control 0.15 M NaCl	Thymulin solution 10^{-9} mg/ml	Thymulin solution 10^{-19} mg/ml
Exp. I	200	51.3 ± 2.3[a]	42.8 ± 6.4	27.1 ± 4.5* [b]
	100	41.7 ± 5.1	33.7 ± 5.5	17.3 ± 4.3*
	50	27.5 ± 4.2	19.5 ± 2.9	15.1 ± 3.6
	25	15.3 ± 2.7	15.5 ± 2.4	7.5 ± 0.2***
Exp. II	200	54.3 ± 1.9	47.1 ± 4.0	42.8 ± 1.7***
	100	48.8 ± 1.0	45.2 ± 4.8	38.5 ± 1.9***
	50	33.0 ± 2.3	27.8 ± 3.2	26.2 ± 1.2*
	25	20.4 ± 0.9	16.5 ± 1.5	17.2 ± 1.1
Exp. III	200	47.8 ± 3.1	31.8 ± 3.9*	33.4 ± 4.2*
	100	30.5 ± 3.5	22.4 ± 3.3	21.2 ± 4.7
	50	19.1 ± 3.2	15.3 ± 2.0	10.0 ± 3.6
	25	11.9 ± 1.7	12.1 ± 1.0	3.8 ± 1.2*

[a] Percent specific lysis ± s.e.m. Each value is the mean of the value for 5 lots of 2 mouse spleens.
[b] Statistical significance : Newman-Keuls multiple comparison test.
* $P < 0.05$, $P < 0.01$, $P < 0.001$.

Table II. Specific humoral immune response of Swiss OF1 mice treated with very low doses of natural mouse $\alpha\beta$ IFN.

IFN/injection [a]	Experiment I	Experiment II	Experiment III	Experiment IV
0	55 ± 5 [b]	209 ± 23	167 ± 13	11 ± 2
2 IU	140 ± 39 $P < 0.05$ [c]	328 ± 32 $P < 0.01$	193 ± 24	17 ± 4
2×10^{-10} IU	164 ± 16 $P < 0.05$	353 ± 14 $P < 0.01$	256 ± 25 $P < 0.05$	58 ± 8 $P < 0.001$

[a] Mice were treated with 4 inj.i.p. 0.2 ml.
[b] Number of PCF/10^6 cells ± s.e.m.
[c] Statistical significance (Newman-Keuls multiple comparison test).

Table III. Immunomodulation of the NK cell response by administration of low dose of mouse $\alpha\beta$ interferon to C57BL/6 mice.

Treatment	Experiment 1	Experiment 2	Experiment 3	Experiment 4
0	21.4 ± 3.0 [a]	36.9 ± 2.3	27.1 ± 2.2	22.4 ± 1.9
2 IU/injection	ND	47.0 ± 2.5* [b]	37.0 ± 2.5**	34.3 ± 3.7**
2×10^{-10}/inj.	26.5 ± 3.2	ND	20.9 ± 1.4	42.2 ± 1.2**

[a] Cytotoxicity of the splenic NK cells measured by the 51-Cr-release and expressed as percent specific lysis ± s.e.m. ; effector cells/target cell = 50.
[b] Statistical significance : Newman-Keuls multiple comparison test or Student's t test (single comparison).
* $P < 0.05$.
** $P < 0.01$.

We evaluated the effect of the same dilutions of interferon on the specific cellular secondary response in C57BL/6 mice immunized with P 815 cells; the mice who had received a dose of 16 x 10^{-10} IU interferon before and after the first injection of P 815 cells showed an increase (P < 0.001) in the cellular response [3, 7, 8]. The non-specific natural killer (NK) cellular response to YAC-1 cells was tested in C57BL/6 mice treated with leucocytary interferon. The results expressed in Table III show the effect of interferon at 2 IU and 2 x 10^{-10} IU/injection (5 injections at day-12, day-7, day-5, day-2 and -16 h).

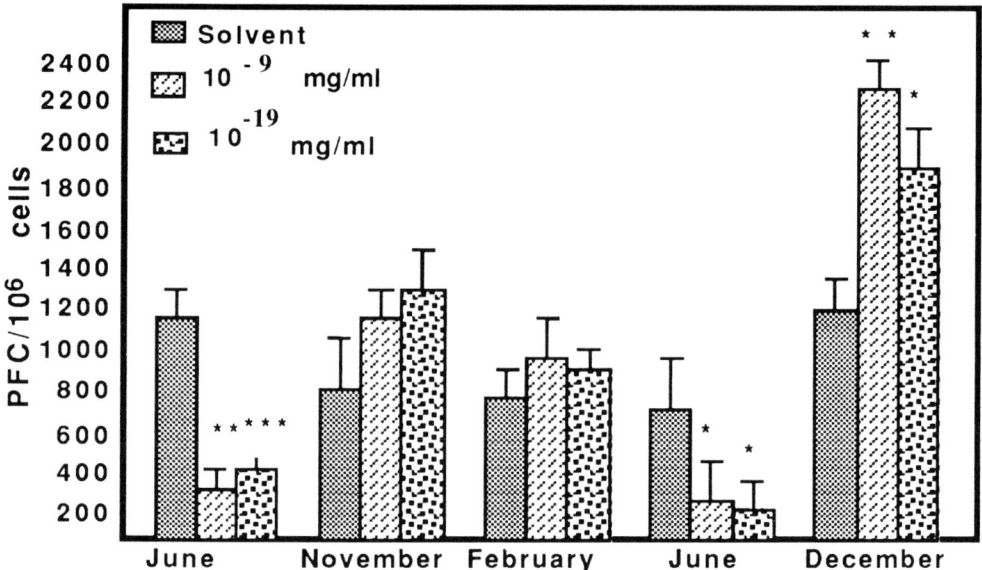

Figure 2. Seasonal variation of the number of PFC from mice treated with very low dose of thymosin fraction /.
* P<0.05 ** P<0.01 *** P<0.001.
Newman Keuls multiple comparison test.

- *Effect of other thymic hormones:* The immunopharmacological effects observed in healthy mice treated with thymic hormones show that they did not affect the synchronizers. We studied thymosin 5 at doses of 10^{-9} and 10^{-19} mg/ml for two years and thymopoietin II peptide 29-41 at the doses of 10^{-9}, 10^{-15}, 10^{-19} and 10^{-23} mg/ml for one year. In both cases, we observed a decrease in PFC of treated mice compared with the control mice in June and an increase in PFC during the cold season (November-December). These seasonal variations were observed over the period of two consecutive years in Swiss mice treated with thymosin 5 (Figure 2) and over the period of one year in thymopoietin-II treated mice (Figure 3). The period of the physiological circannual rhythms was not changed but the amplitude was increased.

- *Effect of IL-2:* We also studied the effect of IL-2 on cellular and humoral immune responses of mice using doses of 2 IU et 2×10^{-10}/injection [2, 7]. Using the same treatment protocole as for the C57BL/6 mice to evaluate the cellular immune response (pretreatment during three weeks before and after the two immunizations with P815 cells and treatment during the last day before the test), we obtained a significant stimulation of the cytotoxicity test in treated mice compared with the control mice (Figure 4). Concerning the humoral immune response, we obtained different results according to the treatment and immunization schedule as shown in Table IV. We did not observe any effect when the mice were pretreated before SRBC immunization ; if the animals were treated before and after the immunization, we observed a significant increase in PFC (primary response). If the treatment was performed after two immunizations (secondary response), we observed a significant suppression of the response. These results can be explained by the fact that modulation of the immune response by IL-2 is dependent on T-lymphocyte activation.

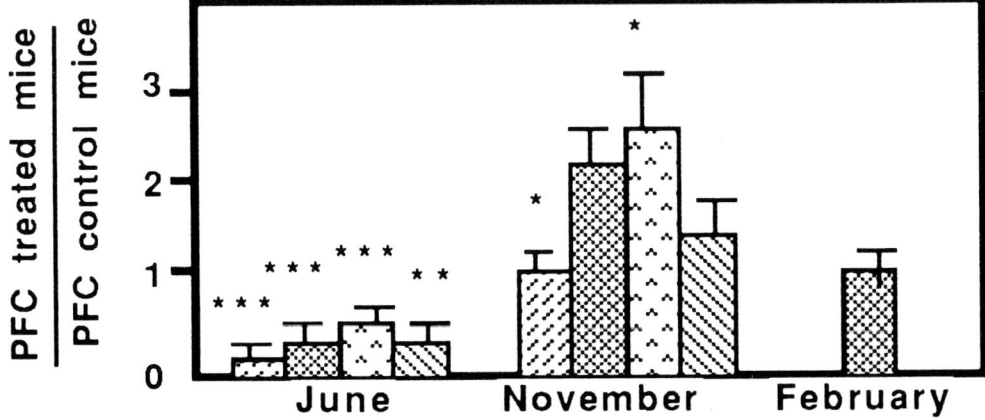

Figure 3. Seasonal variation of the number of PFC from mice treated with very low dose of thymopoietin II 29-41 fragment.

▨ 4×10^{-9}mg ▩ 4×10^{-15}mg ▨ 4×10^{-19}mg ▨ 4×10^{-23}mg/ml

* $P < 0.5$, ** $P < 0.005$, *** $P < 0.001$. Newman-Keuls multiple comparison test.

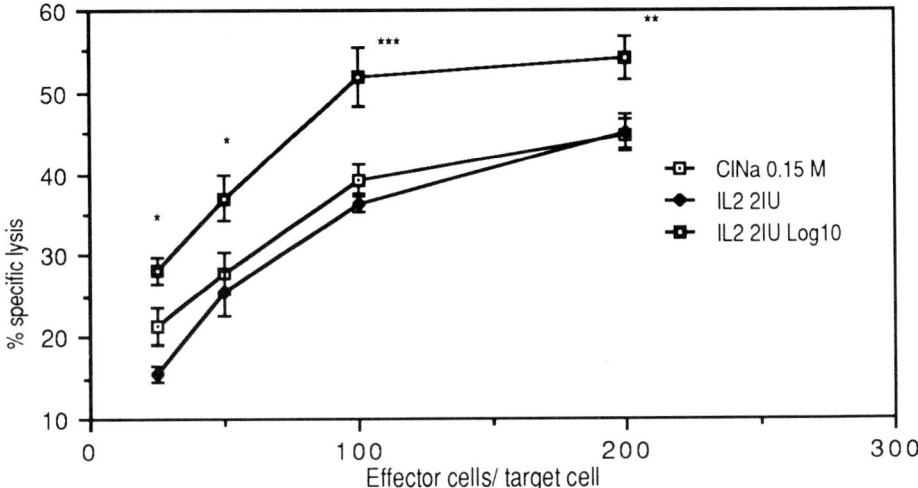

Figure 4. Allospecific cellular immune response of C57BL/6 mice treated with very low doses of IL2.

Table IV. Modulation of the specific humoral response of mice treated with very low doses of IL-2.

IL-2/injection	Before SRBC challenge [a]		Before and after SRBC challenge [b]		Secondary response [c]
	Exp. I	Exp. II	Exp. I	Exp. II	Exp. III
0	340.0 ± 36.1 [d]	53.1 ± 5.3	39.1 ± 4.6	25.0 ± 2.5	235.8 ± 19.7
2 IU	335.7 ± 80.1	87.0 ± 13.5	62.8 ± 6.7 $P < 0.025$ [e]	45.6 ± 2.6 $P < 0.001$	163.2 ± 2.6 $P < 0.01$
2×10^{-10} IU	357.5 ± 80.1	62.9 ± 10.4	68.9 ± 6.7 $P < 0.025$	24.4 ± 3.6	143.2 ± 19.1 $P < 0.01$

[a] OF1 mice were treated i.p. on day 13, 11, 8, 6 before the challenge SRBC were injected on day 4 before the test.
[b] OF1 mice were treated i.p. on day 14, 13, 8, 6 and 3, 2, 16 h before t test ; SRBC were injected on day 4 before the test.
[c] OF1 mice were treated i.p. on day 3, 2, 1 (2 inj./day) between 2 SRI injections (for the secondary response).
[d] Number of PFC/10^6 cells ± s.e.m.
[e] Statistical significance (Newman-Keuls multiple comparison test).

In vitro studies in healthy mice

Mouse peritoneal macrophages from female BALB/c mice aged 4 to 12 weeks were incubated with natural murine $\alpha\beta$ interferon at 1.6 IU and 1.6×10^{-10} IU/ml. The production of reactive oxygen intermediates was evaluated by the chemiluminescence test. The treatment was able to modulate the PMA-induced chemiluminescence of macrophages. The two concentrations tested caused a decrease in the chemiluminescence of adherent cells from mice aged 4 to 5 and 8 to 12 weeks and an increase in the chemiluminescence of adherent cells from mice aged 6 weeks [8].

Experimental results in immunocompromised mice : *ex vivo* studies

It was next decided to determine whether thymulin or interferon at very low doses could have an effect on immunocompromised mice. NZB mice whose thymus undergoes degeneration and who show a decrease in the thymulin secretion as of the age of four weeks were chosen for the study. Female NZB mice aged 6 weeks were treated with 10^{-9}, 10^{-15}, 10^{-19}, 10^{-23} mg/ml of thymulin or with 2 IU and 2×10^{-10} IU/mouse of interferon. All four dilutions of thymulin significantly stimulated the specific humoral immune response. The cellular immune response was evaluated after treatment with 10^{-9} and 10^{-19} mg/ml of the hormone ; the lowest concentration of thymulin significantly stimulated the cellular response against EL4 cells [6, 7]. When the NZB mice were treated with interferon, we obtained a significant decrease in the cellular immune response. As shown in Figure 5, we always observed an opposite effect when we compared the results obtained in healthy mice with those obtained in immunocompromised mice. In addition, a crude extract of thymus at 10^{-9}, 10^{-15}, 10^{-19} and 10^{-23} mg/ml also showed opposite effects on the immune response when administered in healthy and NZB mice [2, 3, 5, 7].

We also tested *ex vivo* the mitogenic response to ConA and PHA of lymphocytes from NZB mice treated with thymulin ; these mice are high responders to these mitogens as we verified in control mice. The female NZB mice treated with 10^{-15} mg/ml thymulin showed a significant decrease in lymphocyte stimulation [5]. Taken together, we conclude that treatment with very low doses of thymulin caused an improvement in the immune response of NZB mice. However, these results have to be considered very carefully since unpublished results of thymulin-treated MRL mice showed an aggravation of their autoimmune pathology.

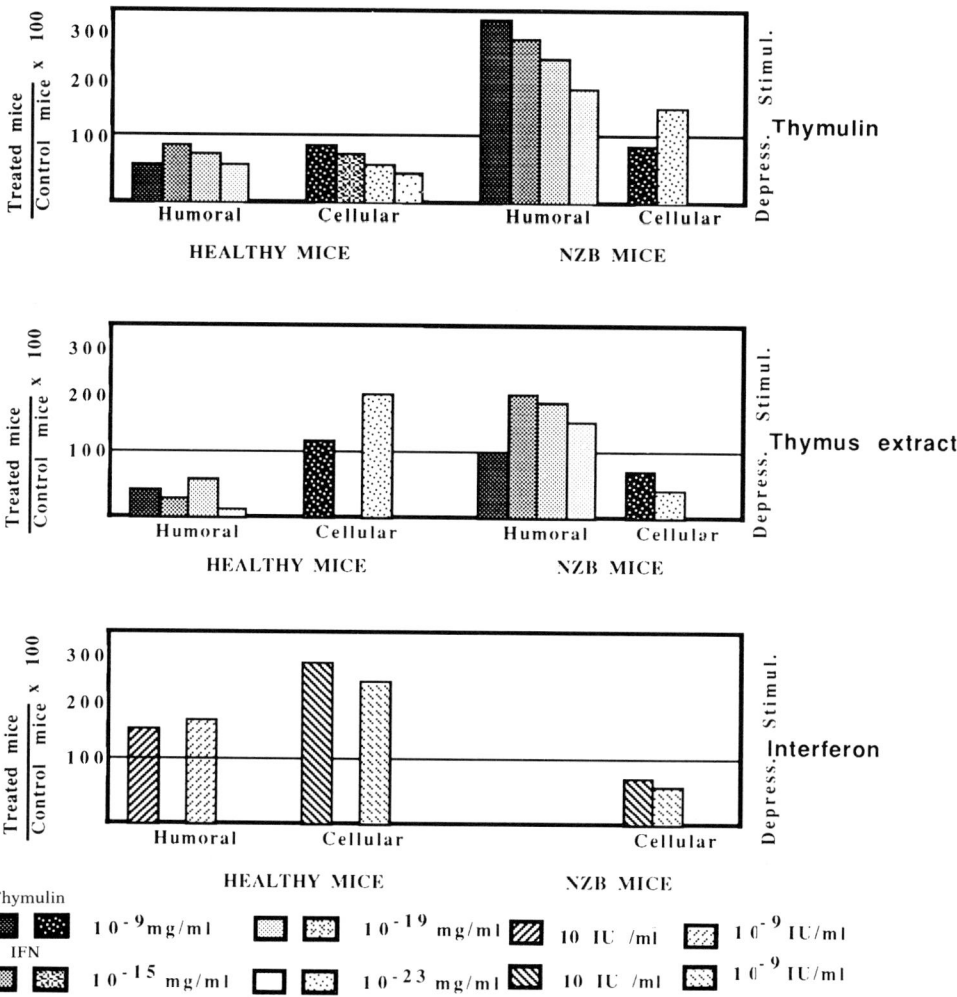

Figure 5. Comparison of the effect of thymulin, a thymus extract and interferon on the immune response of healthy and immunocompromised mice.

Effect of *in ovo* administration of high dilutions of bursin in bursectomized chickens

Chick embryos were surgically bursectomized at 80 h of incubation and then given saline or bursin *in ovo*, a tripeptide isolated from the bursa of Fabricius, at days 6 and 9. Four groups of chicken were tested : one untreated sham-operated control group (N) ; one saline treated bursectomized group (BX+S) ; one 100 fg bursin treated group (BX+fg) ; one 10^{-27}g bursin treated group (BX+ 10^{-27}). The 10^{-27}g bursin solution was prepared by 1/100 serial dilutions according to the homeopathic preparations. The four groups were repeatedly immunized with porcin thyroglobulin (Tg) at days 21, 30, 39 after hatching. Plasma corticosterone levels and serum titers antibodies against thyroglobulin were evaluated on days 20, 29, 38 and 47 after hatching. The immunized N group had high concentrations of corticosterone but not the bursectomized BX+S group. This level was completely restored in the two treated groups (Figure 6). Specific antibodies to Tg remained at very low background in the BX+S group in spite of repeated stimulations, whereas N group produced a strong specific antibody response. *In ovo* administration of very low doses of bursin (100 fg and 10^{-27}g) led to high antibody production (Figure 7). These results support the hypothesis that bursa of Fabricius influences the functional maturation of adrenocorticotropic axis and that the production of specific antibodies operates, at least partly, through bursin-dependent mechanisms. They also demonstrate that a bursin-specific informing structure remains in the highest diluted preparations of bursin [9].

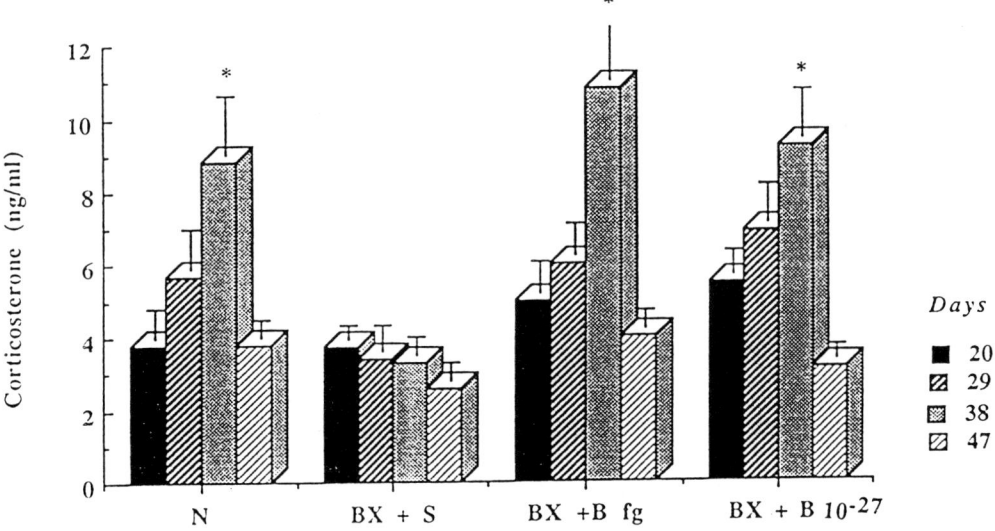

Figure 6. Plasma corticosterone levels as determined 1 day before (D20) the first injection and 8 days after the first (D29), second (D38) and third (D47) immunization.
N = sham-operated control birds ; BX+S = bursectomized birds and saline injection ; BX+B = bursectomized birds and bursin injections (fg = 100fg ; 10^{-27} = 5×10^{-27}g).
Values are given as mean ± sem ; n = 5 to 9.
* Statistically significant (Student's t-test) difference at $p < 0.05$ vs. D20.

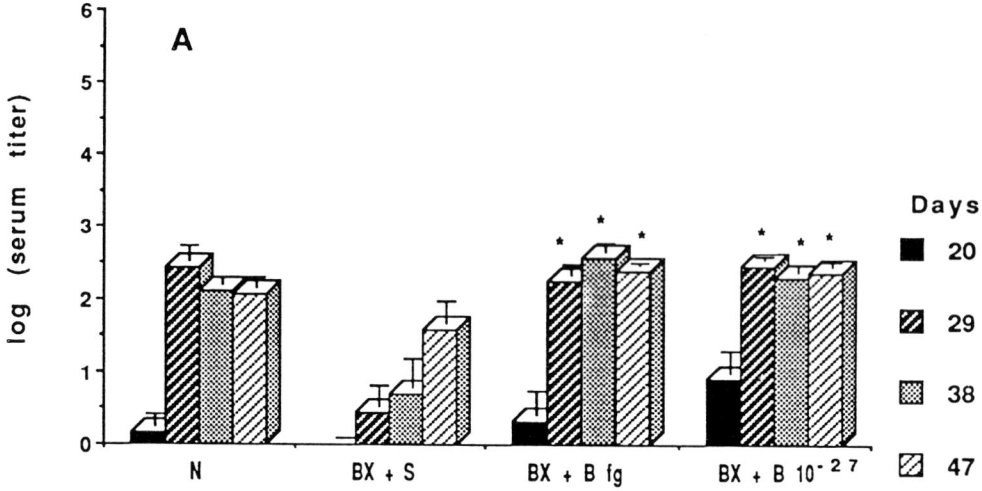

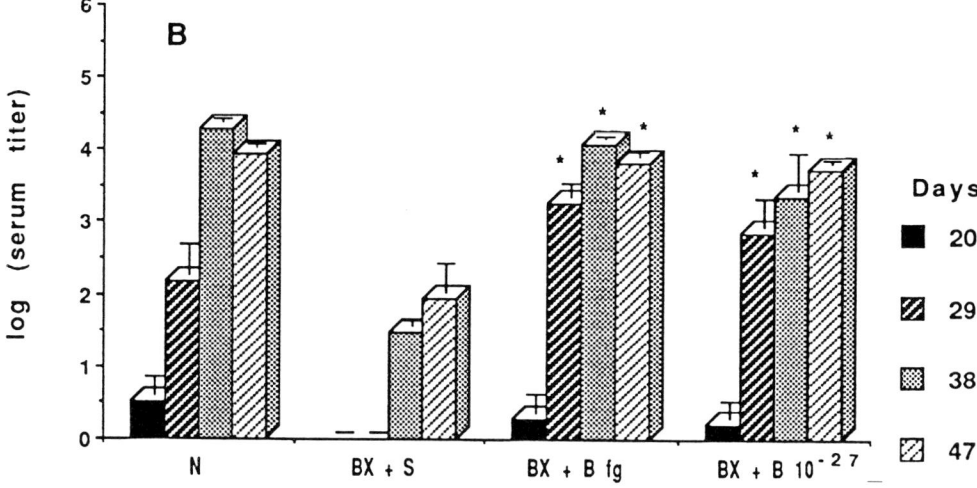

Figure 7. Titers of anti-Tg antibodies (A) IgM and (B) IgG as determined 1 day before (D20) the first injection and 8 days after the first (D29), second (D38) and third (D47) immunization. N = sham-operated control birds ; BX + S = bursectomized birds and saline injection ; BX + B = bursectomized birds and bursin injections (fg = 100fg ; $10^{-27} = 5 \times 10^{-27}$g).
Values are given as mean ± sem ; n = 3 to 9.
* Statistically significant (Student's t-test) difference at $p < 0.05$ vs. BX + S.

Clinical studies

To investigate the clinical relevance of our findings, one clinical study has already been performed and others are in preparation. The first trial was an open one and was performed by private physicians. It was conducted with highly diluted solutions of thymulin during the winter of 1989-1990 on children suffering from recurrent rhino-pharingitis [10]. In the trial, one group of patients received thymulin and the control group received an immunomodulatoring agent used in France for this indication (*Klebsiella* cell wall extracts associated ribosome extracts). For ethical reasons, no placebo was included in the study. Thymulin was administered according to the age of the children. Children younger than two years received 10^{-15} g/ml thymulin, whereas children older than 2 years received 10^{-19} g/ml thymulin, both, once a week during the first two months and then once in two weeks. The control group received the treatment according to the posology indicated by the manufacturer. The children were treated from November throughout the winter. The groups are compared in Table V. The results (Figures 8 and 9) show a similar immunostimulating effect in the two groups with a slight, mostly non-significant advantage of the thymulin group with respect to the duration of the episodes and the length of antibiotherapy.

Table V. Thymulin and reference immunomodulator groups.

Patients	Thymulin	Reference immunomodulator
Boys	25	26
Girls	22	15
Mean age (months)	38 ± 2	38 ± 2

Discussion

In the literature, there are several reports describing the effects of high dilutions (pico- and fento-molar concentrations) in *in vitro* models of biological systems. Protein kinase C isolated from fresh rat brain was found to be activated by picomolar concentrations of lead [11]. Leung-Tack *et al.* [12] demonstrated an inhibitory effect of a synthetic peptide (postin) at a concentration of 10^{-14} M on phagocyte function. Other reports described similar effects [13, 14]. Wagner *et al.* [15, 16] showed the immune stimulating effect of very low doses (10^{-15} g) of cytostatic drugs such as azathioprine, colchicine, methotrexate. Since these experiments were carried out *in vitro*, no pharmacokinetic or tissue diffusion data was reported.

However, recent data [17] have shown a better stimulating effect of very low doses of thymulin (1 ng/kg) compared to a higher concentration (1 µg/kg) in restraint stressed mice.

The experimental results reported here demonstrate the efficacy of highly diluted solutions of hormones, peptides and cytokines in biological systems. They raise the problem of the character of the signal given by thymulin, for example at a concentration lower than 10^{-23} M, or bursin used at the theoretical concentration of 10^{-27} g. This solution contains theoretically no active molecule. There are other experimental results using other models in which similar and lower concentrations have been used, suggesting that our findings are not an artefact and that the biological system indeed receives an information [18-21].

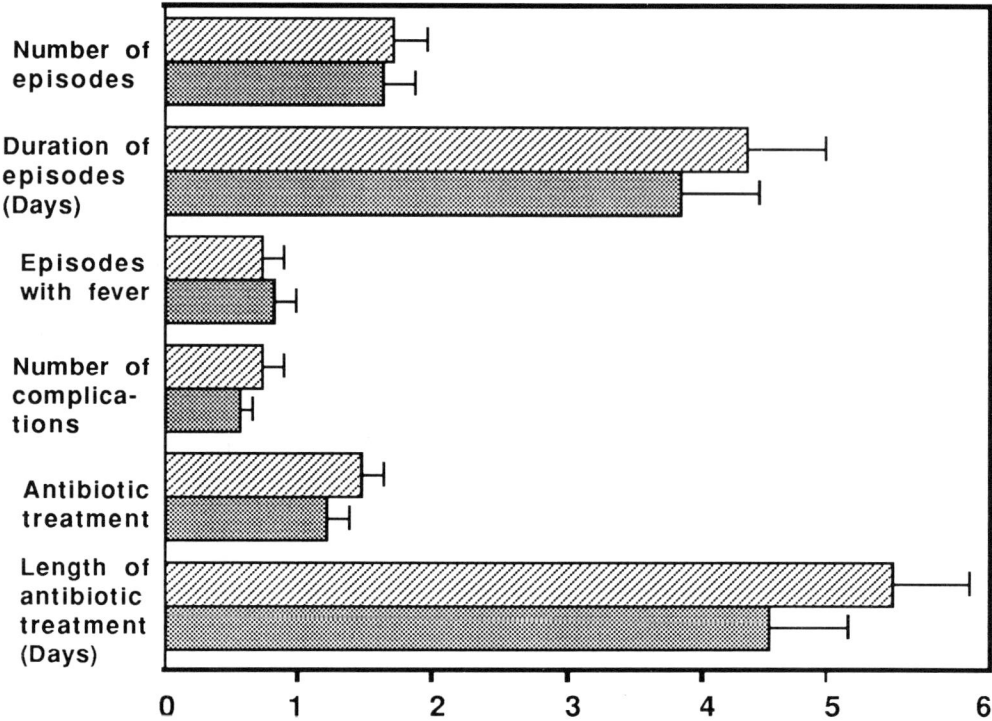

Figure 8. Effect of reference immunomodulator ▨ and Thymulin ▩ on various parameters. Results expressed in terms of mean pourcentage and mean duration to all patients.

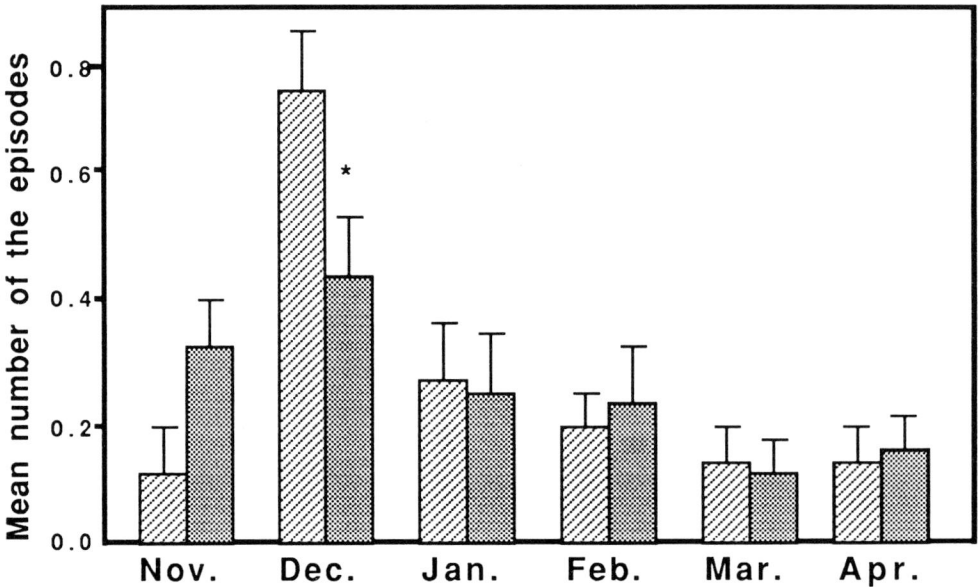

Figure 9. Frequency of the rhinopharingitis during the winter season.
▨ Reference immunomodulator ; ▩ Thymulin. * $P < 0.05$ (Student's t test).

Many problems remain to be solved : among them, what is the nature of this information ? Physicists are now studying the possibility of a physical electromagnetic message. A theoretical approach and experiments are now in process using the mathematical approach supported by the Ethers theory [22, 23]. The physical frame of it is related to the quantum theory of the fields. The mathematical calculation shows, when the particle has disappeared, the appearance of a non trivial physical field with the same unit as the electromagnetic field : it has been called the remanent wawe. This remanent wawe consists in an informing structure : in this procedure, matter has been mediatized to become an information. The organism of the receiver is able to deal with this information and to react. This could deal with a new paradigme of information, different from the mechanistic one [24].

Acknowledgement

The author thanks Dr M. Oberbaum for critical comments. This work was supported by Dolisos Laboratories (Drs M. Tetau and P. Dorfman, Scientific Directors) to whom the author is grateful.

References

1. Bach JF, Dardenne M. Studies on thymus products. II : Demonstration and characterization of a circulating thymic hormone ? *Immunology* 1973 ; 25 : 353-66.
2. Bastide M. Research on very low dose or high dilution effects : a report. In : Bastide M, ed. *Signals and Images*. Paris : Atelier Alpha Bleue, 1991 : 9-26.
3. Bastide M, Doucet-Jaboeuf M, Daurat V. Activity and chronopharmacology of very low doses of physiological immune inducers. *Immunol Today* 1985 ; 6 : 234-5.
4. Doucet-Jaboeuf M, Guillemain J, Piechaczyk M, Karouby Y, Bastide M. Evaluation de la dose limite d'activité du Facteur Thymique Sérique. *CRAcad Sci Paris* 1982 ; 295 : III : 283-7.
5. Doucet-Jaboeuf M, Pélegrin A, Cot MC, Guillemain J, Bastide M. Seasonal variations in the humoral immune response in mice following administration of thymic hormones. *Annu Rev Chronopharmacol* 1984 ; 1 : 231-4.
6. Bastide M, Daurat V, Doucet-Jaboeuf M, Pélegrin A, Dorfman P. Immunomodulator activity of very low doses of thymulin in mice. *Int J Immunother* 1987 ; 3 : 191-200.
7. Daurat V, Dorfman P, Bastide M. Immunomodulatory activity of low doses of interferon α,β in mice. *Biomed Pharmacother* 1988 ; 42 : 197-206.
8. Carriere V, Bastide M. Influence of mouse age on PMA-induced chemiluminescence of peritoneal cells incubated with $\alpha\beta$ interferon, at very low and moderate doses. *Int J Immunother* 1990 ; 6 : 211-4.
9. Youbicier-Simo BJ, Boudard F, Mekaouche M, Bastide M, Baylé JD. Effects of embryonic bursectomy and *in ovo* administration of highly diluted bursin on adrenocorticotropic and immune response of chickens. *Int J Immunother* 1993 ; 9 : 169-80.
10. Hunin M, Tisserand G, Dorfman P, Tetau M. Intérêt de la thymuline dans le traitement préventif des pathologies ORL récidivantes de l'enfant. *Cah Bioth* 1990 ; n° 107 : 77-82.
11. Markovac J, Goldstein GW. Picomolar concentrations of lead stimulate brain protein kinase C. *Nature* 1988 ; 334 : 71-3.
12. Leung-Tack J, Martinez J, Sansot JL, Manuel Y, Colle A. Inhibition of phagocyte functions by a synthetic peptide lys-pro-pro-arg (postin). *Protides Biol Fluids Proc Colloq* 1986 ; 34 : 205-8.

13. Shinoshara N, Watanabe M, Sachs DH, Hozumi N. Killing of antigen-reactive B cells by class II-restricted soluble antigen-specific CD8 cytolytic T lymphocytes. *Nature* 336 : 481-4.
14. Zarling JM, Moran PA, Haffar O, Sias J, Richman D, Spina CA, Myers DE, Kuebelbeck V, Ledbetter JA, Uckun FM. Inhibition of HIV replication by pokeweed antiviral protein targeted to CD4$^+$ cells by monoclonal antibodies. *Nature* 1990 ; 347 : 92-5.
15. Wagner H, Kreher B, Jurcic K. *In vitro* stimulation of human granulocytes and lymphocytes by pico- and fentogram quantities of cytostatic agents. *Arzneim Forsch/Drug Res* 1988 ; 38 : 273-275.
16. Wagner H, Kreher B. Cytotoxic agents as immunostimulators. In : *Signals and images*. Paris : Atelier Alpha Bleue, 1991 : 27-53.
17. Masahiro O, Masatara M Chikako S, Katsuhiko N. Restorative effect of short term administration of thymulin on thymus-dependent antibody production in restraint-stressed mice. *Int J Immunopharmacol* 1993 ; 15 : 757-62.
18. Cal JC, Larue F, Guillemain J, Cambar J. Chronobiological approach of protective effect of Mercurius corrosivus against mercury-induced nephrotoxicity. *Annu Rev Chronopharmacol* 1986 ; 3 : 99-102.
19. Cal JC, Larue F, Dorian C, Guillemain J, Dorfman P, Cambar J. Chronobiological approach of mercury-induced toxicity and of the protective effect of high dilutions of mercury against mercury-induced nephrotoxicity. *Liver Cells Drugs* 1988 ; 164 : 481-5.
20. Davenas E, Poitevin B, Benveniste J. Effect on mouse peritoneal macrophages of orally administered very high dilutions of silica. *Eur J Pharmacol* 1987 ; 135 : 313-9.
21. Davenas E, Beauvais F, Amara J, Oberbaum M, Robinzon B, Miadonna A, Tedeschi A, Pomeranz B, Fortner P, Belon P, Sainte-Laudy J, Poitevin B, Benveniste J. Human basophil degranulation triggered by very dilute antiserum against IgE. *Nature* 1988 ; 333 : 816-8.
22. Conte RR, Berliocchi H, Andras HG. *Nouvelle économie sémiotique*. Paris : Economica Ed., 1993.
23. Berliocchi H. *Théorie des Ethers*. Paris : Economica, 1994.
24. Bastide M, Lagache A. *The paradigm of signifiers*. Paris : Alpha Bleue, 1992.

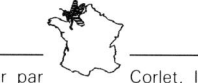

Achevé d'imprimer par Corlet, Imprimeur, S.A.
14110 Condé-sur-Noireau (France)
N° d'Imprimeur : 6920 - Dépôt légal : mars 1995

Imprimé en C.E.E.